ALLE ZEIT WACH
1842

G. Feifel U. Hildebrandt N. J. McC. Mortensen (Eds.)

Endosonography in Gastroenterology, Gynecology and Urology

With Contributions by
J. Beynon, W. H. Cooner, G. Feifel, U. Hildebrandt,
H. Hötzinger, B. Kramann, P. Langenscheidt,
N. J. McC. Mortensen, H.-P. Schwarz, T. L. Tio, J. J. Wild

Foreword by
S. M. Goldberg

With 349 Figures and 19 Tables

Springer-Verlag
Berlin Heidelberg New York
London Paris Tokyo
Hong Kong Barcelona

GERNOT FEIFEL, M.D.
Professor of Surgery
Dept. of Surgery, University of Saarland
D-6650 Homburg/Saar, FRG

ULRICH HILDEBRANDT, M.D.
Dept. of Surgery, University of Saarland
D-6650 Homburg/Saar, FRG

NEIL J. McC. MORTENSEN, M.D.
Consultant Surgeon
University of Oxford, Dept. of Surgery and Gastroenterology,
Clinical School, John Radcliffe Hospital
Headington, Oxford OX 3 9 DU
Great Britain

ISBN-13:978-3-642-74254-5 e-ISBN-13:978-3-642-74252-1
DOI: 10.1007/978-3-642-74252-1

Library of Congress Cataloging-in-Publication Data. Endosonography in gastroenterology, gynecology, and urology/G. Feifel, U. Hildebrandt, N. J. McC. Mortensen (eds.); with contributions by J. Beynon...[et al.]. p.cm.ISBN-13:978-3-642-74254-5 (U.S.:alk. paper) 1. Endoscopic ultrasonography. 2. Gastrointestinal system – Ultrasonic imaging. 3. Generative organs, Female–Ultrasonic imaging. 4. Prostate–Ultrasonic imaging. I. Feifel, G. (Gernot). II. Hildebrandt, Ulrich. III. Mortensen, N. J. McC. (Neil J. McC.). IV. Beynon, J. (John) [DNLM: 1. Gastroenterology. 2. Gynecology. 3. Ultrasonic Diagnosis. 4. Urology. WB 289 E564] RC78.7.E48E54 1990 616.07′543–dc20 DNLM/DLC for Library of Congress 90-9725 CIP

Softcover reprint of the hardcover 1st edition 1990

2121/3130-543210 – Printed on acid-free paper

Foreword

Technical improvements over the past twenty years have made endoscopy the procedure of choice for examination of the hollow organs of the genitourinary and gastrointestinal tracts. The development of electrosurgical techniques, laser technology, injection therapy, and a wide variety of other modalities now allow the endoscopist to treat many problems that in the past required open surgery. The simultaneous development of transcutaneous abdominal sonography has had an equally dramatic impact on the practice of gastrointestinal and genitourinary surgery. The marriage of these proven technologies, known as endoscopic sonography, provides an exciting new modality that promises to further revolutionize the diagnosis and management of many intraabdominal diseases.

Endoscopic sonography opens new frontiers by overcoming the primary limitations of its parent technologies. Fiberoptic endoscopy is limited by the inability to see beyond the luminal surface, this is particularly important when considering neoplastic disease because depth of wall invasion is a key factor in determining treatment. The limiting factor in transcutaneous sonography is the distance between the transducer and the target organ. With endoscopic sonography, the transducer is placed in close proximity to the target organ. This allows the use of high frequency waves (greater than 5 MHz), which provide better tissue resolution and eliminates the image distortion caused by overlying structures. The advantages offered by endoscopic sonography are precise definition of mural structure, high resolution imaging of previously inaccessible organs such as the prostate and pancreas, and the ability to image structures in real time. Real time imaging may be used for dynamic assessment of function, and guidance of biopsy and therapy.

Since the pioneering work of Wild and Reid[1] at the University of Minnesota, many exciting areas of application have been identified. Transrectal ultrasound of the prostate is the most sensitive technique available for the detection of early prostate cancer. Although it is not yet clear that identifying subclinical cancers gives a clinical benefit, early detection is clearly an advantage for studying the natural history of prostate cancer. Endoscopic sonography is also of use for following the

[1] Wild JJ, Reid JM: Echographic tissue diagnosis. Proceedings at the Fourth Annual Conference on Ultrasonic Therapy 1955:1

response of prostatic cancer to treatment, in the diagnosis of chronic prostatitis, the valuation of disorders of the seminal vesicles and ejaculatory ducts, and in the dynamic assessment of bladder emptying. In the gastrointestinal tract, transrectal ultrasound is the most accurate method of preoperative staging of rectal cancer. It is also of use for determining the depth of invasion of esophageal carcinoma, diagnosing early recurrence after esophagectomy or low anterior resection, and evaluating submucosal lesions of the upper gastrointestinal tract or large sessile polyps of the rectum. Endoscopic sonography of the pancreas provides high resolution images that may aid in the vexing problem of early diagnosis of pancreatic cancer.

As experience with this new technology increases, and technical improvements such as the development of miniature probes occurs, we can expect that endoscopic sonography will have an increasing impact on the diagnosis and treatment of gastrointestinal and genitourinary disease in the future. The authors have succeeded admirably in capturing the current state of the art in this rapidly developing field. This work should be of interest to all who treat diseases of the abdominal and pelvic organs.

STANLEY M. GOLDBERG

Preface

Although endosonography is still in its infancy, it is worth remembering that the first instruments, rigid and flexible, were already completed in the mid-1950s. Because of technical shortcomings they were never used clinically, but they inspired further efforts in the development of endosonographic imaging.

Despite major progress in conventional transcutaneous ultrasonography, higher frequencies can be used in endosonography by approaching the area of interest directly via the intestinal lumen. The initial steps were difficult and frustrating, mainly due to the low frequency (3.5 MHz) and other equipment shortcomings. Now that more sophisticated high-quality instruments and frequencies up to 12.0 MHz are available, the interpretation of the intestinal layer structure has become standard.

Endosonography is remarkably accurate in staging esophageal cancer and predicting its resectability. It also makes it possible to differentiate benign smooth muscle tumors from malignant changes. Examination of stomach malignancies, cancer and lymphoma, will predict the curative or palliative nature of a surgical intervention, or indicate that the tumor is nonresectable. By approaching the pancreas directly from the gastric antrum or duodenum with no interfering structures, a very detailed image can be obtained of the pancreatic parenchyma and the ductular system, thus enabling the differentiation of pancreatitis and pancreatic malignancy. Endosonography is of importance in the analysis of the area of the papilla, especially if a decision between local or wide surgical excision of a tumor has to be made.

Staging of rectal cancer has usually been performed with rigid probes. The accuracy rate is high, and the implications for treatment, epecially for small rectal lesions, have now been well defined. However, there are lesions which are present at or just beyond the rectosigmoid junction. Such lesions are better investigated with flexible equipment and may improve patient acceptance in painful disorders. There is still a controversy over the definition of objective criteria for differentiating benign from malignant lymph nodes.

Urology was the first discipline to apply endosonographic techniques widely to screen an asymptomatic population for prostatic cancer. Refined instruments and high frequencies provide access to structures within and around the prostate which previously were inaccessible to examination. In gynecology, endosonography has gained wide acceptance. The spectrum of indications ranges from inflammatory disease, via pregnancy definition, follicle puncture, and fetal biometry, to tumor screening and staging as well as follow-up examination.

There remains the issue of who should perform endosonography. This is not a matter of controversy for gynecologists and urologists. For gastroenterologists and surgeons, however, it will undoubtedly depend to a large extent on the local situation. Experience in endoscopy and ultrasonography will remain a prerequisite for successfully applying the new technique. Especially in hospitals where surgeons are engaged in minimal invasive surgery, endosonography will necessarily be in their hands.

GERNOT FEIFEL
ULRICH HILDEBRANDT
NEIL J. McC. MORTENSEN

Contents

List of Contributors

BEYNON, JOHN, M.S., University of Bristol, Dept. of Surgery, Bristol Royal Infirmary, Bristol BS2 8WH, Great Britain

COONER, WILLIAM H., M.D., Mobile Urology Group, Professional Center of Mobile, Suite 103, 1720 Center Street, Mobile, Alabama 36690, USA

FEIFEL, GERNOT, M.D., Professor of Surgery, Dept. of Surgery, University of Saarland, D-6650 Homburg/Saar, FRG

HILDEBRANDT, ULRICH, M.D., Dept. of Surgery, University of Saarland, D-6650 Homburg/Saar, FRG

HÖTZINGER, HARALD, M.D., University of Bochum, Dept. of Radiology and MRI, Marienhospital, Hölkeskampring 40, D-4690 Herne 1, FRG

KRAMANN, BERNHARD, M.D., Professor of Radiology, Dept. of Radiology, University of Saarland, D-6650 Homburg/Saar, FRG

LANGENSCHEIDT, PHILIPP, Dept. of Surgery, University of Saarland, D-6650 Homburg/Saar, FRG

MORTENSEN, NEIL J. McC., M.D., Consultant Surgeon, University of Oxford Clinical School, Dept. of Surgery and Gastroenterology, John Radcliffe Hospital, Headington, Oxford OX3 9DU, Great Britain

SCHWARZ, HANS-PETER, Ph.D., Fraunhofer-Institute, Dept. of Medical Engineering, D-6670 St. Ingbert, FRG

TIO, T. LOK, M.D., Acad. Med. Centre, University of Amsterdam, Div. of Gastroenterology-Hepatology, Meibergdreef 9, NL-1105 AZ Amsterdam, The Netherlands

WILD, JOHN J., M.D., Ph.D., The Medico-Technological Research Institute, 4262 Alabama Avenue South, St. Louis Park, Minnesota 55416-3105, USA

1 A Historical Review of the Genesis and Early Development of Intrusive Pulse-Echo Ultrasound

J. J. Wild

1.1 Introduction

The development of semi-invasive instrumentation arose as a logical step to overcome frequency-range resolution and other basic acoustic limitations. These limitations, emerging as the work progressed in laboratory and clinic, followed two primary basic scientific discoveries reported in 1949. These discoveries were (a) sonic energy reflection from both gross and fine histological structure of soft tissues [6] and (b) observation of differential sonic reflection and acoustic properties of cancerous tissue [7]. Follow-up of these fundamental observations founded the field of diagnostic ultrasound and set the stage for early cancer detection at accessible sites on a screening basis [8–10].

1.2 Basic Proof of Echo Production by Biological Tissues

In the spring of 1949, a piece of World War II ultrasound radar training equipment operating at 15-MHz frequency was used to determine the feasibility of clinically gauging the thickness of intact, functioning human gut. Dog bowel was used to demonstrate successfully the slight difference in thickness between the point of attachment of the mesentery and the opposite wall. Difficulties in working within the large radar tank necessitated the construction of a small, self-contained, water-filled echo chamber sealed with a thin rubber membrane.

At this point, a conveniently available fresh biological specimen was needed to readjust the naval electronics gear for each series of biological experiments after each of its routine, long-range military radar training operations. Fresh beef muscle and fat were placed upon the small, water-filled chamber. Attenuation of the sonic energy at 15 MHz was found to be much greater in fresh beef muscle than in structural beef fat. Varying thicknesses of fat and naturally attached muscle were tried for through transmission of the sonic energy. The final standard test specimen which emerged was approximately 9 mm fat thickness and 1 mm muscle thickness. Thus, the naturally attached fat-muscle interface was asymmetrical relative to the tissue-air interfaces of the test specimens.

Two important observations were made with this first biological standard test specimen: the gross fat-muscle interface was identifiable, and, most importantly, echoes from within the 1-mm-thick sliver of beef muscle were observed. The proof of echo production by the standard test phantom was obtained by turning

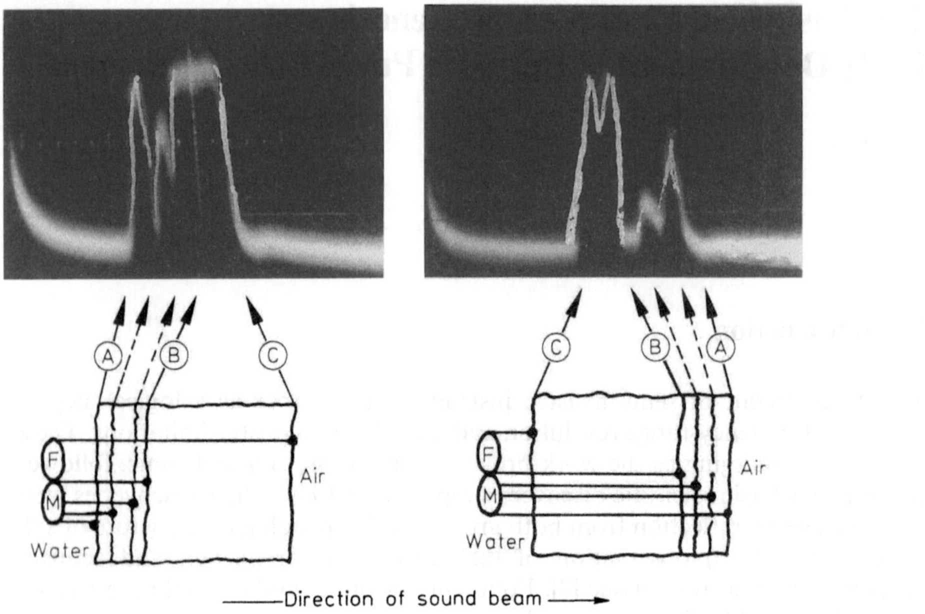

Fig. 1.1. The time-amplitude traces of reciprocal transmission through a 1-cm-thick composite specimen of beef fat (*F*) and muscle (*M*). The *left trace* shows echoes from 1 mm beef muscle followed by no echoes from the 9 mm beef fat. The *right trace* shows a transposition of the trace configuration; it also shows the beef-fat interface clearly. The baseline of this trace shows that about equal time is required to traverse 9 mm structural beef fat and 1 mm beef muscle. This means that fat attenuates ultrasound energy to a lesser degree than beef muscle. This experiment proved echo reflection by soft tissues and founded the field

the specimen through 180° to produce transposition of signals in the A-mode, time-amplitude, trace (Fig. 1.1). The resolution of muscle fasciculi at 15 MHz meant that, in addition to gross anatomical interfaces, fine histological structure could be seen with this system. Further experiments with ground-up beef muscle and fat demonstrated the destruction of the fat-muscle interface, as evidenced by an unchanged A-mode echo pattern in all planes of a 1-cm cube of ground beef. These fortuitous experiments, demonstrating the resolution of sonic reflections from both gross interfaces, and fine histological structure, were the first scientific proofs of echo reflection by pulse-echo ultrasound.

1.2.1 Proof of Bowel-Bowel Interfaces

Interfaces between layers of fresh dog bowel could also be resolved through a rubber membrane (Fig. 1.2), which would be necessary when the projected intraluminal endosonographic instrument was introduced into the living bowel (Fig. 1.3). One more check had to be made with human bowel. This experimental imperative led to the serendipitous discovery that malignant tumor tissue could be detected with the equipment. Human bowel was not obtainable when time be-

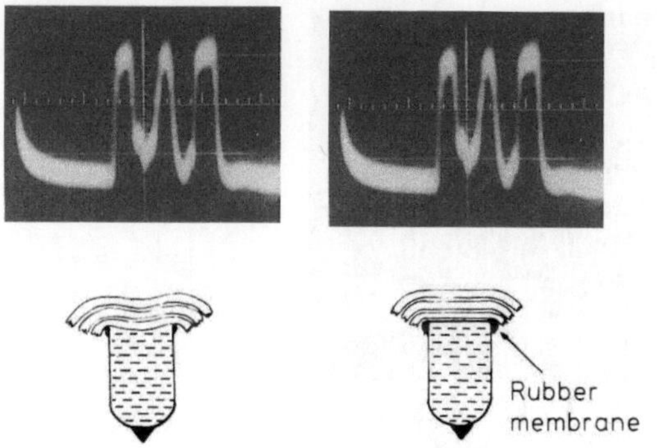

Fig. 1.2. The interfaces between three layers of fresh dog bowel are clearly discernible both without (*A*) and with (*B*) a thin rubber membrane closure. It was not known whether the rubber membrane would transmit sonic energy

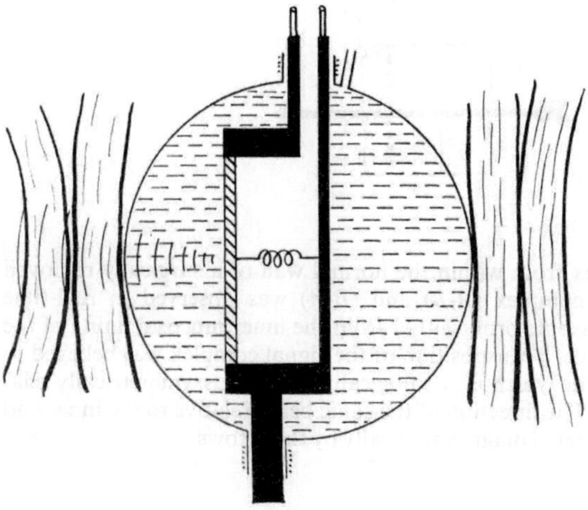

Fig. 1.3. The proposed instrument for measuring changes in thickness of living, intact bowel. A water-filled balloon is shown inflated after introduction into the mouth and bowel

came available to the assisting technicians at the military base. Instead, a fresh slice of an operative specimen of human stomach containing a carcinomatous ulcer was used. A natural asymmetrical structure, the lamina muscularis mucosae, within the stomach wall was identified by again turning the specimen through 180°, providing further proof of echo production from histological structure (Fig. 1.4).

1.3 Discovery of Potential of Pulse-Echo Ultrasound for Tumor Detection and Diagnosis

Further examination of the specimen revealed greater sonic attenuation by the stomach wall close to the ulcer, which had not increased in thickness but which was palpably infiltrated with malignant growth. In addition, many echoes were seen when the sonic beam was directed through the ulcer edges (Fig. 1.5). This discovery prompted the hope that pulse-echo ultrasound would prove to be a much-needed tool for early cancer detection. There was now no doubt that the then formidable task of building clinical instrumentation for clinical assessment of bowel-wall thickness, the original objective of the work, could be justified. Even greater justification lay in the hope that neoplastic growth could be

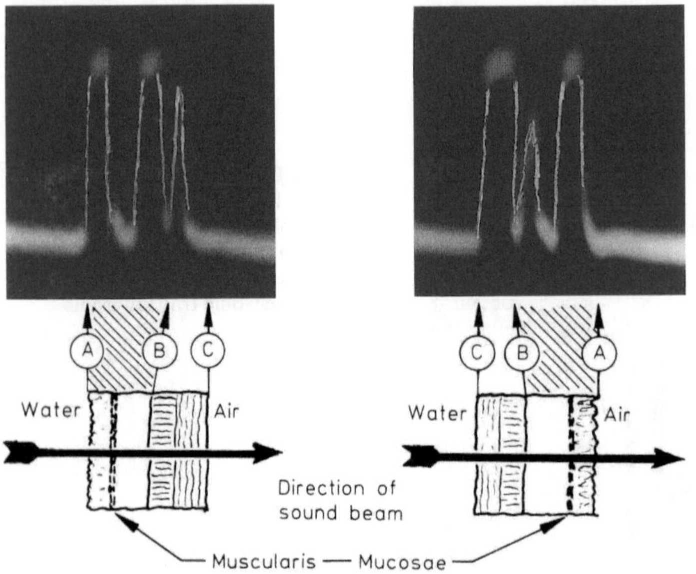

Fig. 1.4. Transposition of signal complex from within the normal wall of a surgically removed stomach. Transposition of the signal complex (*A-B*) and (*B-A*) was observed in real-time depending upon application of the ultrasonic probe either from the inner mucosal lining of the stomach or from the outer serosal surface. Transposition of the signal complex was believed to arise from the lamina muscularis mucosae which is histologically situated assymmetrically relative to the surfaces of the stomach wall. The direction of the sonic beam relative to the inner and outer surfaces of the stomach wall is indicated diagrammatically by the arrows

detected at an early, asymptomatic stage. The problem now was how to deal with the completely new type of information coming from tissues in order to demonstrate its use to medicine unequivocally. The biological technique used was to compare the sonic reflection properties of abnormal tissue with those of comparable normal (control) tissue under conditions of unchanging variables. With this technique, subjective differences were observed between A-mode traces of tumor and those of controls.

1.4 Detection of Soft Tissue Neoplasia

Unfixed whole brains, immediately post mortem, were used to demonstrate that both obvious and occult cancerous brain tumors reflected sonic energy as A-mode, time-amplitude, traces to a greater extent than did normal (control) brain tissues at comparable gain settings of the instrumentation [2, 3].

1.4.1 Preliminary Studies

Experimental attempts to produce clinical and histological damage failed [4] and paved the way toward direct clinical examination of brain and breast tumors.

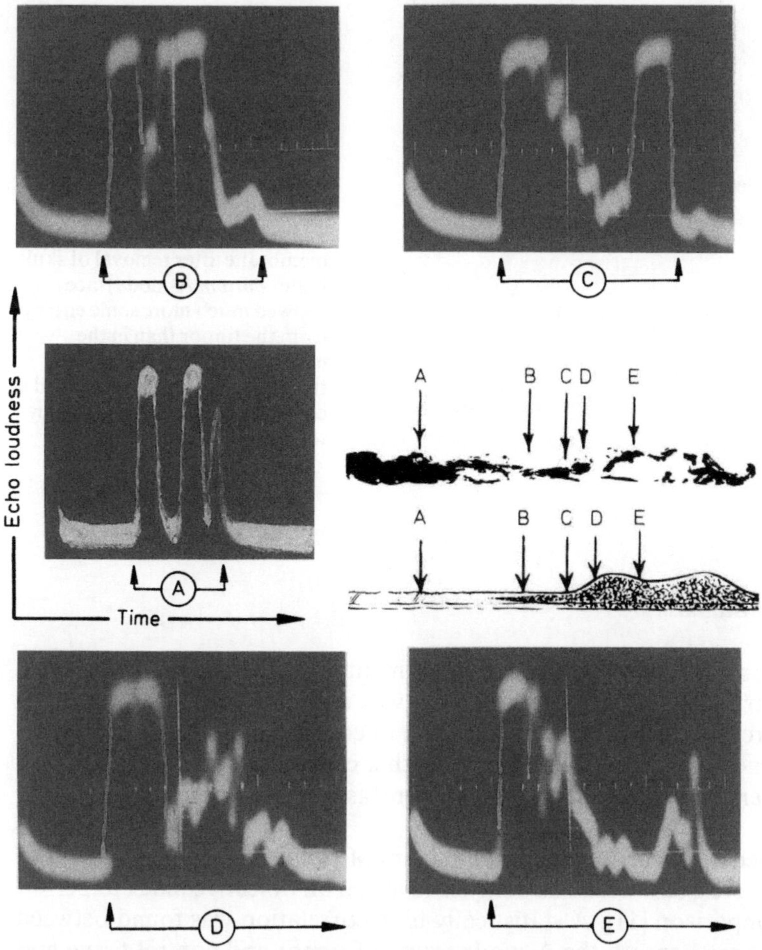

Fig. 1.5. Examination of an operative specimen containing a carcinomatous ulcer. The time base for normal stomach wall, shown at *A*, is greatly widened at *B*, where the stomach wall was not increased in thickness but was infiltrated with cancer growth. At position *C*, just next to the ulcer, more signals can be seen arising from within the infiltrated stomach wall. At *D* and *E* signals from within the ulcer are demonstrated

Subjective examination of A-mode traces of tumors and comparable normal tissue of origin was again used.

1.4.2 Living Brain

The first clinical use of localization of brain tumors at operation was recorded on 30 June 1951 [12]. The tumor was 1.5 in. in diameter, and a preoperative diagnosis of meningioma (benign) was made. The A-mode traces of tumor and control (Fig. 1.6) differed to such a degree that a correct diagnosis of malignancy was confidently made in the operating room.

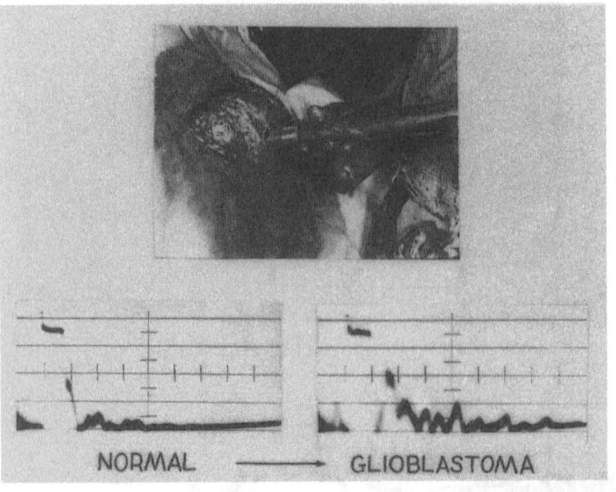

Fig. 1.6. *Top* A sound head was applied to the brain surface with a sterile wand sealed by a rubber membrane after removal of skull bone. *Bottom* A-mode trace showed much more sonic energy from the tumor than in the normal trace at the same electronic gain setting; this enabled a correct diagnosis of malignancy to be made

1.4.3 The Breast

1.4.3.1 A-Mode Studies

Since construction of endosonographic instruments presented greater technical problems, construction of a breast instrument was undertaken. The breast was a convenient source of small tumors from which to confirm and develop optimum acoustic instrumentation and techniques for other cancer sites. Differential sonic reflection properties of neoplastic growth were assumed to be common to all sites.

An unselected series of 21 comparable pairs of prebiopsy A-mode traces of breast nodules were examined. The analysis revealed an objective index to permit case-to-case comparison [11]. A statistically high correlation was found between the ratio of the area beneath the A-mode traces of tumor and control tissue and the histological diagnosis of the tumors in terms of malignancy and benignity. Malignant tumors of various types were found to have an "area-ratio" greater than unity, and nonmalignant tumors less than unity. This finding was confirmed with a sector B-mode "radar" image of a portion of a small malignant nodule (Fig. 1.7).

The existence of a natural, differential, sonic energy return between neoplastic tumors and surrounding tissues heralded the possibility of real-time visual location by natural contrast imaging. By that time, sufficient evidence of the potential of pulse-echo ultrasound for direct visual imaging of neoplastic tissue had been collected to justify construction of a multipurpose clinical display unit. This display unit would accommodate the multiple short-range clinical cancer detection instruments deemed necessary to circumvent the basic range limitations due to acoustic attenuation at 15-MHz frequency. At the time, the only commercial transducer assemblies operating at the high frequency necessary for resolution of fine histological detail were supplied to the United States Navy. In spite of this limited choice of transducer assemblies, the feasibility of B-mode clinical in-

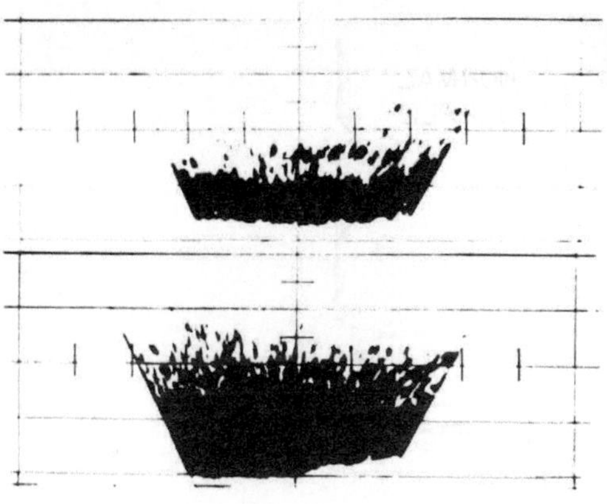

Fig. 1.7. Sector B-mode scans of a malignant breast tumor. The difference in the *amount* of sonic energy between normal tissue (*top*) and the tumor (*bottom*) at the same gain setting can be seen

strumentation at important short-range cancer sites (such as the breast, cervix uteri, prostate, and upper and lower gastrointestinal tract) was demonstrated.

1.4.3.2 B-Mode Studies

Attenuation of breast tissue at 15-MHz frequency limited the range to 4 cm, which required examination of the patient in the supine position to produce breast flattening under the influence of gravity and tissue compression by the instrument. Operation in real time, considered essential to obviate the effects of physiological movement of the breast, was also invaluable for adjustment of electronic amplifier gain to produce maximum visual contrast between the tumor and surrounding tissue. As predicted from the A-mode area-ratio work, this instrument produced the first images of a malignant breast tumor (Fig. 1.8; May 1953) and of a cyst (September 1953) and was immediately put to clinical use, primarily to determine whether all histological types of small neoplasms could be detected.

Preoperative histological diagnosis was attempted in a series of 117 cases in order to encourage clinical interest in, and acceptance of, this completely new field [5]. Diagnostic success soon brought patients for examination. Two types of contrast between solid tumors and surrounding tissue were observed; positive, or *sonescent*, where the tumors stood out from the normal background at a suitable gain setting, adjusted in real time while observing the tissue image; and negative, or *lacunary*, where the tumor was less echoic, as compared with the echo patterns of contiguous tissue, again at a gain setting adjusted to produce maximum contrast. The hope based on the A-mode area-ratio findings that the positive type of tumor image would prove malignancy and the negative type benignity was not realized. But further technical improvement in clarification of tissue speckle believed to come from diffuse backscatter did permit histological diagnosis of both the negative and positive types of tumor image. It was found that the speckle pattern was condensed or "filled in" in proximal parts of the image (Fig. 1.9). This absence of tissue speckle was considered to be due to infiltration by malig-

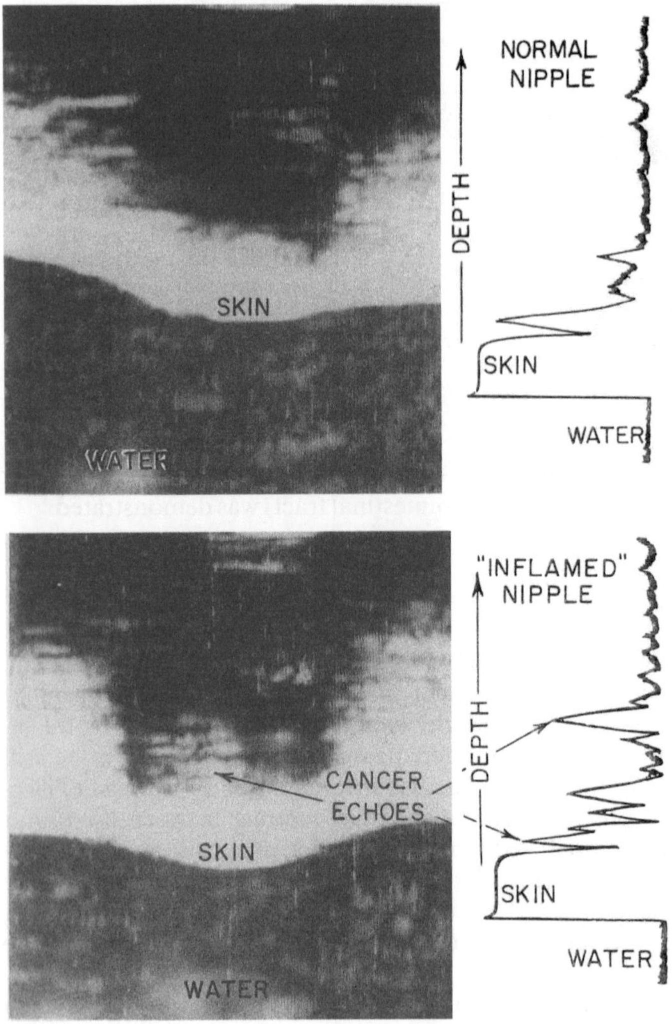

Fig. 1.8. A composite representation of the first cancer imaged in real-time linear B-mode in May 1953. The normal contralateral nipple image (*top left*) shows few signals within the anechoic (*black*) portion. The *lower* image shows a dense cluster of signals (*white*) within the nipple. These signals were produced in maximum (black/white) contrast from a clinically unsuspected 7-mm malignancy. The diagnosis was made from an objective numerical index of the area subtended by the A-mode traces (*right*). The ratio was 1.34:1. This figure correctly indicated cancer, which was confirmed at biopsy. This image is still unique in the literature

nant cells surrounding cancerous tumors. The breast cancer detection and screening objective to determine whether all types of small tumors could be revealed) was realized, down to the size of a 1-mm cancer in the naturally anechoic nipple-areola area.

Processing the objective area-ratio electronically for instantaneous, numerical readout was considered essential for population screening in cancer detection.

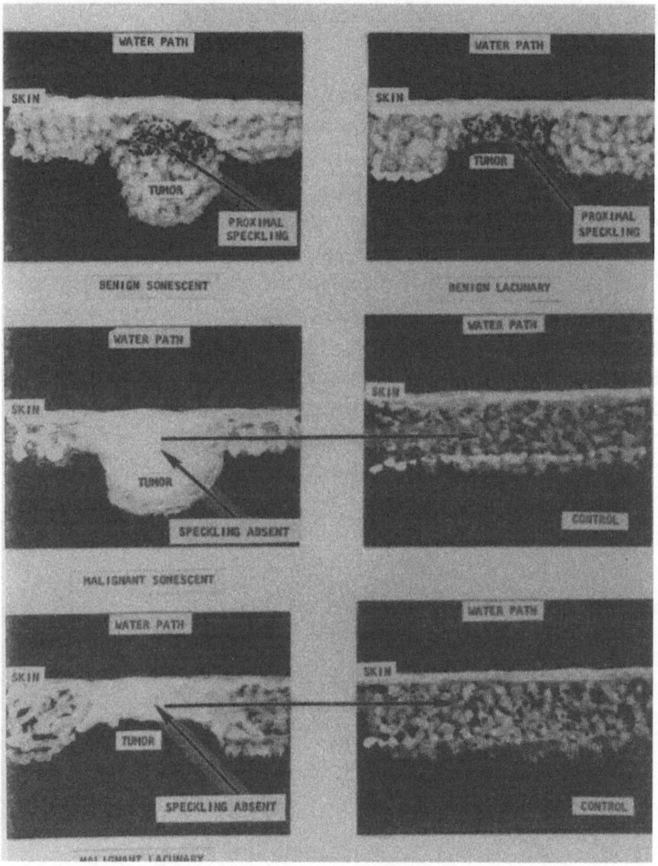

Fig. 1.9. Positive- and negative-contrast images of benign and malignant tumors. The *top* pair shows sonescent (*left*) and lacunary (*right*) benign types, in which tissue speckle is present in the proximal part of the image. (Tissue speckle is not to be confused with noise speckle.) The malignant positive and negative types are shown (*middle left* and *bottom left*). The "fill-in" of proximal tissue speckle as compared with the controls (right) is thought to be due to infiltration by malignant growth

This ongoing research effort continued over many years and was finally successful in December 1963 [9].

1.4.4 Application of Experimental Breast Techniques to Internal Sites

Both visual maximum-contrast imaging and quantitative numerical readout techniques are applicable to internal sites of neoplasia. The quantitative numerical instantaneous readout is the more favorable of the two techniques where suspect tissue forms a very small part of the total volume of tissue to be interrogated at sites such as the colon.

1.5 Development of Endosonographic Instrumentation

The high-frequency operation necessary for resolving small volumes of abnormal histological growth could best be realized for some important deep-seated cancer sites by placement of sonic interrogating heads as close to the target tissue as possible. As with the breast, priority in the choice of site, from the medical point of view, was determined by the incidence of cancer and the ease of accessibility. Access to these deep sites could be obtained from the anus, the mouth, and the vagina. Mechanical and acoustic design for these confined body spaces presented a challenge. Since commercial supply of natural transducer material was limited – ceramic transducers were only just appearing – the United States Navy 15-MHz transducer capsules were adapted, where possible, for clinical study. Real-time operation was again deemed obligatory for clinical study. In 1951, instrumentation for cervix, uterus, prostate, rectum, and colon was designed within the existing technical limitations and with the available materials, and construction was started.

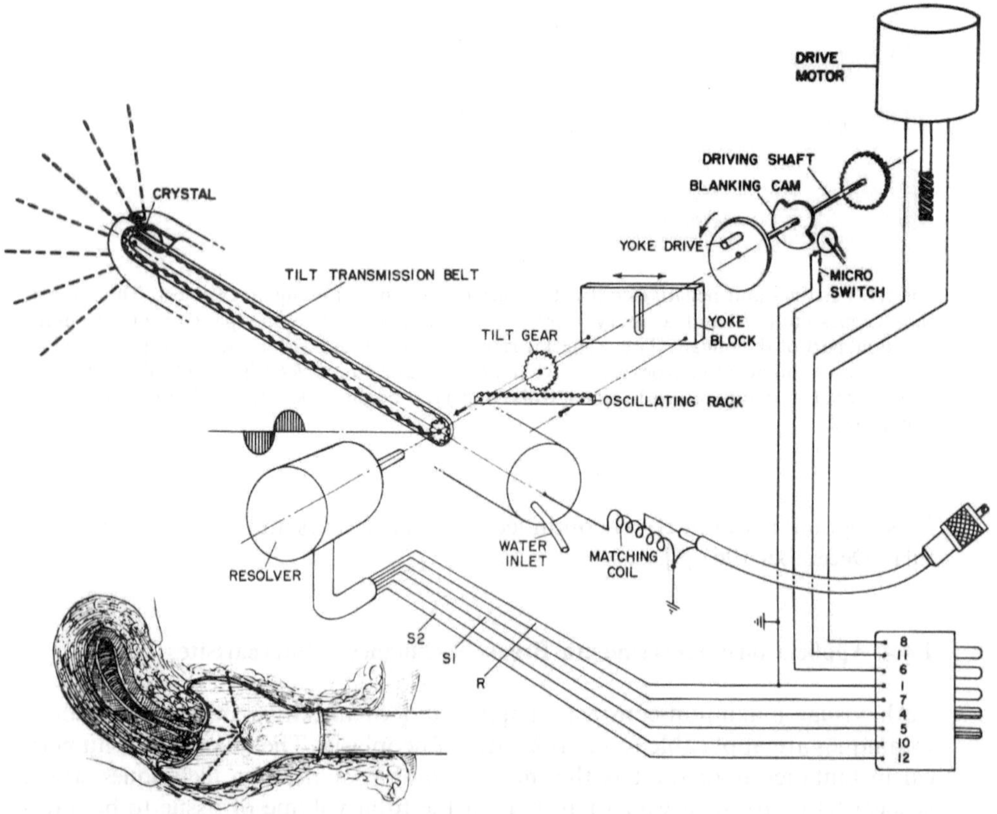

Fig. 1.10. The first vaginal sector scanning instrument, designed in 1953

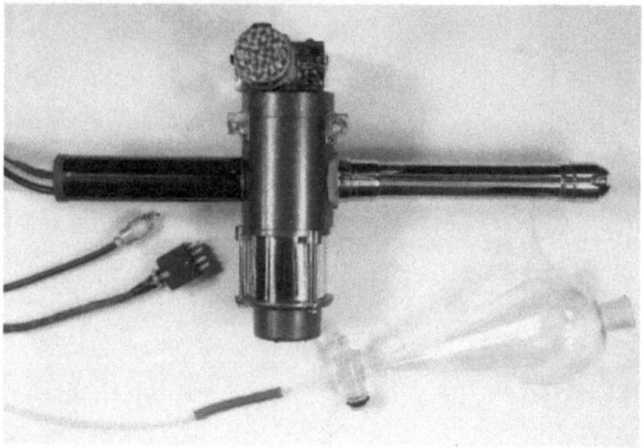

Fig. 1.11. The finished vaginal sector scanning instrument, completed in 1954

1.5.1 Vaginal Approach

Figure 1.10 shows a schematic drawing of the self-contained instrument designed to produce a sector B-mode scan of the cervical area and beyond. This instrument, completed in 1953 (Fig. 1.11), was never used clinically because of transducer difficulties; however, practicability was demonstrated.

1.5.2 Anal Approach

A preliminary drawing of the rigid rectosigmoid-prostatic instrument (June 1953) is shown in Fig. 1.12. The automatic operation necessary for complete serial tomographic imaging was realized by provision of an automatic withdrawal mechanism, with sequential photographic recording of the radial time-base scan images (Fig. 1.13). A schematic drawing of the final version is shown in Fig. 1.14. In use, the colonoscope (Fig. 1.15) was inserted with bowel inflation,

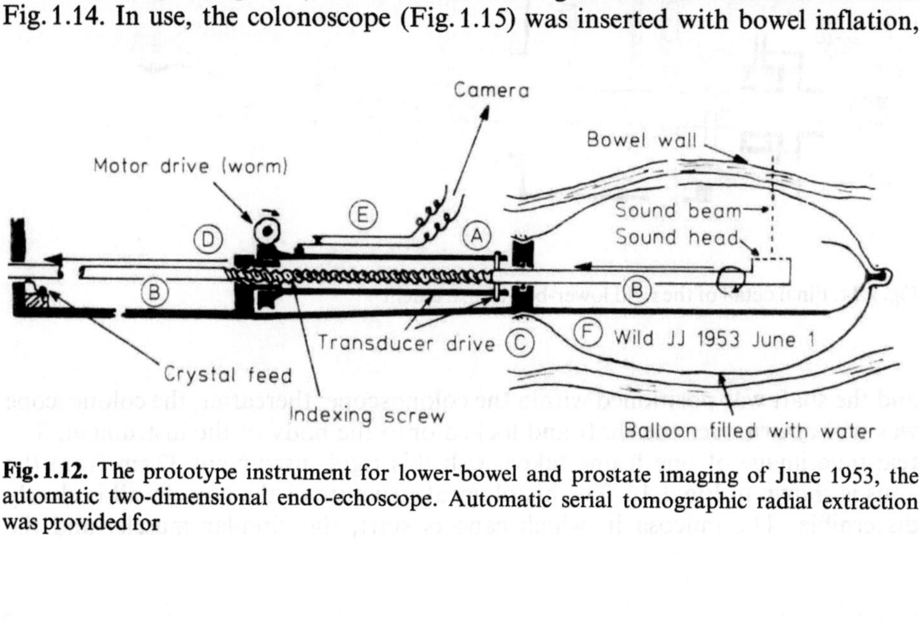

Fig. 1.12. The prototype instrument for lower-bowel and prostate imaging of June 1953, the automatic two-dimensional endo-echoscope. Automatic serial tomographic radial extraction was provided for

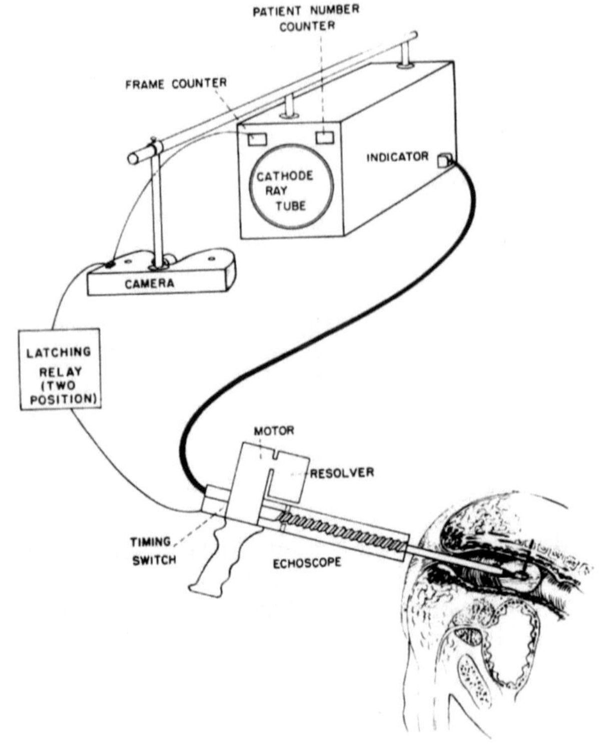

Fig. 1.13. The prototype instrument shown in Fig. 1.12 as used in three-dimensional mass rectal scanning

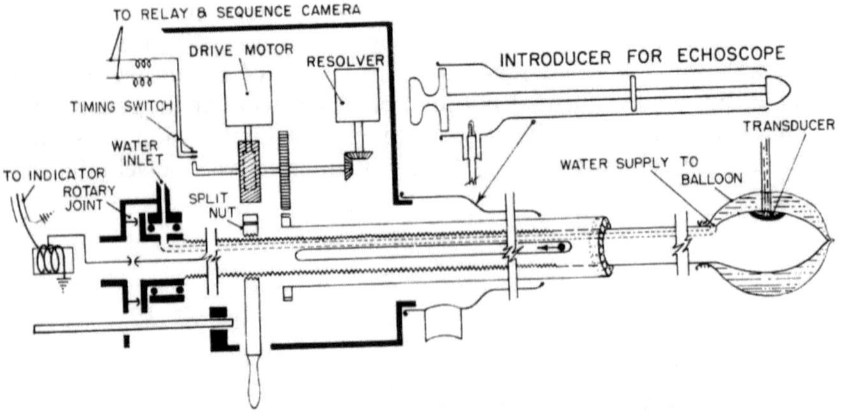

Fig. 1.14. Final detail of the rigid lower-bowel instrument

and the shaft was positioned within the colonoscope; thereafter, the colonoscope was withdrawn over the shaft and locked onto the body of the instrument. The real-time image of one frame taken with this rigid instrument 32 cm from the anus is shown in Fig. 1.16. The histological structure of the bowel wall is clearly discernible. The mucosa in which cancers start, the circular muscle, and the

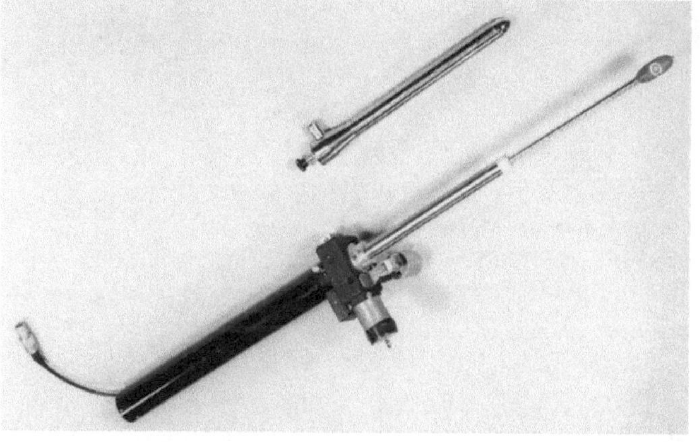

Fig. 1.15. The finished rigid lower-bowel instrument. The total length of the probe portion was 32 cm, with 20 cm of automatic extraction being provided

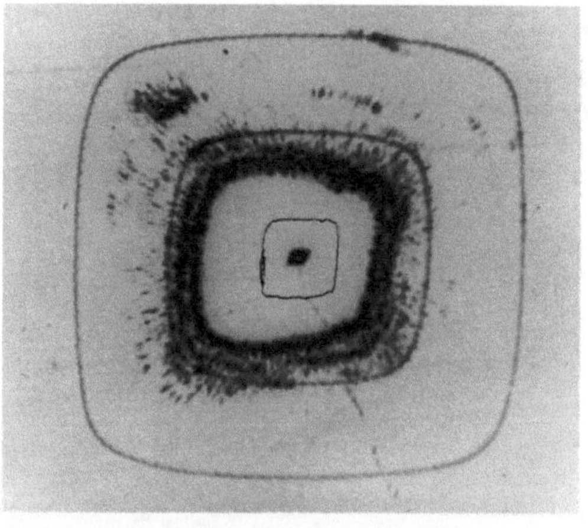

Fig. 1.16. The first radial time-base image taken at 30 cm within normal colon at 15-Mc frequency. The range marks are 1 cm apart. The histological layers of the bowel wall are resolved. The mucosa, the circular layer of muscle, and the three longitudinal muscle bands are shown. The square shape is due to a failure in the resolver windings. The images were made in 1955–1956

bands of longitudinal muscle are easily identified. This first pulse-echo image of the bowel was published in June 1955 [14]. A second prostatic linear B-mode instrument was constructed, but it was not completed, again because of transducer difficulties.

1.5.3 Flexible Instrumentation for Colon and Lower Bowel

For the colon, a flexible instrument was necessary. This first instrument, completed in 1953, was self-contained and hand-held. It was driven by the coaxial

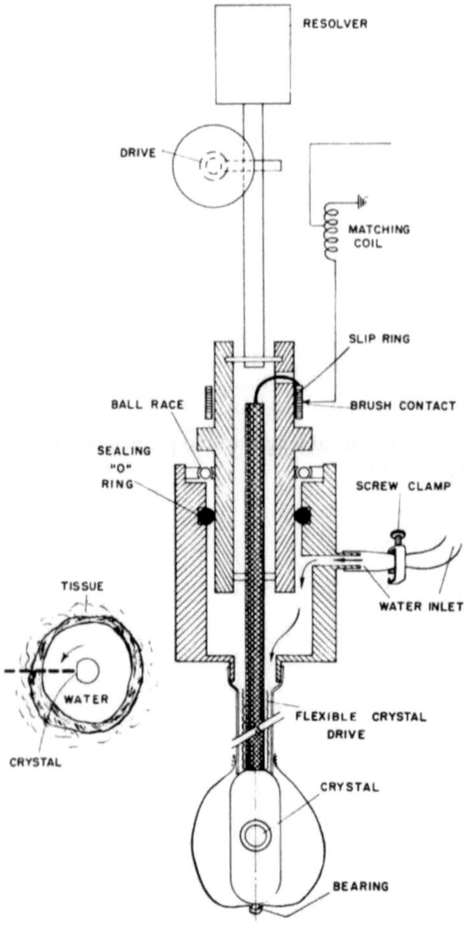

Fig. 1.17. The first flexible colon instrument design (1954). The coaxial wire connection to the transducer was used to drive the sound head

cable supplying the transducer (Fig. 1.17). Figure 1.18 is a photograph of the completed instrument. No means was provided for automatic extraction. The instrument was never used clinically because of the jerky drive discernible in Fig. 1.19.

When this instrument was being tested, a shubunkin goldfish was allowed to swim freely in the tank. The tripartite tail and other diaphanous fins were seen to be resolved whenever presented in the line of sight of the revolving sound beam. This revelation inspired further efforts to develop a smooth, circular, radial transducer drive and instrumentation suitable for automatic lower-bowel imaging.

Figure 1.20 shows a sectional drawing of the second flexible sound head designed for the necessary "blind" insertion into the lower bowel. The problem of jerky drive was solved by use of an "O" ring with a frictional fit on the drive shaft. A photograph of the completed unit is shown in Fig. 1.21. In order to obtain a constant water path, a water cavity sealed by a replaceable rubber membrane was provided within the sound head. This design ensured constant contact

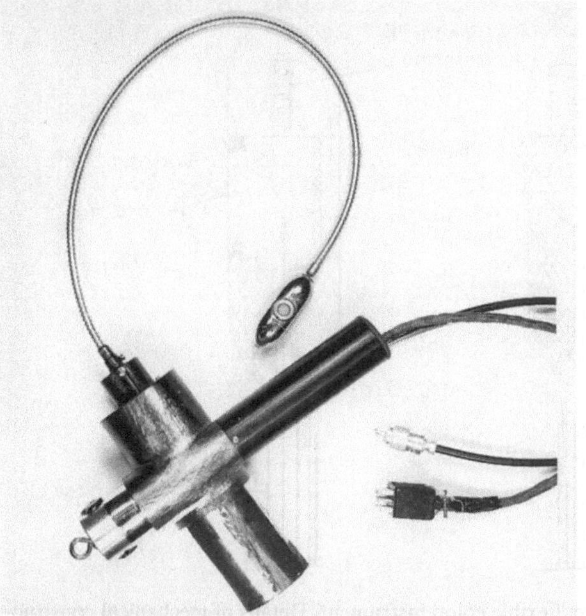

Fig. 1.18. The final version of the self-contained, hand-held instrument shown in Fig. 1.17, which had a length of 60 cm. No automatic withdrawal was provided

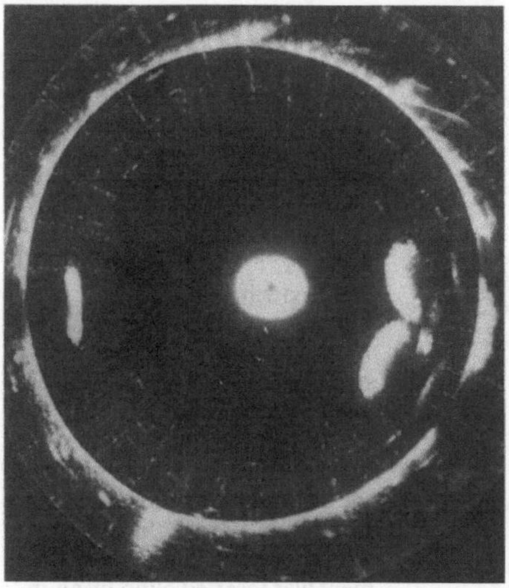

Fig. 1.19. The images of two finger palps (*right*), taken when the instrument shown in Fig. 1.19 was tested in a cylindrical tank of water. The radial lines arose from jerkiness of the drive shaft

with the bowel lining during extraction. Two consecutive frames of normal bowel are shown in Fig. 1.22. A radiograph of the instrument in place is shown in Fig. 1.23. Serial radial tomograms of the normal colon were recorded automatically as the sound head was withdrawn. The fine histological structure of the normal colon and signals believed to arise from the prostate were observed as the instrument was nearing complete withdrawal.

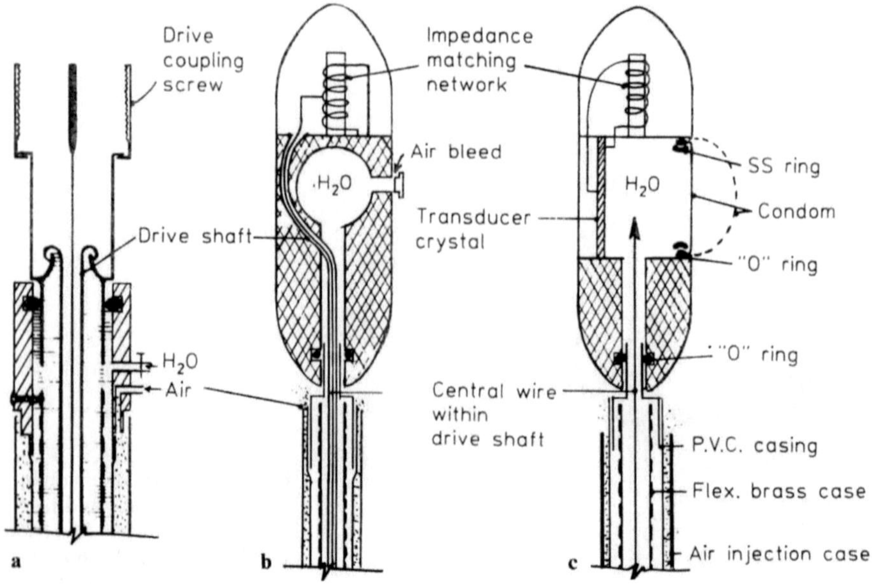

Fig. 1.20 a–c. The final smooth-drive, flexible colon instrument. Details of mechanical construction are shown, but the drawing is not to scale

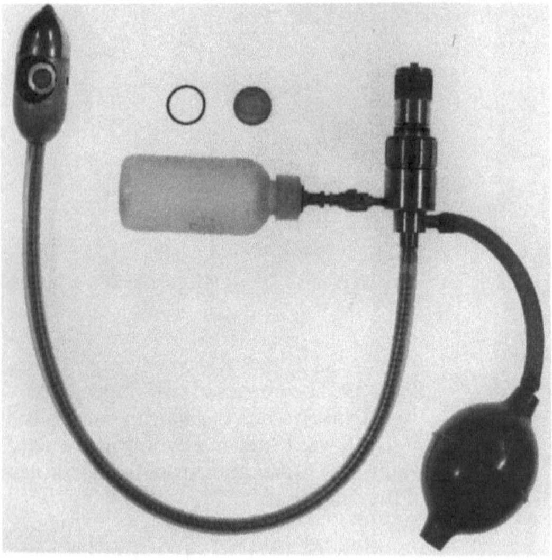

Fig. 1.21. The instrument depicted schematically in Fig. 1.20, which was completed in 1956. The rubber membrane, stretched over a ring and held by an O ring, is pushed into the transducer chamber. The latter is filled with degassed water from the plastic bottle to form a domed membrane, which is in contact with the bowel lining. The instrument was inserted blind by air inflation. The length was 48 cm

A recurrent carcinoma of the colon, where the rectum had been removed and the colon surgically attached to the anal region, was examined with the instrument shown in Fig. 1.21. A series of radial time-base images (Fig. 1.24) showed destruction of the normal histological structure by the cancer as the instrument neared the anal region. Large-bowel screening for neoplasia had become possible.

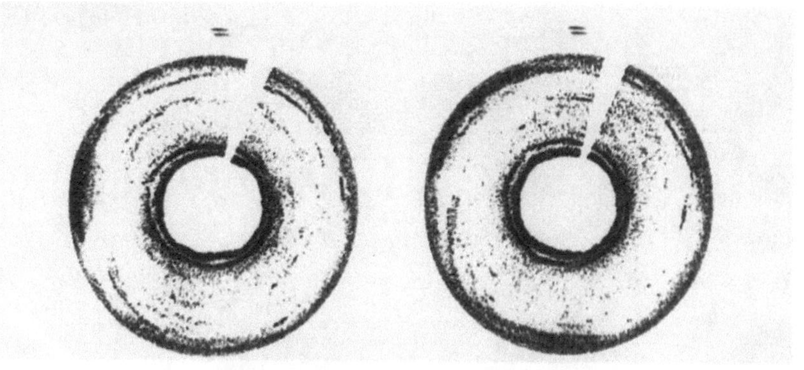

Fig. 1.22. Two of the automatic serial real-time images of the normal colon at high gain, taken as the sound head neared the anus. The mucosa is clearly resolved, together with the circular muscle layer. In addition, signals from the prostate are defined

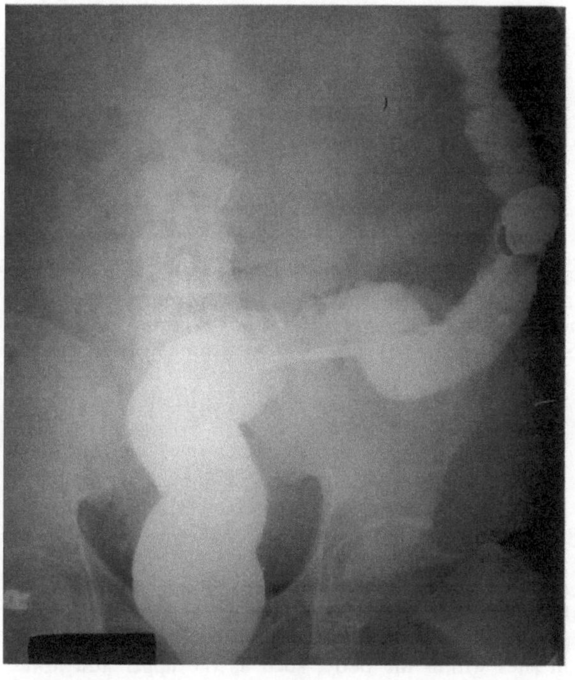

Fig. 1.23. Radiograph of the instrument shown in Fig. 1.22, which was used early in 1956

We looked into the future and hoped that for mass screening purposes, the use of flexible sound head units would permit time-saving "blind" insertion by air inflation into several waiting patients, prior to connection with the extraction instrumentation. Employment of several flexible examination units would also facilitate efficient cleaning and sterilization to prevent cross-infection. These flexible units could even be disposable.

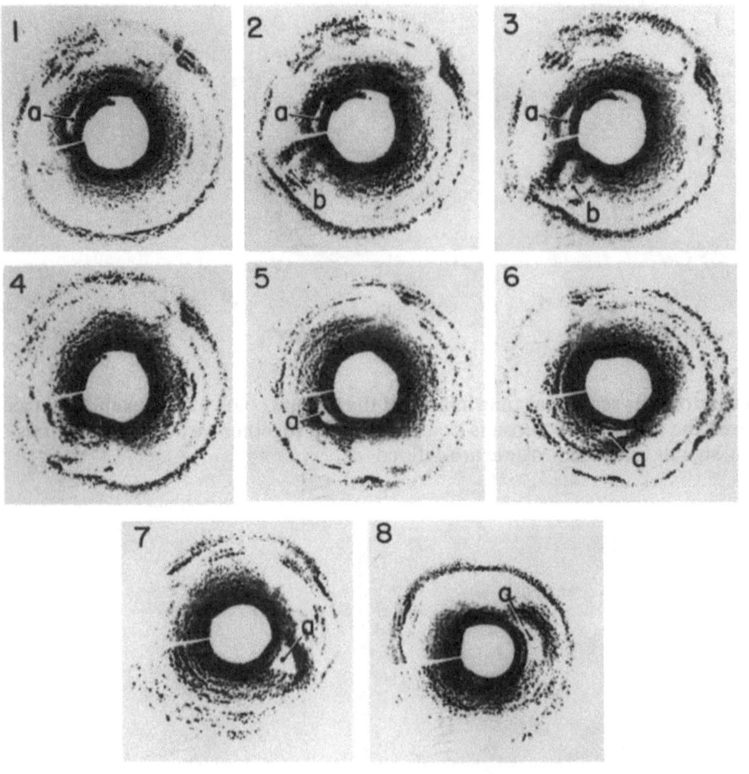

Fig. 1.24. Radial time-base images of a case of recurrent carcinoma of the colon. The gain of the system was approximately the same as that in Fig. 1.23. The bowel is shown surrounded with malignant infiltration. Frames 1–4 show an ulcer protruding into the bowel lumen. At *a*, negative contrast (lacunae) was thought to be due to necrotic tissue. At *b*, the peripheral signals were thought to arise from the prostate

1.6 Discussion

In 1954, Wild and Reid [13, p. 282] stated:

> By selecting the highest available frequency (15 megacycles) as a starting point for studies in spite of apparent range limitations, the authors believe that they have made possible the early detection and diagnosis of irregularities of tissue structure of sufficiently small size to be of value in the control of cancer, at common sites within the body, such as the upper and lower gastrointestinal tract, accessible from the mouth and anus, respectively, the cervix uteri, and prostate.

Each site presents special problems, depending on the range. In the colon, advantage can be taken of the occurrence of neoplasms at minimal range to obtain an optimally increased frequency. Because of the great internal surface area to be interrogated, instantaneous numerical readout would be desirable and possible, together with automatic withdrawal of the sound head. The tissue comparison techniques described for the breast can also be applied to the prostate, ovaries, uterus, and cervix uteri where the range is comparable.

Results produced with these systems continue to be unique in the field because the techniques used are different in concept from conventional radiology, which is set on defining an anatomical map. The superior images are believed to result primarily from reflection of the diffuse backscattered sonic energy from cellular structure at high frequency, together with the technique of producing maximum black/white visual contrast. The method is capable of adaptation to the instantaneous electronic readout necessary for screening.

A useful, somewhat loose, analogy to distinguish between the two visual ultrasound techniques (subjective visual scrutiny of cartographic images and instantaneous, high-contrast readout) for tumor detection is that of looking for the proverbial needle in a haystack. The interpretive visual scrutiny approach has to distinguish the needle by minute examination of the signal pattern of the hay matrix; in the high-contrast readout approach, the interrogating transducer simulates a magnet passed over the hay maxtrix, which ignores the hay until the needle comes into range and is immediately revealed as it attaches itself to the magnet with a click.

Perhaps it is time to reexamine these early successful techniques, developed many years ago, more closely – a sentiment echoed recently by Dempsey [1], who sees future ultrasound research focusing on some of these original efforts.

References

1. Dempsey PJ (1988) Breast sonography: historical perspective, clinical application, and image interpretation. Ultrasound Q 6:73
2. French LA, Wild JJ, Neal D (1950) Detection of cerebral tumors by ultrasonic pulses. Cancer 3(4):705–708
3. French LA, Wild JJ, Neal D (1951) The experimental application of ultrasonics to the localization of brain tumors. J Neurosurg 8:198–203
4. French LA, Wild JJ, Neal D (1951) Attempts to determine harmful effects of pulsed ultrasonic vibrations. Cancer 4:342–344
5. Reid JM, Wild JJ (1956) Current developments in ultrasonic equipment for medical diagnosis. Proc Natl Electron Conf 12: (Also IRE Trans Ultrason Eng 1957) 5:44
6. Wild JJ (1949) Report on the use of ultrasonic pulses for the measurement of biological tissues. Department of Surgery, University of Minnesota, Nov
7. Wild JJ (1950) The use of ultrasonic pulses for the measurement of biologic tissues and the detection of tissue density changes. Surgery 27:183–188
8. Wild JJ (1978) The use of pulse-echo ultrasound for early tumour detection: history and prospects. In: Hill Cr, McCready VR, Cosgrove DO (eds) Ultrasound in tumour diagnosis. Pitman, Kent, pp 1–26
9. Wild JJ (1983) Review of the ultrasonic examination of the breast. In: Jellins J, Kobayashi T (eds) Ultrasonic examination of the breast. Wiley, New York, pp 21–30
10. Wild JJ (1985) The potential of pulse-echo ultrasound for breast screening. Proceedings, Ultrasonics International, 1985, pp 958–963
11. Wild JJ, Reid JM (1952) Further pilot echographic studies on the histological structure of tumors of the living intact breast. Am J Path 28:839–861
12. Wild JJ, Reid JM (1953) The effects of biological tissues on 15mc pulsed ultrasound. J Acoust Soc Am 25:270–280
13. Wild JJ, Reid JM (1954) Echographic visualization of lesions of the living, intact human breast. Cancer Res 14:277–283
14. Wild JJ, Reid JM (1957) Progress in the techniques of soft tissue examination by 15 M.C. pulsed ultrasound. Proceedings, symposium on ultrasound in medicine and biology, June 1955. Publication no 3, 1957, American Institute of Biological Sciences

2 Endosonography: Physical Basics and Instrumentation

H.-P. SCHWARZ

2.1 Introduction

"Ultrasound" is the name given to a class of mechanical pressure waves that can be propagated to liquids, solids, and, to some extent, gases [1]. Mechanical waves have frequencies which range from little more than 0 Hz up to several hundred million. For convenience, this vast range may be represented in the form of an *acoustic spectrum,* which is analogous to the more familiar spectrum of electromagnetic radiation. A typical frequency spectrum of mechanical waves is represented in Fig. 2.1, where a logarithmic scale has been chosen so that each tenfold increase in frequency is represented by an equal distance. The spectrum can be seen to consist of three broad regions, which overlap at their boundaries. The central region encompasses the audible spectrum from about 20–30 Hz up to about 16 Hz, these frequencies being the approximate lower and upper frequency limits of the average human ear. The region below about 20 Hz is designated *infrasound*, while frequencies greater than about 16 kHz are called *ultrasound* (US).

US makes it possible to produce cross-sectional images of organs and parts of the body. But US examination of a patient is fundamentally different from most other diagnostic procedures [2, 3]. In the X-ray department, the radiologist or technologist prepares the patient and sets up the instrument; if the proper adjustments are made, a useful picture will be produced automatically. In the nuclear medicine laboratory, the technician sets up the scanner, aligns the patient, and injects the bolus of isotope; the machine does the rest. In both of these techniques, there is little interaction among operator, instrument, and patient once the actual procedure starts. By contrast, the final result of all US procedures, good or bad, depends on the operator's knowledge and ability to use the instrument in an interactive way on the subject. The operator must be able to interpret the dynamic echo patterns as the procedure progresses in order to control the direction of the US beam to secure the desired result. The information patterns produced must be optimized by movement of the transducer and manipulation of the instrument controls to achieve a scan or image that coincides with established standards and techniques. In all these applications, there are appropriate acoustic or dynamic landmarks serving as references in generating images that must be learned and understood.

This interactive process must become second nature if the physician or technologist is to be really effective. This means that the operator of the equipment should have an almost intuitive understanding of all the elements of this complex interactive detection and measurement system. To understand the function and

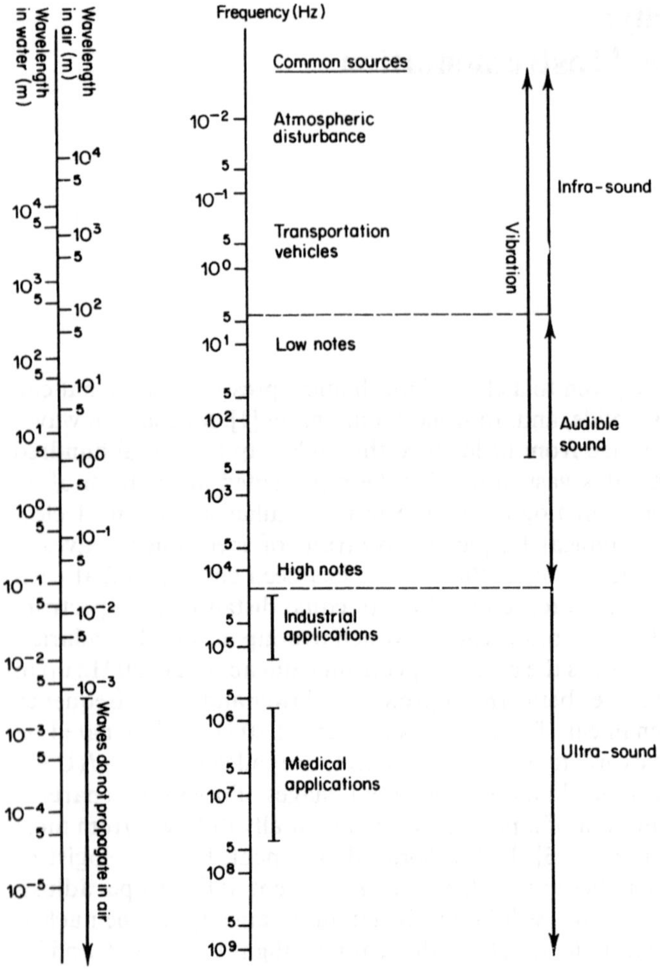

Fig. 2.1. An acoustic spectrum illustrating the range of frequencies of mechanical waves and some common sources of generation and fields of application. (From [8])

the role of the technical aspects of these procedures, one may consider the processes depicted in Fig. 2.2. There are three principal components involved in these interactive procedures: the physician or technologist, the instrument, and the patient. The instrument serves as a coupler or converter to transform acoustic information from the subject into a form interpretable by a qualified operator. The machine is not automatic; therefore, the results that it presents to the user depend on its design and on how it is operated.

The basic instrument has two principal interfaces. First, the electroacoustic interface, called the transducer, converts electronic signals into acoustic pulses or continuous waves, which are transmitted into the tissue of the patient. These same transducers serve as receivers to detect the reflected pulses from within the subject. Second, an audiovisual-electronic interface converts the detected or

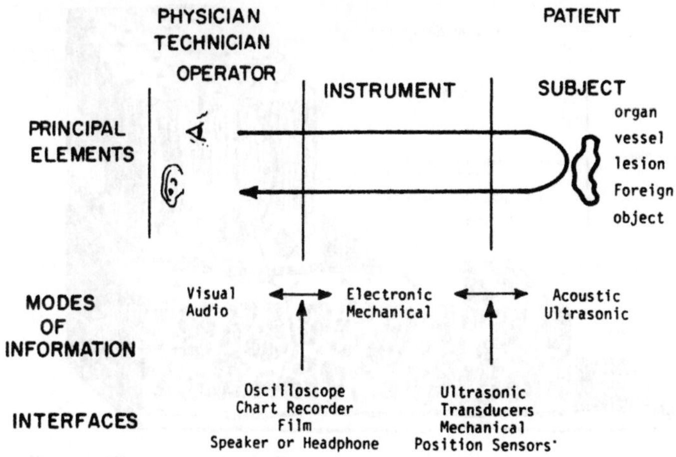

Fig. 2.2. Electronics, acoustics, and mechanics are used to transform information in a physical form within the subject into a form that the operator or physician can interpret. The optimal instrument permits the most efficient transfer of information through the two interfaces. (From [4])

processed echo signals, which pass through the electronics of the instrument, into a form that the technologist can evaluate. This interface may be the screen of an oscilloscope, a chart recorder, a camera, or a speaker in Doppler sonography [4].

2.2 Special Problems

Endosonography is a special examination and makes great demands both on the physician's technical knowledge and on the technical equipment used. One important example in the field of endosonography is the identification and differentiation of single layers in adjacent organs, such as the rectal, bladder, or stomach wall. This is essential for accurate so-called sonographic staging. But in fact, the differentiation of layers and the correspondence between US images and anatomical topologies represents one of the central problems in endosonography [5].

To illustrate this problem, Figs. 2.3–2.6 show the anatomical structure and some corresponding US images of the rectal wall. In Fig. 2.3, seven anatomical layers can be recognized, with four bigger layers (mucosa, submucosa, muscularis, and serosa). In Fig. 2.4, these four important layers are represented again schematically. The thickness of the individual layers ranges from 0.1 mm to a few millimeters. The total thickness is about 4 mm. The physician expects to see the various layers in the US image. Figures 2.5 and 2.6 show US images of the rectum. In the first picture, recorded with older technical equipment (3.5-MHz transducer), a lesion on the left side is to be seen, but no layers can be separated or differentiated, and so clinical staging is not possible. In Fig. 2.6, recorded with newer equipment (5-MHz transducer), another rectum is depicted, and here three white lines, separated by two dark lines, are perceptible.

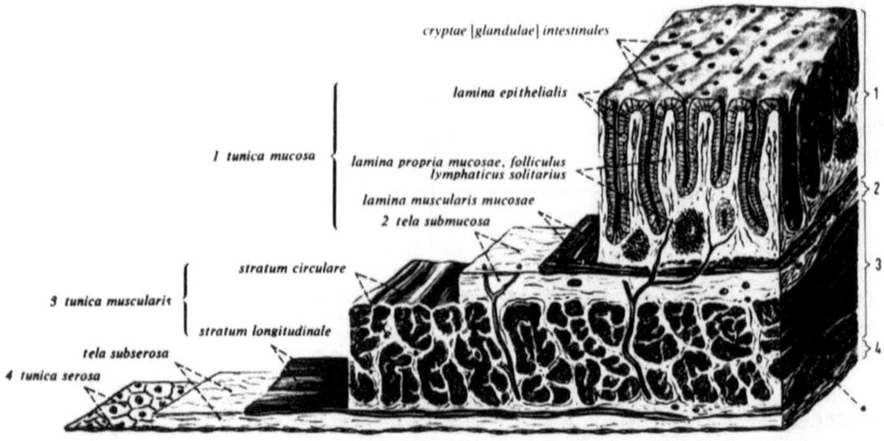

Fig. 2.3. Anatomical layers of the rectal wall. Numbers *1–4* indicate the larger layers. (From [15])

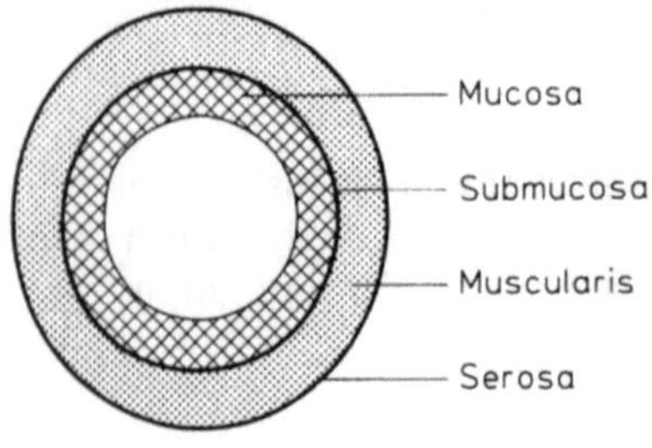

Fig. 2.4. The four important layers of the rectal wall

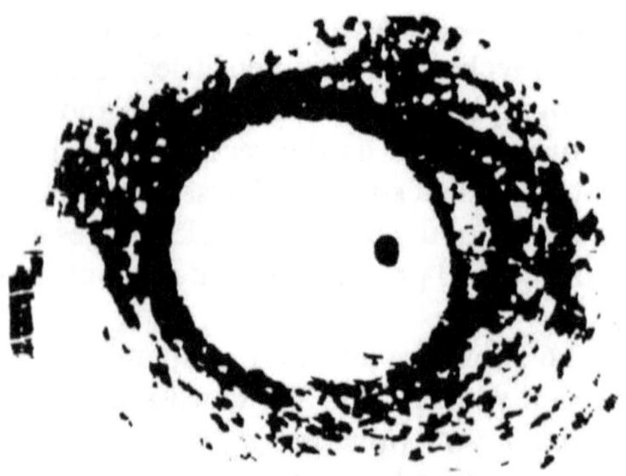

Fig. 2.5. Sonogram of a rectum, recorded with older equipment (3.5 MHz)

The following questions arise from these images:

1. What is the meaning of the white and dark lines in an US image of the rectum? Do they represent layers such as mucosa or muscularis?
2. In general, what is the correspondence between US images and anatomical topologies?

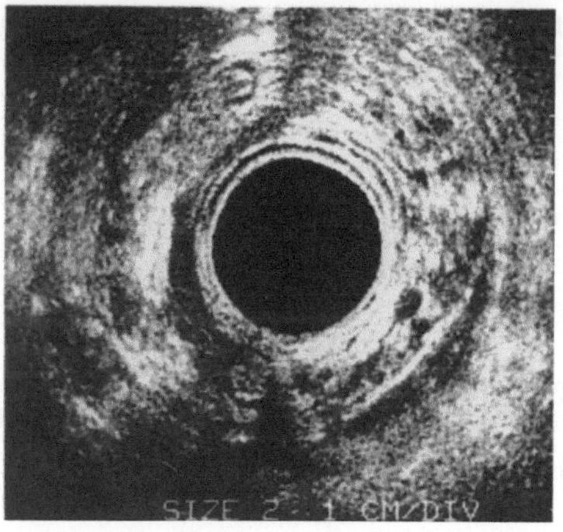

Fig. 2.6. Sonogram of a rectum, recorded with a newer ultrasound system (7.5 MHz)

3. Why are sometimes only one or two lines seen and sometimes two or more lines?
4. Why do the lines arise only at the top of Fig. 2.6, and not at the bottom, too?

To answer these questions, we have to go into a little bit of theory.

2.3 Basic Principles

First, we must make clear how an US image is generated. Nearly all of the US imaging methods are based on the so-called pulse-echo method, whereby an US pulse is generated by a transducer and transmitted into an adjacent medium, e.g., a human body in medical applications or a steel specimen in nondestructive applications. If the US pulse reaches an interface, it is reflected, and the reflected pulse is received by the transducer again. Another kind of imaging is US computer tomography (CT), similar to X-ray CT. But as US CT has not the same importance in medicine as X-ray CT, we shall only discuss pulse-echo methods.

2.3.1 A-Scan

An US pulse is only reflected when it reaches an interface (Fig. 2.7). An interface is a boundary between two different media with different acoustic impedance values, the impedance being defined as

$$Z = \varrho c$$

where Z is the acoustic impedance, ϱ is the density of the medium, and c is the sound velocity of the medium. The latter is defined as

$$c = \lambda \nu$$

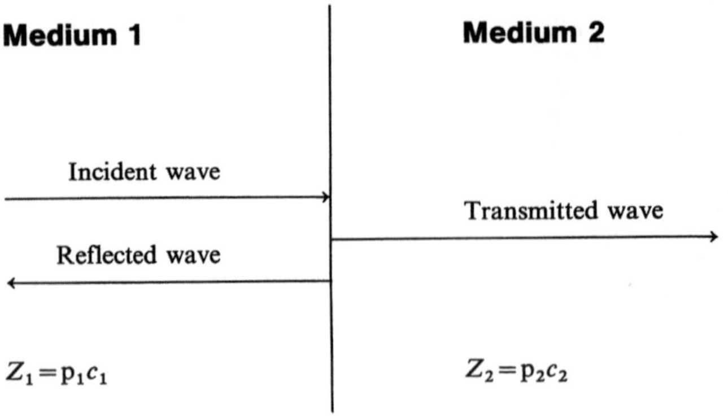

Fig. 2.7. Reflection and transmission of an ultrasound pulse at an interface

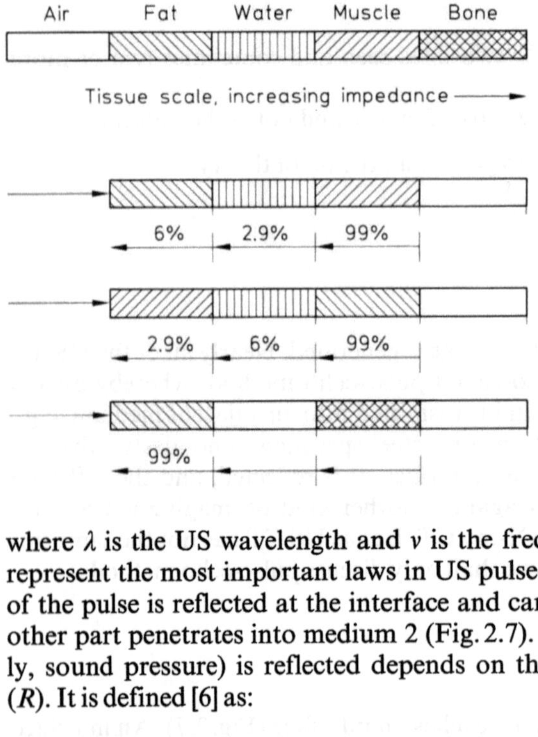

Fig. 2.8. Examples of reflected pressure amplitudes (expressed as percentages) at different tissue interfaces. *Arrows* (*left*) indicate incident waves

where λ is the US wavelength and ν is the frequency. These physical quantities represent the most important laws in US pulse-echo imaging methods. One part of the pulse is reflected at the interface and can be received by a transducer; the other part penetrates into medium 2 (Fig. 2.7). How much energy (more precisely, sound pressure) is reflected depends on the so-called reflectivity coefficient (R). It is defined [6] as:

$$R = \frac{Z_2 - Z_1}{Z_2 + Z_1}.$$

In medicine, the impedances of the different tissues (liver, kidney, spleen, muscles, fat, collagen etc.) only vary in a very small range, and so the factor R only has a value of about 0.01–0.06. This means that only 1%–6% of the sound amplitude is reflected at such an interface. In Table 2.1, some typical values of US parameters for various tissues are shown. Figure 2.8 shows schematically the reflected pressure amplitudes at several tissue interfaces.

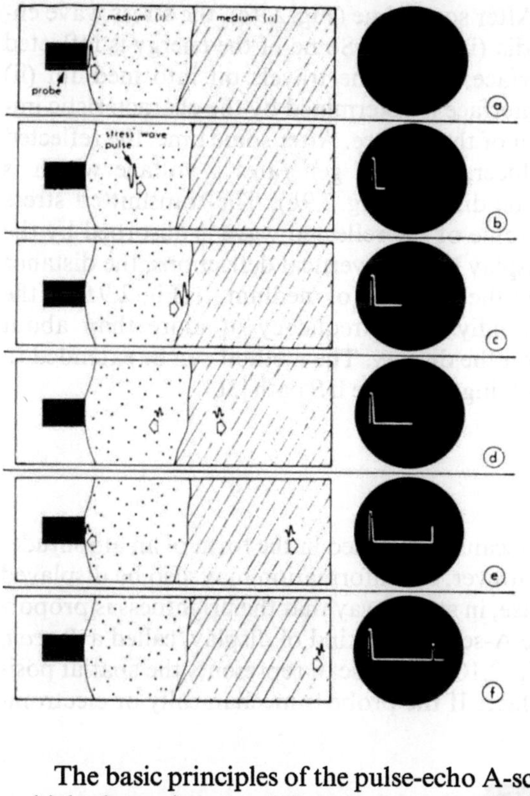

Fig. 2.9 a–f. Basic principles of the pulse-echo system. For details see text. (From [3])

The basic principles of the pulse-echo A-scan system are illustrated in Fig. 2.9, which shows how an US pulse may be used to measure the depth of an echo-producing interface. The US probe is arranged to emit a short-duration stress wave into medium (i) in response to an electrical excitation. At the same instant, the luminescent spot on the screen of a cathode-ray tube display begins to move at a constant velocity from left to right. The vertical-deflection plates of the cathode-ray tube are connected to the output from an amplifier, the input of which is derived from the US probe. Therefore, the luminescent spot is deflected vertically at the instant that the stress wave is transmitted because the exciting voltage is also applied to the amplifier (Fig. 2.9 a). The stress wave travels at a constant velocity through medium (i), and the luminescent spot traces a horizon-

Table 2.1. Typical values of ultrasound parameters in various media

Parameter	Medium								
	Water	Blood	Connective tissue	Fat	Liver	Kidney	Muscle	Lung	Bone
ϱ (g/cm^3)	1.00	1.06	1.06	0.92	1.06	1.04	1.03	0.40	1.60
v (mm/μs)	1.50	1.57	1.54	1.45	1.55	1.56	1.54	0.65	4.08
$z (\times 10^6\ \mathrm{kg\,m^{-2}\,s^{-1}})$	1.50	1.66	1.63	1.33	1.64	1.62	1.59	0.26	6.53
$\lambda_{5\,\mathrm{MHz}}$ (mm)	0.30	0.31	0.31	0.29	0.31	0.31	0.31	0.13	0.82

tal line on the display (Fig. 2.9 b). After some time (Fig. 2.9 c), the stress wave encounters the interface between media (i) and (ii). Some of the energy is reflected back into medium (i) at the interface, and some travels on into medium (ii) (Fig. 2.9 d); the reflectivity of the interface is determined by the characteristic impedance ratio and the configuration of the surface. After some time, the reflected stress wave returns to the transducer, where it generates a voltage which is amplified to deflect the trace on the display (Fig. 2.9 e). The transmitted stress wave travels on into medium (ii), some of the reflected wave is absorbed by the transducer, and the trace on the display has two vertical deflections, the distance between these being proportional to the thickness of medium (i) (Fig. 2.9 f). If the process is repeated sufficiently rapidly (at a frequency of more than about 20 Hz), a steady trace is observed on the display. The method can be extended to the examination of many interfaces lying along the US path [3].

2.3.2 B-Scan

The information obtained by an A-scan is presented in the form of an amplitude-modulated time base (Fig. 2.9). However, the information may also be displayed on a brightness-modulated time base, in such a way that the brightness is proportional to the echo amplitude of the A-scan. This kind of display, called a *B-scan*, is compared with the A-scan in Fig. 2.10. The B-scan represents the spatial position of each echo-producing interface. If the probe is mechanically or electroni-

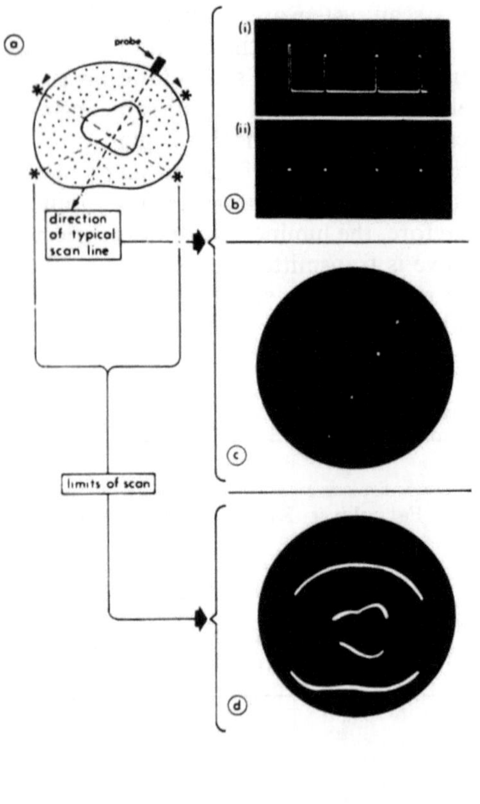

Fig. 2.10 a–d. A-scope and B-scope methods for displaying ultrasound pulse-echo information. **a** A section through a patient. **b** A-scope presentation (*i*) of a typical scan line and B-scope presentation (*ii*) of the same scan line. **c** B-scan as in **b** (*ii*), but with the direction of the time base linked to the direction of the ultrasound beam. **d** Compound B-scan, integrated from many individual scans, each one similar to **c**. (From [3])

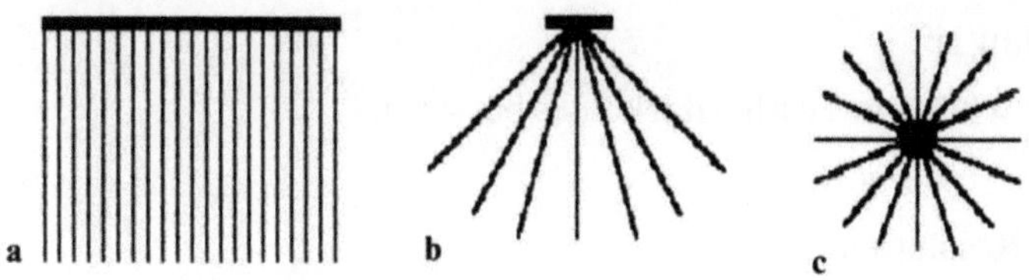

Fig. 2.11 a–c. Real-time scanning methods. **a** Linear scan. **b** Sector scan. **c** 360° scan

cally moved around the patient, and if all the separate B-scans (each one similar to that shown in Fig. 2.10c but corresponding to a different transducer position and beam direction) are integrated, e.g., on a photographic plate, then an image such as that shown in Fig. 2.10d is produced. This is a compound B-scan, and it represents a two-dimensional section through the patient in the plane of the scan.

Several two-dimensional US scanning systems are possible. The better known methods (where the probe is moved mechanically or electronically are (Fig. 2.11) (a) linear scan, (b) sector scan, and (c) 360° scan. The scanning method used, in endosonography is the 360° scan (Fig. 2.11).

2.3.3 Correspondence Between Morphologic Stratification and B-Scan Representation

Let us consider a very simplified layer model of the rectal wall (Fig. 2.12). This model consists of two layers and three interfaces. Each of the interfaces produces a peak in the A-scan representation, and if the probe is moved, three white lines appear in the two-dimensional B-scan representation. This fact is very important; many people misinterpret US images because, as this example shows, only interfaces are represented by US; i.e., one layer, always bounded by two interfaces, is generally represented in a B-scan device by two white lines with one dark line between them (if we omit scattering effects). We are now able to recognize a general law:

1 layer produces 2 white lines with 1 dark line between.
2 layers produce 3 white lines with 2 dark lines between, and so on.

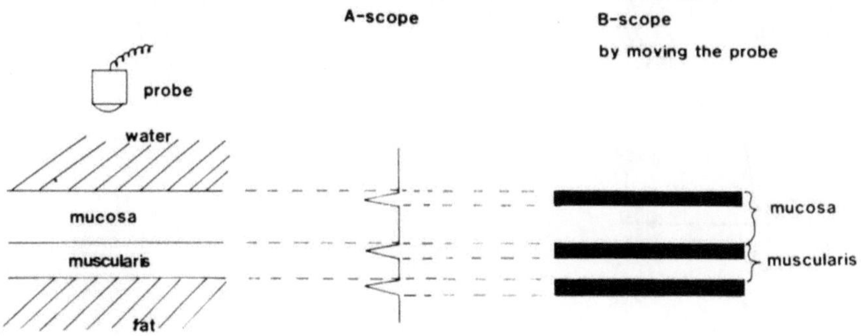

Fig. 2.12. Correspondence between morphologic stratification (*left*) and ultrasound B-scope representation (*right*)

The general form of this law is:

n layers produce $n+1$ white lines with *n* dark lines between.

2.3.4 Lateral and Range Resolution

A further requirement must be met: the range resolution of the US equipment has to be good enough to separate the layers in the way described above. This fact is elucidated in Fig. 2.13: the upper part shows two surfaces or interfaces which can be separated by the US pulse. In the lower part, the interfaces are too close together, and the two signals melt into one signal, which means that separation is no longer possible. This illustrates the problem of US imaging: sometimes, if the layer is thick enough, it is represented by two white lines, and at other times, if it is too small, it is represented by only one line. That is to say, a sufficiently high resolution capacity is a necessary condition for accurate differentiation of rectal layers, or accurate clinical staging.

The range resolution itself, defined as the ability to separate two points or interfaces lying one behind the other in the direction of the sound propagation, depends on the following physical quantities:

1) The length of the electrically transmitted pulse
2) The damping of the probe
3) The frequency
4) The presetting of the gain

The range resolution is improved when:

1) The length of the electrical impulse decreases.
2) The damping of the probe increases.
3) The frequency increases.
4) The gain of the amplifier is decreased as much as possible.

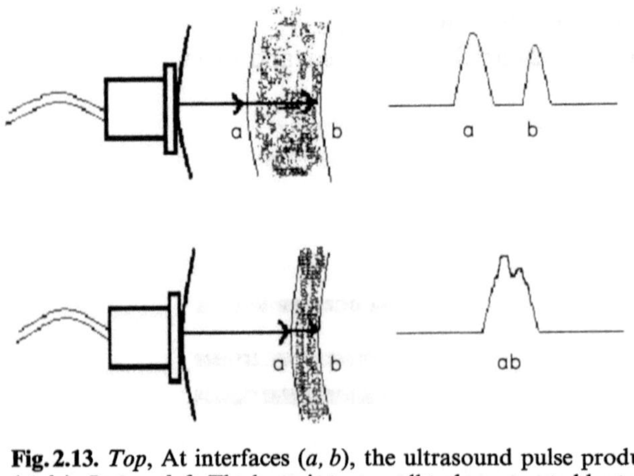

Fig. 2.13. *Top*, At interfaces (*a*, *b*), the ultrasound pulse produces two separate A-scan signals (*right*). *Bottom left*, The layer is too small to be separated by two A-scan signals. *Right*, There is only one A-scan signal. Artifacts due to insufficient range resolution.

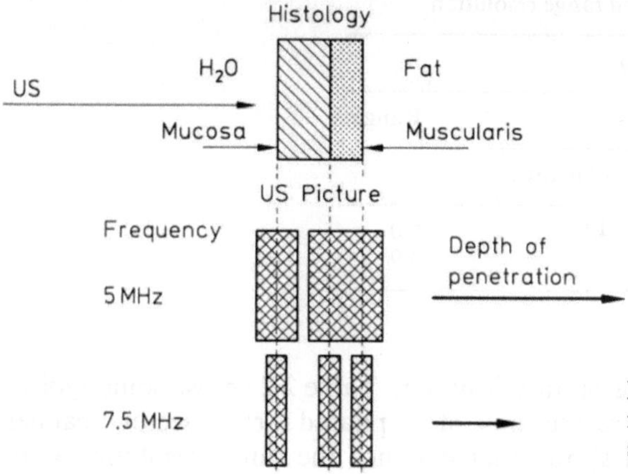

Fig. 2.14. Improvement of the range resolution by increasing the ultrasound frequency

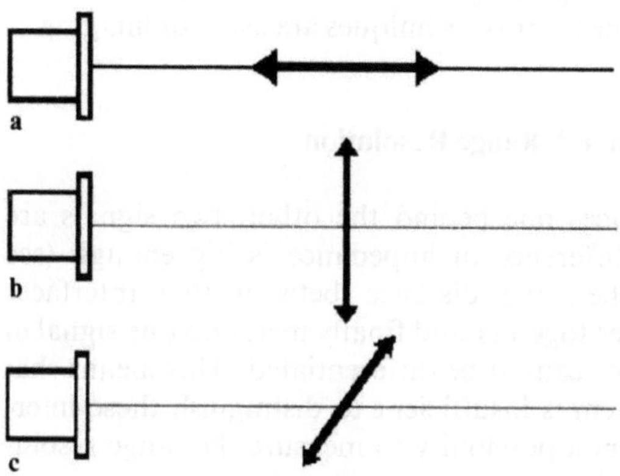

Fig. 2.15 a–c. The three types of resolution: range (**a**), elevative lateral (**b**), and azimuthal lateral resolution (**c**)

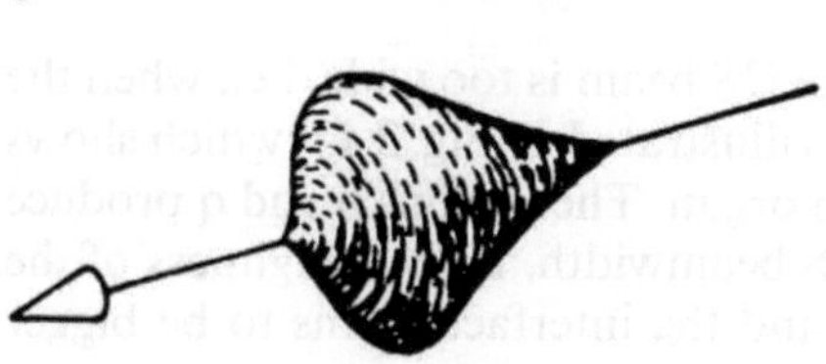

Fig. 2.16. The resolution cell of a typical pulse-echo system. (From [7])

Figure 2.14 makes this clear in a simple way: the performance of interface differentiation increases with higher frequencies; however, the depth of penetration decreases with increasing frequency.

Another type of resolution is the lateral resolution. We have to differentiate between two forms, elevative and azimuthal lateral resolution. The lateral resolution is defined as the ability to separate two points or interfaces lying on a line perpendicular (either azimuthal or elevative) to the direction of sound propagation.

The three types of resolution are depicted in Fig. 2.15. Together, they form the resolution cell, in which the interaction between US and medium (human tissue, materials, water) occurs (Fig. 2.16) [7]. The resolution cell or the three types of resolution represent one important parameter among the many which define

Table 2.2. Typical values for lateral and range resolution

Distance	Resolution (mm)		
	Lateral		Range
	Azimuthal	Elevative	
50 mm	1.8	4.5	1.0
100 mm	3.3	5	0.9

the quality and the performance of an US system. Table 2.2 shows some typical values for lateral and range resolutions of a phased array sector scanner (3.5 MHz). The example given shows that it is not the range resolution (1.0, 0.9 mm), but the lateral resolution, especially the elevative lateral resolution, which is a problem when phased or linear array techniques are used for imaging.

2.3.5 Artifacts Due to Insufficient Lateral/Range Resolution

If an US pulse reaches two interfaces one behind the other, two signals are produced (occur) as long as the difference in impedance is big enough (see Sect. 2.3.1; Figs. 2.7, 2.13). But when the distance between the interfaces decreases, the two signals move closer together and finally melt into one signal in the A-scan, so that the two interfaces cannot be differentiated. This means that the range resolution of our US system is insufficient to distinguish these interfaces in the B-scan image. This offers a possibility to measure the range resolution of an US system using the B scan image.

We find another type of artifact when the US beam is too wide, i.e., when the lateral resolution is insufficient. This effect is illustrated in Fig. 2.17, which shows schematically a wavelike surface of a human organ. The regions p and q produce two separate echoes because of the finite US beamwidth. If the roughness of the surface increases, the echo only broadens, and the interface seems to be bigger than it is in reality.

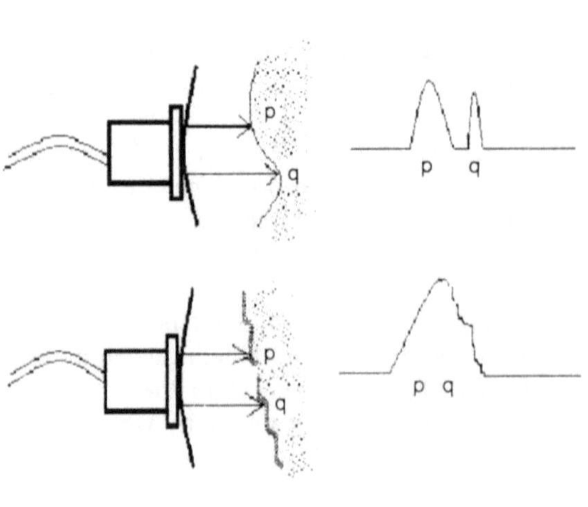

Fig. 2.17. Artifacts due to finite beamwidth. For details see text

2.3.6 Focusing Sound

It is possible to use the properties of reflection or refraction to cause the wave energy distributed along the entire wave front to be concentrated at one small point in space, known as a *focus*. This means that the lateral resolution improves, and with it the US B-image. Focusing has no direct influence on the range resolution capability.

But why do we have to focus an US wave in general? The answer is that the US field of a transducer is very inhomogeneous in the near field (Fig. 2.18). The nearfield (N), defined as

$$N = \frac{D^2}{4\lambda},$$

where D is the aperture of the transducer and λ is the wavelength of the US beam, is the distance from the transducer to the point where the last pressure maximum occurs (in Fig. 2.18, the distance O–N). For example, if we use a transducer with a 7-mm aperture (diameter) and with a driving frequency of 7.5 MHz (a very suitable frequency in endoscopy), the transducer has a near-field length of about 61 mm. But in the near field, an examination is not possible because of the alternating sound pressure.

The simplest device for bringing a plane wave front to a focus is a curved reflector (this is analogous to the use of a curved mirror to focus a beam of light). Figure 2.19 shows two rays from a plane progressive wave being brought to a focus at point F after reflection from a curved surface, which is a portion of a sphere. As in optics, one only obtains a point focus if the rays are close to the

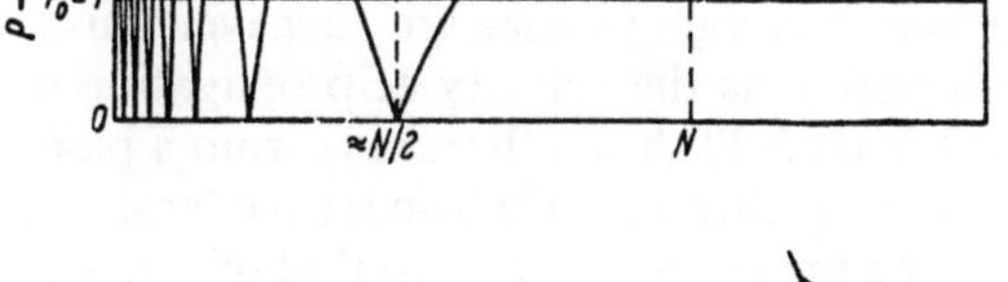

Fig. 2.18. Near and far field of a transducer, or sound pressure (P) on the acoustic axis. (From [8])

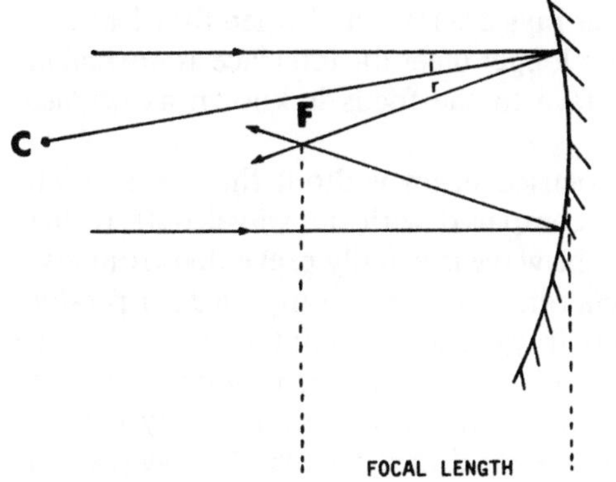

Fig. 2.19. Reflection from a curved surface to generate a point focus (F) of sound. As in optics, the point C represents the center of the sphere from which the curved reflector has been cut. The angle of incidence (i) is equal to the angle of reflection (r), so that the focal length is half the radius of curvature (From [8])

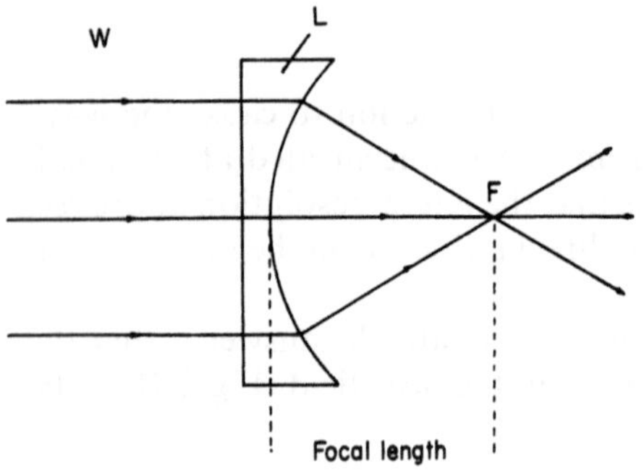

Fig. 2.20. The path of a plane acoustic beam through a converging lens (*L*) suspended in water (*W*), which concentrates the sound at the focus (*F*). (From [8])

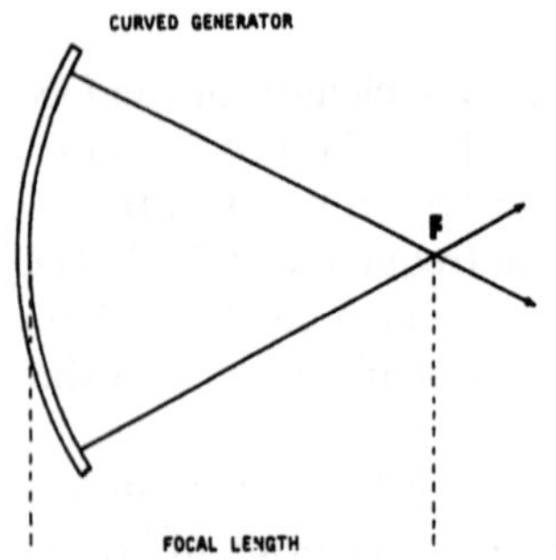

Fig. 2.21. A curved transducer generates a focus (*F*) whose dimensions depend upon the aperture of the transducer relative to the wavelength (i.e., a large transducer having a spherical surface must generate a large focal volume because of spherical aberration). (From [8])

focus, i.e., if it is a reflector of small aperture. But this type of focusing is not usual in endoscopic US imaging.

A plane wave may also be brought to a focus by refraction through a lens, which may be made of any material whose velocity of propagation is different from that of the bulk medium. In general, solid lenses have propagation velocities greater than that of water, and therefore converging lenses are concave. This is the opposite of the situation found in optics, as the velocity of propagation of light in glass is lower than that in air. Figure 2.20 shows three rays from a plane progressive mechanical wave striking the flat face of a plano-concave lens. The lens material is chosen to have an acoustic impedance similar to that of water so that most of each wave enters the lens; the rays are not refracted, as they enter at normal incidence. However, the two outer rays are refracted when they leave the lens and reenter the water because they no longer meet the interface at normal incidence. The distance from the lens surface to the focus is known as its *focal length.*

A curved generator can produce a focused beam without the use of a lens (Fig. 2.21). The generator must be large compared with the wavelength (otherwise it would act as a point source), and the wave is usually prevented from leaving the back of the generator. Curved generators are commonly used for producing focused fields of US waves [8]. But in practice, a point focus cannot be achieved, and the situation illustrated in Fig. 2.22 exists. According to Wells [7], the focal volume is roughly ellipsoidal. The diameter of the intensivity volume, being reduced by 3 dB (see Sect. 2.6) from the maximum value in the x-y plane, is

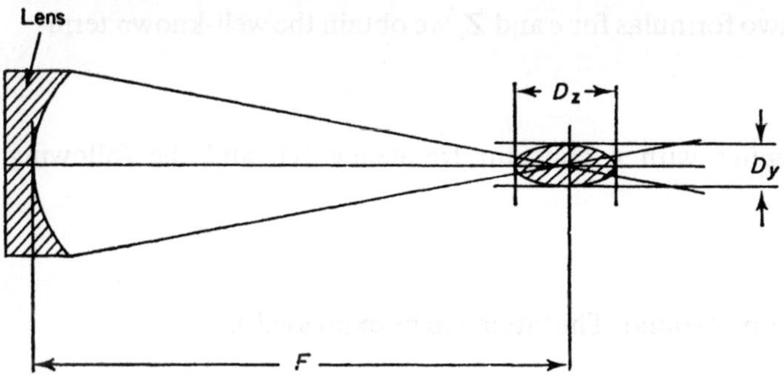

Fig. 2.22. The focal region of a focusing system. *F*, focal length; *D*, diameter. For details see text. (From [7])

given by

$$D_y = D_x \sim \lambda F/D$$

where λ is the wavelength in tissue and D is the aperture, i.e., the diameter of the probe. The diameter of the focal volume in the x-z plane or y-z plane [7] is given by

$$D_z \sim 15\, D_y$$

which means that there is a small focal range in the x-y plane and a large focal range in the x-z or y-z plane.

2.3.7 Ultrasound Interactions with Media

Two forms of US interactions can be distinguished: (a) elastic interactions and (b) nonelastic interactions [9].

2.3.7.1 Elastic Interactions

Some of the elastic interactions have already been discussed, e.g., reflection. In addition, elastic sound propagations belong to this group of interactions. The sound propagates in a medium with a certain velocity (c), which is defined as

$$c = \sqrt{(K/\varrho)}$$

where K is the elasticity modulus and ϱ is the density of the medium. But the propagation is disturbed by interfaces of tissue, organs, bones, and cancer nodes, according to the different impedances of the various tissues (see Sect. 2.3.1). The impedance (Z) is given as

$$Z = \sqrt{(K\varrho)}.$$

If we combine the two formulas for c and Z, we obtain the well-known term

$$Z = \varrho c.$$

The sound propagates with a constant frequency (ν), and the following relationship exists:

$$c = \lambda \nu$$

where λ is the wavelength of sound. The latter can be expressed as

$$\lambda = c/\nu$$

This means that the velocity (c) and the wavelength (λ) are not constant and vary according to the tissue in which the wave is propagating. The frequency has a constant value if we neglect the frequency-dependent attenuation.

In Fig. 2.23, the sound velocities in various tissues are shown. One can see that even the sound velocity in a given tissue varies within a certain range, and so it is obvious that tissue differentiation based solely on the parameter of sound

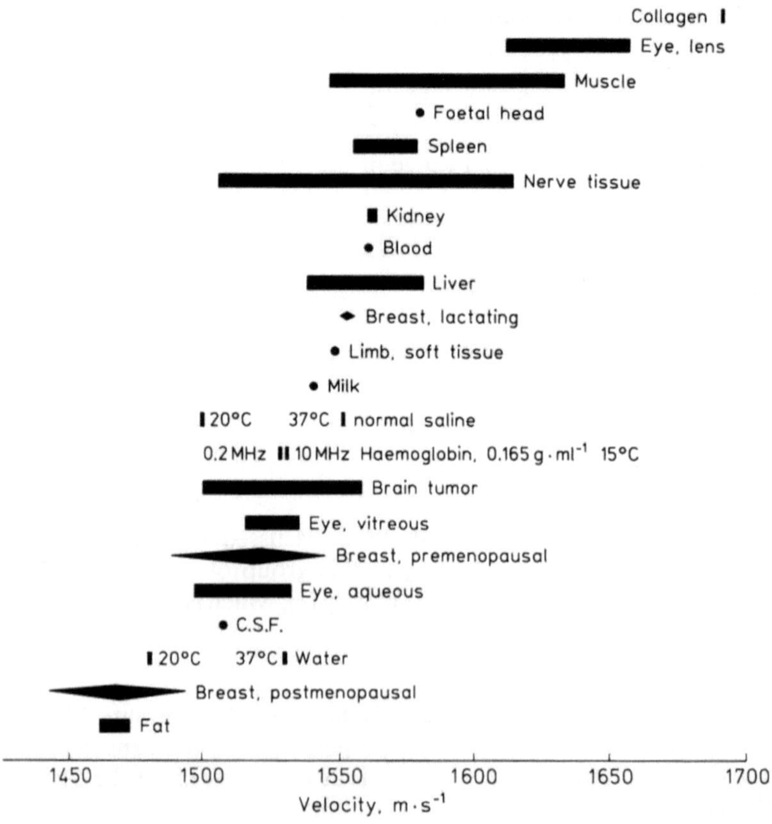

Fig. 2.23. Sound velocity values for various tissues. ■, total range; ◆, mean ± 1 SD; ●, single estimate. (From [7])

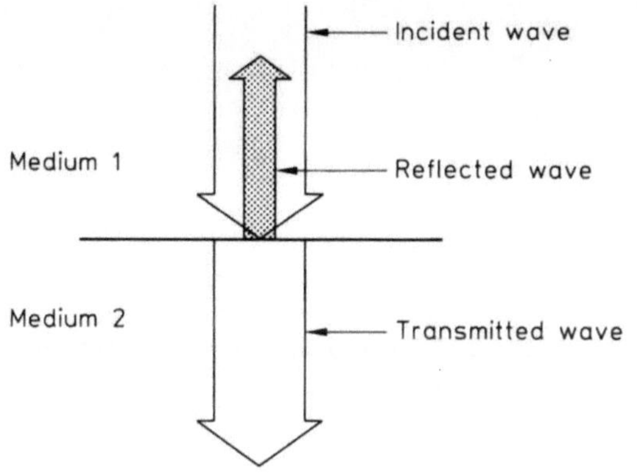

Fig. 2.24. Reflection of ultrasound at a large interface

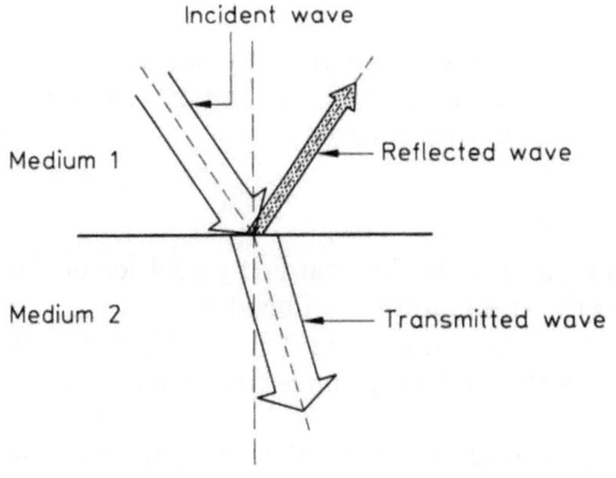

Fig. 2.25. Refraction of ultrasound at a large interface

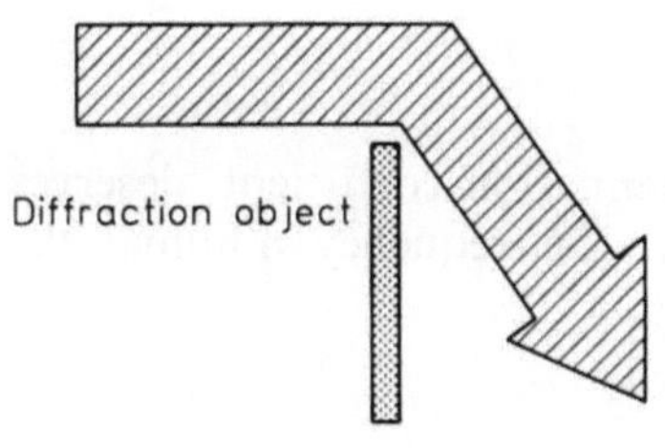

Fig. 2.26. Diffraction of an ultrasound wave at a small diffraction object

velocity is not possible, given the overlapping velocity values for the various tissues.

The above formulas are the most important relations in elastic wave propagation (if we omit velocity effects such as the Doppler effect). The propagation of sound is further disturbed by reflection, refraction, and diffraction (Figs. 2.24–2.26). Reflection and refraction occur when the object of disturbance is large compared with the US wavelength (e.g., large organ boundaries). Diffraction occurs when the object of disturbance is comparable with the US wavelength (e.g., point reflectors such as edges and tips).

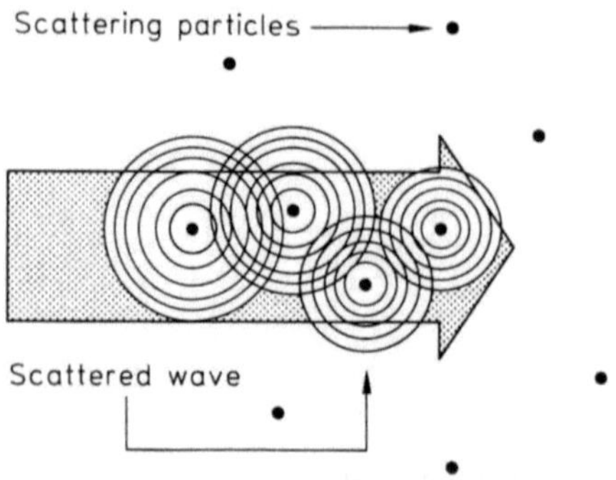

Fig. 2.27. Ultrasound wave scattered by small particles

2.3.7.2 Nonelastic Interactions

The most important effect in nonelastic wave propagation is attenuation; the intensity of the sound wave decreases exponentially with an attenuation coefficient (α) which consists of an absorption and a scattering portion:

$$\alpha = \alpha_A + \alpha_S$$

where α_A is the absorption coefficient and α_S is the scattering coefficient. In medicine, the more significant factor is the attenuation coefficient α_A.

The scattering effect is represented schematically in Fig. 2.27: the US energy is scattered omnidirectionally by particles that are very small compared with the US wavelength (λ).

In summary, the following physical formula expresses the attenuation of the US sound pressure amplitude along the path $X\,[A(X)]$:

$$A(X) = A_0 e^{-[\alpha_A(\nu) + \alpha_S]X}$$

where A_0 is the initial amplitude.

The factor $\alpha_A(\nu)$, the frequency-dependent attenuation coefficient, deserves special attention. This factor increases linearly with the frequency in human tissue:

$$\alpha_A \sim \nu$$

This means that the higher the frequency, the higher is the damping of the US in tissue; i.e., with high-frequency US, penetration of large distances is not possible. But in endoscopic US, only small distances need be penetrated, and so high-frequency US is applicable.

2.4 Instrumentation

2.4.1 Basic Information

The possible applications in the field of endosonography are various. First, we have to differentiate between four types of endosonography: (a) transesophageal, (b) transrectal, (c) transvaginal, and (d) transurethral endosonography. In all these types, the same techniques are used to generate US images.

In general, the following kinds of US systems are available on the market:

1) Mechanical 360° scanners [used in (a), (b), (c), and (d)]
2) Mechanical 90°–110° sector scanners [used in (c)]
3) Electronic linear arrays [used in (a), (b), and (c)]
4) Electronic phased arrays [used in (a)]

The first US scanners (1957) were mechanical, and even today, most of them are still mechanical. The rectal, transurethral, and vaginal scanners have a rigid rod, at the tip of which the one-element transducer is mounted. The transducer can be turned, rotating at about 0–15 cycles/s (Fig. 2.28) [10].

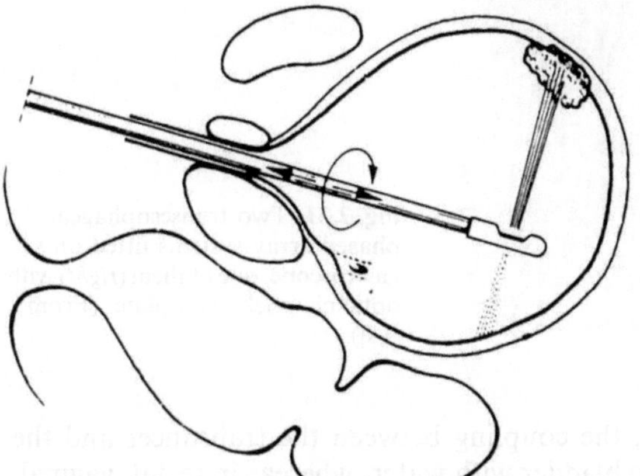

Fig. 2.28. Transurethral ultrasonography: operation of a mechanical scanner. (From [10])

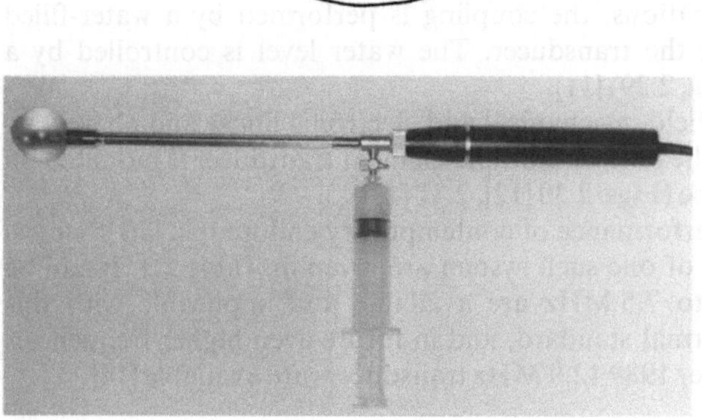

Fig. 2.29. Transrectal mechanical 360° scanner, with rubber balloon and water syringe. (From [11])

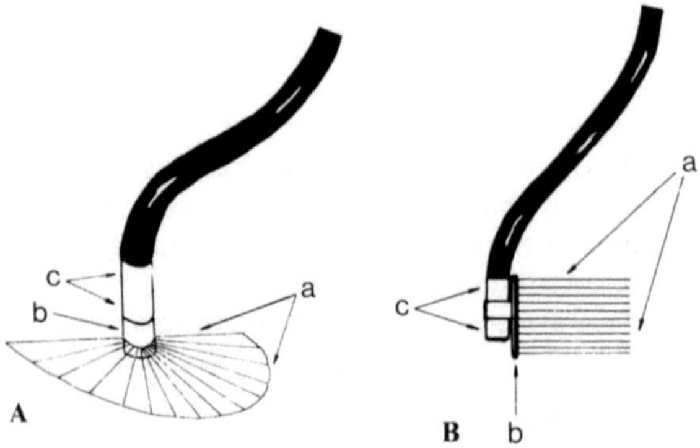

Fig. 2.30 A, B. Transesophageal endoscopic systems. **A** Mechanical sector scanner. *a*, scanning plane; *b*, transducer; *c*, endoscopic part. **B** Electronic linear array system. *a*, scanning plane; *b*, transducer; *c*, instrument tip. (From [12])

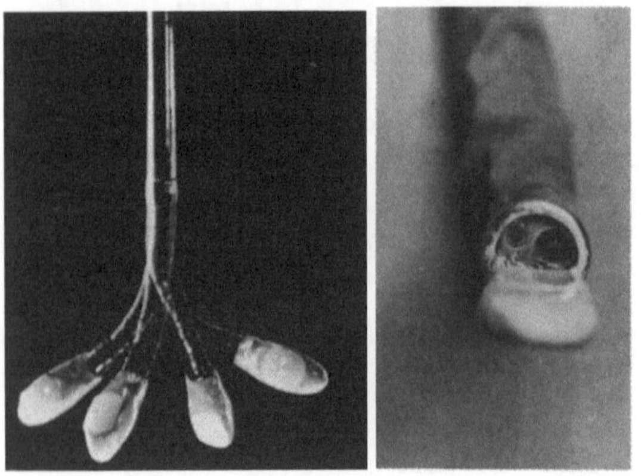

Fig. 2.31. Two transesophageal phased array systems fitted on a gastroscope, one of them (*right*) with optic channels on a plate. (From [13])

In transurethral applications, the coupling between the transducer and the bladder wall is made by filling the bladder with water, whereas in rectal, vaginal, and transesophageal applications, the coupling is performed by a water-filled rubber ballon surrounding the transducer. The water level is controlled by a syringe from the outside (Fig. 2.29) [11].

In the transesophageal field, mechanical and electronic linear and phased array systems are available. The one- or multiple-element transducer is mounted on the tip of a flexible endoscope (Figs. 2.30 [12], 2.31 [13]).

As an example of the performance of contemporary endoscopic US systems, the technical specifications of one such system are given in Table 2.3. It can be seen that transducers up to 7.5 MHz are available and applicable with this system. Today, this is a normal standard, and in future even higher frequencies are conceivable since October 1989 12.0 MHz transducers are available [14].

Table 2.3. Technical specifications of an endoscopic ultrasound system. (From [14])

Item	Specification
Display mode	B-mode
CRT scan method	Standard TV system
Monitor	
Viewing	High-resolution, 9-in. TV monitor
Photography	Built-in 5.5-in. TV monitor
Diagnostic field	6, 9, 12, or 18 cm selectable
Gain control	Overall gain and STC
STC adjustment	8-point slide controls (0, 1, 2, 3, 4, 6, 8, and 10 cm)
Dynamic range	7-step change-over from 20 to 80 dB
Image direction	Lateral inversion possible
Image polarity change-over	Negative/positive inversion possible
Image processing	3 steps: AGC off, 1, and 2
Automatic display	Year, month, day, hour, minute, second; filed size; scanning frequency; grey scale
Parameters measured	Distance, area, and circumference
Power consumption	Ca. 270 W
Dimensions (maximum)[a]	69 × 140 × 100
Weight	110 kg
Photographic equipment	Built-in Polaroid camera
VCR recording	Possible
Frequency	7.5 MHz
Diameter of transducer/focus	7 mm × 30 mm
Scanning method	Radial scanning
Drive method	DC motor with flexible-shaft transmission
Scanning direction	At right angles to direction of insertion
Contact methods	Balloon attachment method, deaerated water immersion method
Outer diameter of distal end	13 mm
Length of rigid distal tip	42 mm
Angulation range	Up-down 130°, left-right 90°
Working length	1300 mm
Viewing direction	70° forward oblique
Angle of view field	80°
Channel diameter	2 mm (does not accommodate forceps)
Photographic equipment	OM-1N Camera with adapter SM-2S

AGC, automatic gain control; CRT, cathode-ray tube; STC, slide time gain control; VCR, videocassette recorder.
[a] Weight × height × depth in millimeters.

2.4.2 Functions of Instrument Controls

The pulse-echo instrument is the principal interface between the operator and the patient. The process of locating, detecting, and evaluating echo patterns depends on close interaction between the operator, the equipment, and the subject. The positioning of the transducer is based on the display results, which the operator can observe and interpret. The signals that appear on the display depend both upon the settings of the various controls on the instrument and on the direction in which the transducer is pointed. Decisions to move the transducer are based on these interactive judgements. Details of the basic pulse-echo system are given in

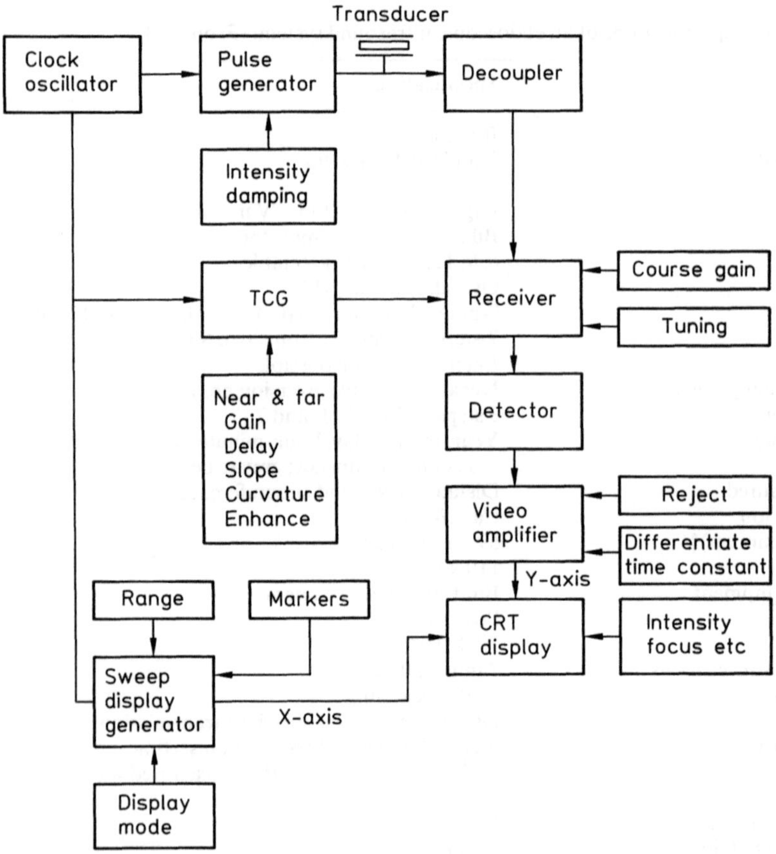

Fig. 2.32. The important control functions of a basic pulse-echo system, which modify the operation of the principal functional elements. *TCG*, time-compensated gain; *CRT*, cathode-ray tube

the form of a block diagram in Fig. 2.32. The control functions indicated in various blocks are the principal knob adjustments that the operator will use to modify the display.

Signals detected from the transducer are amplified in the receiver, detected, further amplified by the video amplifier, and then presented to the cathode-ray tube display. Almost all of the controls with which the operator is concerned have to do with this amplifying and detecting sequence. The first of these are the receiver and time-compensated gain functions. The receiver is used to amplify weak echoes up to the point at which they will be displayed. This amplifier must be capable of compensating for attenuation of the echo, which becomes more pronounced with increasing depth. The compensation is accomplished with a time-compensated gain unit coupled to the receiving amplifier. Without compensation, the echoes will fall in amplitude, as shown in Fig. 2.33. The rate of fall-off of the echo amplitude depends on the transmitted frequency, attenuation characteristics of the tissue, and transducer design (i.e., focused versus non-focused).

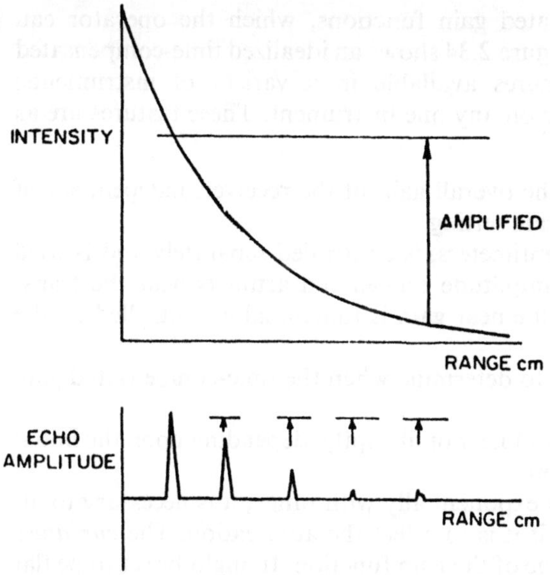

Fig. 2.33. Echoes from distant interfaces need to be amplified more than near echoes in order to produce equal amplitudes on the A-scan display. (From [4])

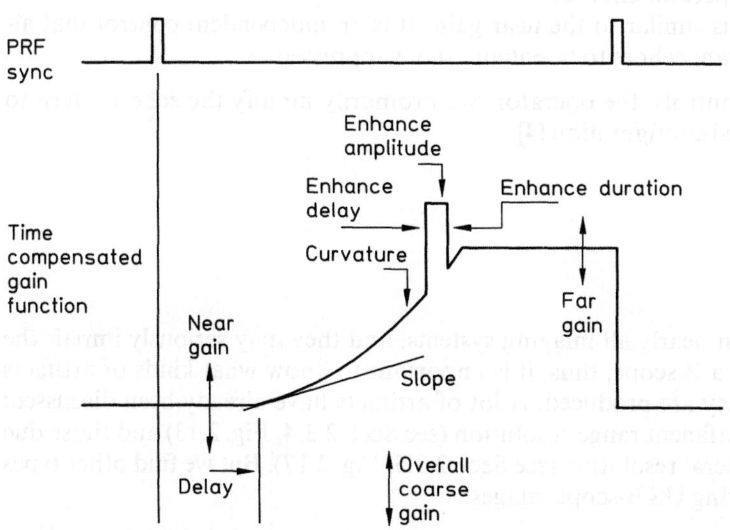

Fig. 2.34. The time-compensated gain function, mastery of which is a very important step in learning to use pulse-echo techniques. *PRF*, pulse repetition frequency; *Sync*, synchronization. (From [4])

Basically, the time-compensated gain unit is designed to increase the echo amplitude with range by an amount sufficient to offset the depth-dependent attenuation. The result is that the echoes from far targets have the same amplitude (deflection) as those from near targets. However, since the attenuation properties of tissue are not necessarily well behaved and known in advance, it is necessary to offer a variety of time-compensated gain functions, which the operator can modify to optimize the display. Figure 2.34 shows an idealized time-compensated gain function that includes features available in a variety of instruments; however, they may not all appear on any one instrument. These features are as follows:

1) The *coarse gain* control sets the overall gain of the receiver, independent of range. It is used for the initial gain setting.
2) *Near gain*, for the first few centimeters, is controlled separately and is used primarily to attenuate large-amplitude echoes and artifacts near the transducer. The depth over which the near gain is functional is controlled by the delay.
3) The *delay* setting can be used to determine when the time-compensated gain function actually begins.
4) The gain functions can start gradually or abruptly, depending upon the initial *slope*, set by the slope adjustment.
5) Since the echo amplitude falls exponentially with range, it is necessary to increase the gain exponentially if it is to affect the attenuation. The *curvature* control varies the rate of change of the gain function. It might be set to be flat or to increase exponentially, or it may actually fall in some cases, depending on what the operator chooses.
6) The *far gain* is similar to the near gain. It is an independent control that allows very distant echoes to be enhanced or suppressed.

With these controls, the operator can ordinarily modify the echo pattern to almost any desired configuration [4].

2.5 Artifacts

Artifacts occur in nearly all imaging systems, and they may seriously impair the image quality of a B-scope; thus, it is important to know what kinds of artifacts exist and how they are produced. A lot of artifacts have already been discussed: those due to insufficient range resolution (see Sect. 2.3.4, Fig. 2.13) and those due to insufficient lateral resolution (see Sect. 2.3.5, Fig. 2.17). But we find other types of artifacts affecting US B-scope images:

1) Artifacts due to *diffraction*. If an US beam penetrates an interface or two media with different sound velocities at an angle of incidence not equal to 90°, the beam is deflected. This is illustrated in Fig. 2.35: an object (A), reflecting the US beam, produces an echo, which, however, appears on the screen at the point B; i.e., B is an artifactual echo.
2) Artifacts due to *reverberation*. Sometimes, the US echo is repeatedly reflected between two interfaces (e.g., tunica mucosa and muscularis or muscularis and fat) before reaching the transducer again; thus, the signal travels further than the distance between the transducer and the interfaces, and artifactual (virtual) interfaces appear on the screen (Fig. 2.36).

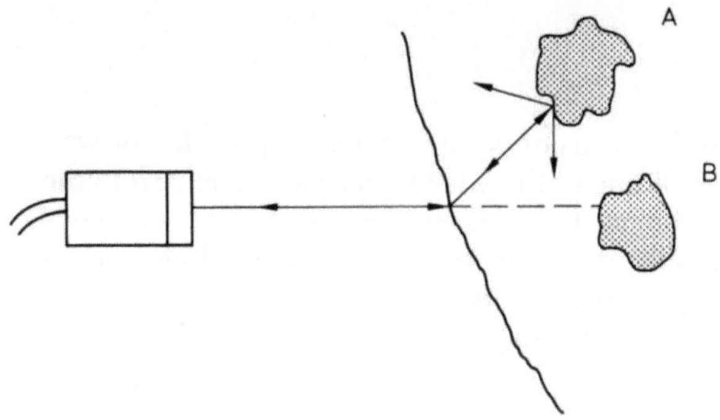

Fig. 2.35. Artifacts due to diffraction, For details see text

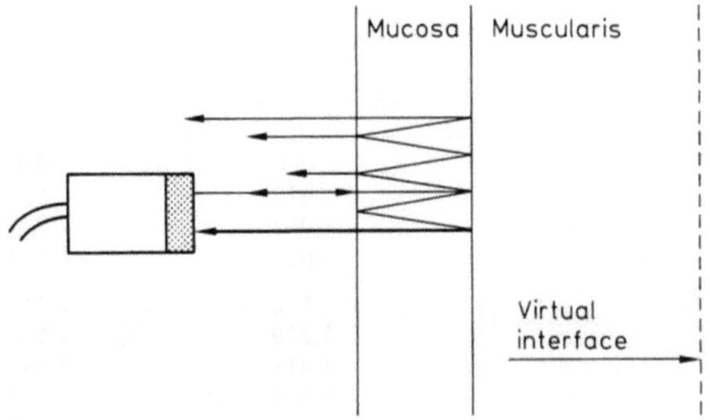

Fig. 2.36. Artifacts due to reverberations

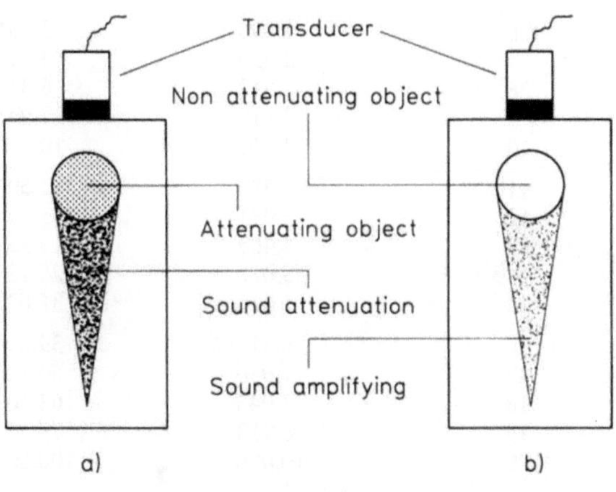

Fig. 2.37 a, b. Artifacts due to sound amplifying

3) Artifacts due to *sound amplifying*. When an US beam passes through an area of nonattenuation (e.g., cysts and water-filled bladder), the structures lying behind this area are represented as lighter than structures not lying behind this area; this effect is called sound amplifying. The reason is that the sound is not attenuated in the normal way, and the US system, compensating for the normal attenuation of the tissue, amplifies the echoes too much (Fig. 2.37 b). The opposite occurs when the sound passes through a region of high attenuation (e.g., bones or air-filled intestine). The structures lying behind this region are represented as much darker than those not so lying (Fig. 2.37 a).

2.6 Decibel Notation

It is often convenient to measure the ratios of pairs of wave amplitudes, or wave intensities, particularly if the level of one of these is taken as a reference for comparison with others. In this way, the need for absolute measurement is avoided, and because US waves are generally both generated and detected electrically, relative wave amplitudes can be expressed as ratios of voltages.

Two advantages accrue if such ratios are expressed as logarithms. Firstly, this affords a simple method of expressing numbers which extend over many orders

Table 2.4. Decibel levels corresponding to various power and amplitude ratios. (From [7])

Negative decibels			Positive decibels	
Amplitude ratio	Power ratio	dB	Amplitude ratio	Power ratio
1.000	1.000	0.0	1.000	1.000
0.989	0.977	0.1	1.012	1.022
0.977	0.955	0.2	1.023	1.047
0.944	0.891	0.5	1.059	1.122
0.891	0.794	1	1.122	1.259
0.794	0.631	2	1.259	1.585
0.708	0.501	3	1.413	1.995
0.631	0.398	4	1.585	2.512
0.562	0.316	5	1.778	3.162
0.501	0.251	6	1.995	3.981
0.447	0.200	7	2.239	5.012
0.398	0.159	8	2.512	6.310
0.355	0.126	9	2.818	7.943
0.316	0.100	10	3.162	10.000
0.282	0.0794	11	3.584	12.59
0.251	0.0631	12	3.981	15.85
0.224	0.0501	13	4.467	19.95
0.200	0.0398	14	5.012	25.12
0.178	0.0316	15	5.623	31.62
0.159	0.0251	16	6.310	39.81
0.141	0.0200	17	7.080	50.12
0.126	0.0159	18	7.943	63.10
0.112	0.0126	19	8.913	79.43
0.100	0.0100	20	10.000	100.00
0.0562	0.00316	25	17.78	316
0.0316	0.00100	30	31.62	1000
0.0178	0.00032	35	56.23	3162
0.0100	0.00010	40	100.00	10000
0.0056	0.00003	45	177.80	31620
0.0032	0.00001	50	316.20	100000
0.00100	10^{-6}	60	1000	10^{6}
0.00032	10^{-7}	70	3162	10^{7}
0.00010	10^{-8}	80	10000	10^{8}
0.00003	10^{-9}	90	31620	10^{9}
0.00001	10^{-10}	100	100000	10^{10}

of magnitude. Secondly, the arithmetic product of two or more quantities is obtained by addition of their logarithms (and, similarly, by subtraction in the case of division). The logarithmic unit which is most commonly used is the decibel, defined as follows:

$$\text{(relative level in decibels)} = 10 \log_{10}(P_2/P_1) = 20 \log_{10}(A_2/A_1)$$

where P_1 and P_2 are the two powers, and A_1 and A_2 are the corresponding wave amplitudes. The decibel levels corresponding to a wide range of power and amplitude ratios are listed in Table 2.4.

In the literature, reference is frequently made to the *neper*: this is a logarithmic ratio, defined as follows:

$$\text{(relative level in nepers)} = \log_e(A_2/A_1)$$

Hence, 1 neper = 8.686 dB [7].

References

1. Hueter TF, Bolt RH (1955) Sonics. Wiley, New York
2. Grossman CC et al. (eds) (1966) Diagnostic ultrasound. Plenum, New York
3. Wells PNT (1969) Physical principles of ultrasonic diagnosis. Academic, New York
4. Donald W, Baker BS (1974) Physical and technical principles. In: King D (ed) Diagnostic ultrasound. Mosby, St Louis
5. Gebhardt W, Schwarz H-P (1982) Untersuchungen zur Blasenwanddickenmessung und Gewebedifferenzierung mit einem transurethralen Scanner, Untersuchungsprotokoll für das Urologische Städtische Klinikum, Karlsruhe, May
6. Krautkrämer J (1975) Werkstoffprüfung mit Ultraschall. Springer, Berlin Heidelberg New York, p 20
7. Wells PNT (1977) Biomedical Ultrasound. Academic, London
8. Roy Williams A (1983) Ultrasound: biological effects and potential hazards. Academic, Medical Physics Series, London
9. Goebbels K (1984) Vortrag: Arbeitskreistagung Intercavitäre Sonographie, Universitätsklinik Homburg/Saar, Oct 6
10. Schueller J et al. (1981) Beurteilung von Blasenveränderung mit der intravesikalen Ultraschalltomographie. Urologe [A] 20:204–210
11. Frentzel-Beyme B et al. (1982) Die transrektale Prostatasonographie. Computertomogr Sonogr Juni 2 (2):58–112
12. Heyder N (1987) Endoscopic ultrasonography of tumors of the oesophagus and the stomach. Surg Endosc 1:17–23
13. Souquet J (1982) Phased array transducer technology for transesophageal imaging of the heart. In: Hanrath P et al. (ed) Cardiovascular diagnosis by ultrasound. Nijhoff, The Hague, p 256
14. Prospect US: GF-UM2/EU-M2. Olympus Optical Co. (Europe)
15. Ferner H, Staubesand J (eds) (1982) Sobotta Atlas der Anatomie des Menschen, vol 2. Urban and Schwarzenberg, Munich
16. McElroy JT (1966) Focused ultrasonic beams. Automation Industry, Inc., Material Evaluation Group, Research Division, Boulder
17. Frey WJ, Dunn F (1962) Ultrasound: analysis and experimental methods in biological research. In: Nastuk WL (ed) Physical techniques in biological research, vol 4. Academic, New York, pp 261–394
18. Recorded by Dr. Hildebrandt, Department of Surgery, University of Saarland, FRG

3 Endosonography in the Detection and Staging of Intra- and Extramural Lesions in the Upper Gastrointestinal Tract

T. L. Tio

3.1 Introduction

Nonendoscopic and endoscopic-guided transintestinal sonography, generally known as endosonography, have been developed to improve the diagnostic accuracy of ultrasound by direct imaging of target lesions via the intestinal lumen with a high-frequency ultrasound beam [2, 3, 6, 8, 14, 18]. This diagnostic procedure allows clear imaging of the gastrointestinal wall architecture and of biliopancreatic abnormalities together with adjacent periintestinal lymph nodes [13–15, 18–21]. In addition, the real-time dynamic properties allow detailed visualization of vascular structures adjacent to the primary lesion, which appears essential in assessing the resectability of tumors and in differentiating vascular lesions from nonvascular abnormalities (e.g., lymph nodes). This technique has been effective in the staging of gastrointestinal tumors. The purpose of this chapter is to describe the accuracy, limitations, clinical usefulness, and future prospects of endosonography in the field of gastroenterology.

3.2 Instruments and Methods

All studies were performed either with a commercially available Olympus echoendoscope EU-M2 or the latest model EU-M3. The echo probe is fixed to the tip of a side-viewing gastroscope. The diameter of the echo probe is 13 mm, and the length of the rigid tip is 4.2 mm. The ultrasound frequency is 7.5 MHz, with a penetration depth of approximately 10 cm and an axial resolution of 0.2 mm (Fig. 3.1 A). More recently, a prototype Olympus echoendoscope with a frequency of 10 MHz has been used. The penetration depth of this instrument is approximately 5 cm with an axial resolution of 0.1 mm. An echoendoscope with a switchable frequency of 7.5 MHz or 12 MHz incorporating a biopsy channel for cytological puncture or biopsy has now become available. In cases of extensive esophageal stenosis, which cannot be passed with this instrument, a prototype Aloka flexible nonfiberoptic instrument with a frequency of 7.5 MHz is used. The diameter of this instrument is 10 mm and the length of the echo probe is 3 cm (Fig. 3.1 B). A catheter echo probe with an outer diameter of 3 mm and a frequency of 7.0 MHz has recently become available which can be passed through the biopsy channel of a large-caliber gastroscope (GIF-IT10 or GIF-

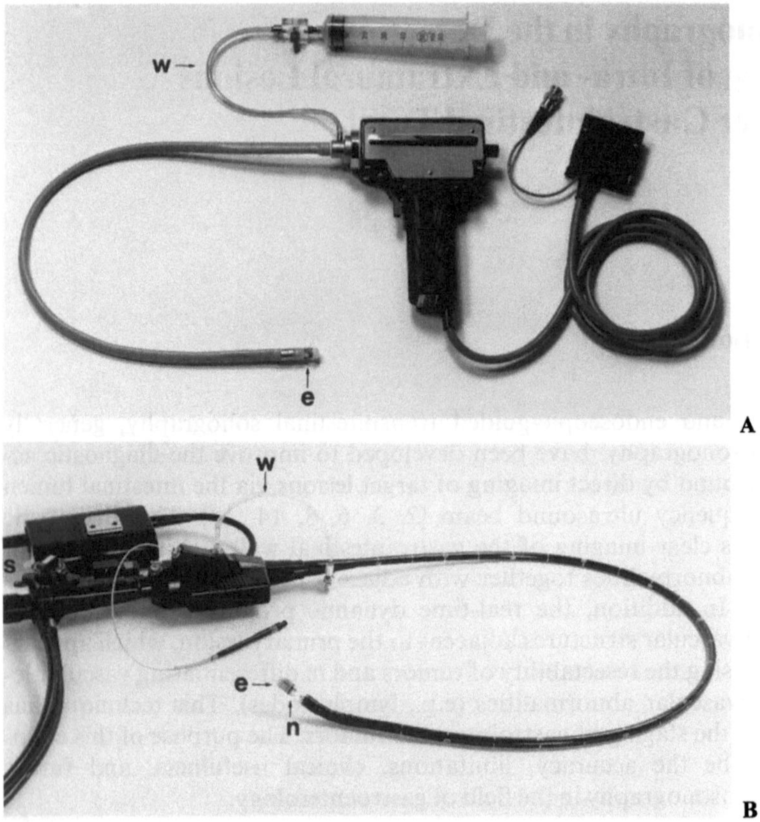

Fig. 3.1. A Prototype Aloka flexible nonfiberoptic instrument, with a small echo probe (*e*) at the tip and a water channel (*w*) for filling the balloon (*b*) with water. **B** Olympus echoendoscope EU-M2, with an echo probe (*e*) covered with a balloon and a water channel (*w*) for filling the balloon and the gastrointestinal lumen with water and a sclerosing needle (*n*) passing through the biopsy channel. *S* = switch for changing the frequency

IT20). In this manner, endoscopic-guided sonography can be performed during a routine endoscopy. Table 3.1 summarizes the technical data of these instruments. In terms of method the examination is like any other kind of upper intestinal endoscopy after local pharyngeal anesthesia and intravenous injection of diazepam. The instrument is introduced slowly and carefully into the stomach. The ultrasound unit should not be switched on while the instrument is being maneuvered into the esophagus in order to protect the rotating unit of the echo probe from any damage. In order to correlate the endosonographic findings with computed tomography (CT), the descending aorta can be placed on the lower left quadrant and/or the liver may be placed on the right quadrant and the spleen on the left quadrant of the screen.

Table 3.1. Technical data of various Olympus echoendoscopes

Echoendo-scope	EU-M2	EU-M2	EU-M3	VU-M2 (video)	Catheter echoprobe
Endoscope	Side-viewing	Side-viewing	Side-viewing	Side-viewing	Forward-fewing (GIF-IT10/ GIF-IT20)
Echoprobe	Mechanical sector or radial scanning (180° or 360°)	Mechanical sector or radial scanning (180° or 360°)	Mechanical sector or radial scanning (180° or 360°)	Mechanical raditor or radial scanning (180° or 360°)	Catheter echo-probe (radial scanning) (360°)
Length	42 mm	42 mm	42 mm	44 mm	In total 140 cm with the catheter
Diameter	13 mm	13 mm	13 mm	10.4 mm	3 mm
Frequency	7.5 MHz	10 MHz	7.5 MHz/ 12 MHz[a]	7.5 MHz	7 MHz
Depth of penetration	10 cm	5 cm	10 cm/3 cm	10 cm	3 cm
Axial resolution	0.2 mm	0.15 mm	0.2 mm/ 0.12 mm	0.2 mm	−0.2–0.3 mm
ES-guided puncture/ biopsy	No	No	Yes	No	No

[a] switchable, frequency

3.3 Gastrointestinal Lesions

By directly approaching target lesions via the intestinal lumen, using water as the transmitting medium for the ultrasound beam, the intestinal wall architecture can be clearly visualized. In vitro (endosonography of fresh autopsy and resection specimens) and in vivo (preoperative endosonography) the intestinal wall is imaged as a five-layer structure. The first, hyperechoic and the second, hypoechoic structure correspond to the border echo (interface) and the mucosa respectively. The third, hyperechoic structure corresponds to the submucosa including the border echo; the fourth, hypoechoic structure to the muscularis propria; and the fifth, hyperechoic structure to the adventitia, or subserosa and serosa, together with the periintestinal fat tissue and the border echo (Fig. 3.2). The interface echos between two different ultrasonic media should, however, be taken into consideration. Abnormalities are visualized as partial or total destruction of this five-layer intestinal wall architecture.

3.3.1 Esophageal Lesions

An ulcer is visualized as a hypoechoic intramural echo pattern usually covered with some hyperechoic structures extending into the submucosa. Extensive ulcers

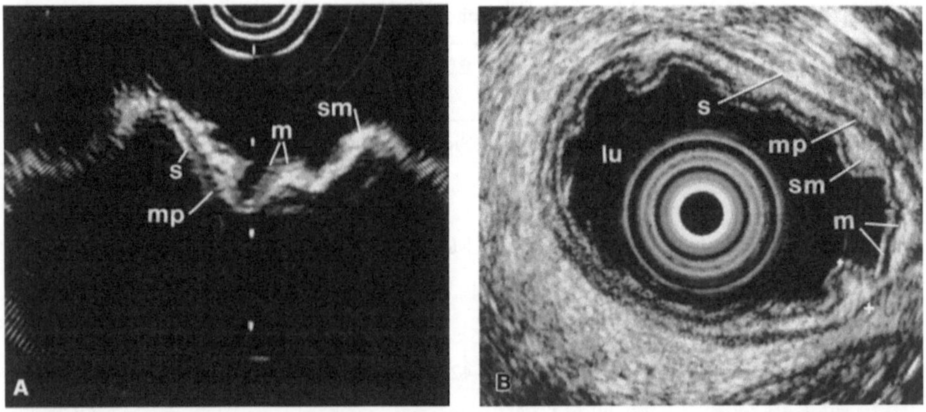

Fig. 3.2 A, B. Endoscopic sonograms. **A** Five-layer structure of intestinal wall. Note the clear transition between the intact wall and the area where the various layers were partially removed. The dark line (*mp*) and the white line (*s*) disappear in the area where they were removed. **B** Normal gastric wall seen as a five-layer structure after the lumen (*lu*) had been adequately filled with water. *m*, mucosa; *sm*, submucosa; *mp*, muscularis propria; *s*, subserosa and serosa

are characterized by a crater with directly adjacent hypoechoic intramural abnormalities, which usually extend into or even through the muscularis propria. In the latter cases, sonographic differentiation between a benign and a malignant ulcer is difficult or even impossible. Supplementary findings such as adjacent lymph node abnormalities are often not very helpful because lymph nodes (with a sonographically suspicious appearence) are usually found adjacent to an ulcerative lesion. A deeply penetrating ulcer with submucosal infiltration of the hypoechoic abnormality into the adjacent wall is strongly suggestive of malignancy. Disappearance of the hypoechoic intramural abnormality during follow-up is suggestive of benign lesions. In contrast, persistence of abnormalities is highly suggestive of malignancy.

3.3.1.1 Benign Lesions

The commonest benign esophageal tumor is leiomyoma, which is usually visualized as a bulging mass covered with smooth mucosa (occasionally associated with a central ulcer) when viewed endoscopically or radiographically [1, 5, 9, 11, 25]. Endoscopic biopsy is rarely helpful in ascertaining the diagnosis or in ruling out malignancy [4, 10]. Generally, the submucosal lesion cannot be reached with a standard biopsy forceps, but with a giant biopsy forceps multiple samples may be obtained from the same suspected area [7]; however, this technique also has limitations, particularly in the esophagus, because of the risk of bleeding. With endosonography, a leiomyoma is visualized as a sharply demarcated lesion with a homogeneous hypoechoic echo pattern, usually covered with normal overlying mucosa (Fig. 3.3). In extensive leiomyomas, a central ulcer within the tumor mass can occasionally be visualized. Moreover, such an extensive lesion may compress but does not penetrate the surrounding tissues.

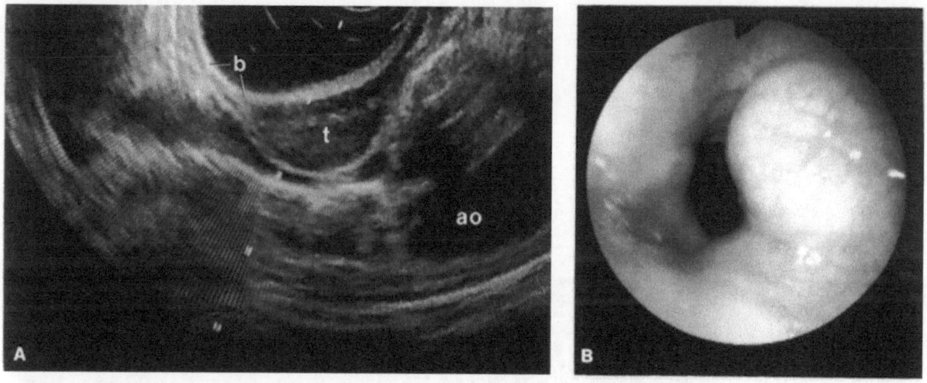

Fig. 3.3. A Endoscopic sonogram showing an ellipsoid, homogeneous hypoechoic echo pattern with sharply delineated borders (*t*) below normal mucosa adjacent to the descending aorta (*ao*). *b*, water-filled balloon. **B** Corresponding endoscopic image showing bulging of the esophageal wall covered with normal mucosa

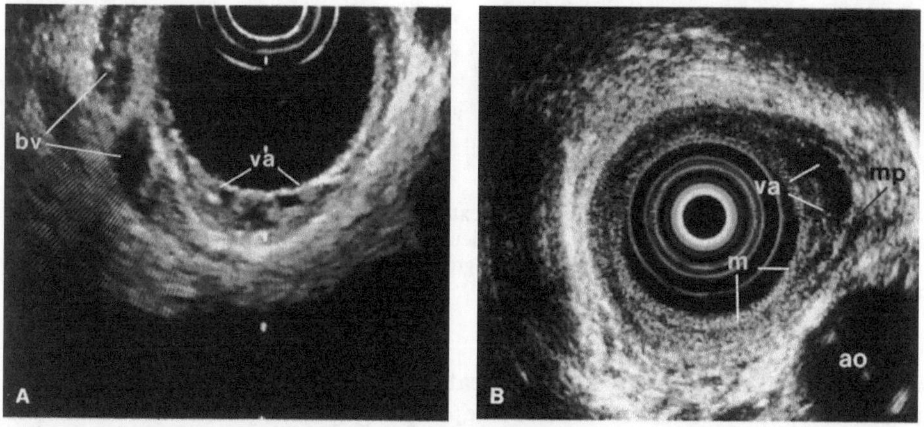

Fig. 3.4 A, B. Endoscopic sonograms. **A** Ellipsoid anechoic structures (*va*) in the submucosal layer compatible with esophageal varices, together with periesophageal collateral veins. *bv*, blood vessel. **B** Ellipsoid anechoic structure (*va*) in the submucosal layer not penetrating the muscularis propria (*mp*). *m*, mucosa; *ao*, aorta

With endosonography, achalasia is visualized as narrowing of the distal esophagus with no evidence of abnormalities of the wall. In contrast, pseudo-achalasia is visualized as a hypoechoic tumor mass immediately adjacent to the narrowed area of the esophagus. Therefore, achalasia and pseudoachalasia can readily be differentiated. Occasionally, aneurysm of the aorta may simulate the presence of achalasia due to compression of the adjacent esophagus. Because of the real-time dynamic properties of endosonography an aneurysm can readily be identified as an anechoic cavity with turbulent blood flow directly adjacent to a calcified aortic wall. In patients with distal esophageal narrowing after surgical repair of hiatal hernia, endosonography visualizes a hyperechoic echo pattern directly adjacent to the narrowed area compatible with fibrotic changes. An

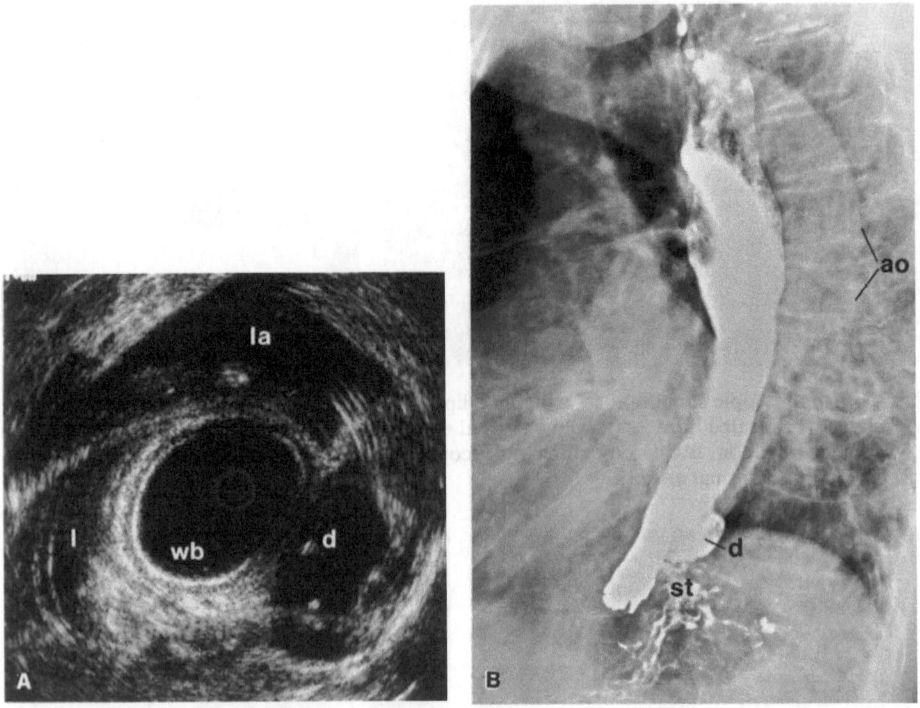

Fig. 3.5. A Endoscopic sonogram showing an extensive anechoic structure (*d*) directly adjacent to the water-filled balloon (*wb*) after the diverticulum (*d*) had been adequately filled with water. *l*, liver; *la*, left atrium. **B** Corresponding radiogram, revealing the diverticulum (*d*) adjacent to the vertebrae and aorta (*ao*). *st*, stomach

Angelchik prosthesis inserted for the treatment of hiatal hernia is visualized as an anechoic circular structure around the esophagogastric junction, because the silicon content of the prosthesis seems to have an impedance similar to that of water.

Esophageal varices are visualized as anechoic or hypoechoic structures localized especially in the submucosa, with or without periesophageal collateral veins (Fig. 3.4). After initial sclerotherapy, thickening of the esophageal wall can be identified, with or without obliteration of the an- or hypoechoic intramural lesions. In the early phase after sclerotherapy, a hypoechoic transmural abnormality may be seen. A sclerotherapy-induced ulcer is visualized as a hyperechoic area on the surface. Long-term success of sclerotherapy can be documented by disappearance of the varices with reappearance of the normal five-layer structure, or by thickening of the wall with the presence of periesophageal collateral veins, particularly in more distal parts of the esophagus or even in the proximal stomach. An esophageal diverticulum is visualized as an anechoic excavation immediately adjacent to the lumen (Fig. 3.5).

3.3.1.2 Malignant Lesions

The commonest malignant esophageal tumor is carcinoma, which is visualized as a hypoechoic intramural lesion with partial or total destruction of the normal five-layer architecture of the wall. An "early" esophageal carcinoma is diagnosed when a hypoechoic echo pattern is limited to the mucosa and/or submucosa with no evidence of penetration into the muscularis propria. Some Japanese surgeons claim that early esophageal carcinoma can be associated with regional lymph node involvement, comparable with early gastric cancer. In contrast, some Chinese surgeons state that lymph node involvement must be ruled out when diagnosing early malignancy because of the poor prognosis of esophageal cancer. Advanced esophageal carcinoma is visualized as a hypoechoic echo pattern penetrating into the muscularis propria with or without lymph node involvement.

In the past we used resectability as the criterion for the preoperative assessment of esophageal carcinoma, as follows: Group I (local resection with curative intent): endosonography visualizes a clearly demarcated hypoechoic tumor that does not penetrate through the organ boundaries (muscularis propria), with no evidence of lymph node involvement (Fig. 3.6).

Group II (palliative resection): endosonography visualizes a clearly demarcated hypoechoic tumor mass penetrating through the muscularis propria into the adventitia or adjacent fat tissue usually associated with regional lymph node involvement (Fig. 3.7).

Group III (nonresectable): endosonography visualizes deep penetration of a hypoechoic tumor mass into the surrounding tissues (e.g., tracheobronchial tree, diaphragm, pericardium) or major blood vessels (e.g., aorta, pulmonary vessels) or liver metastasis (Figs. 3.8, 3.9). Some surgeons claim that an involved lymph node at the celiac axis indicates nonresectability because of the poor prognosis of esophageal cancer.

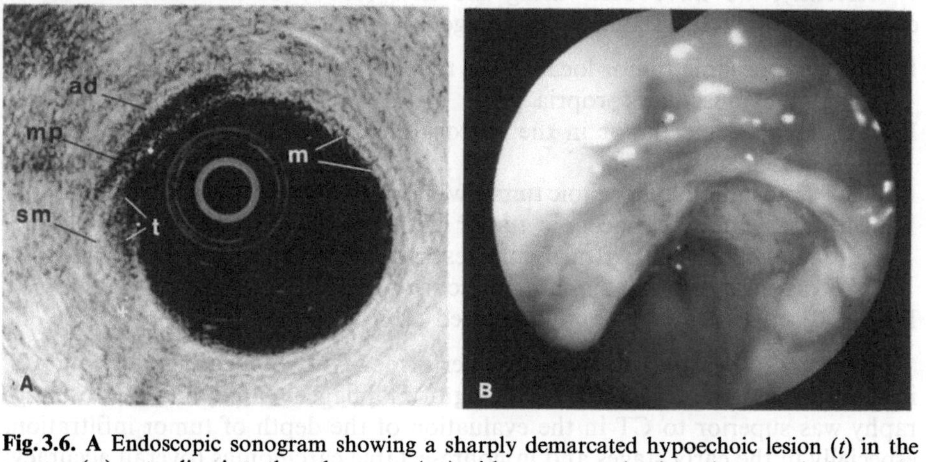

Fig. 3.6. A Endoscopic sonogram showing a sharply demarcated hypoechoic lesion (*t*) in the mucosa (*m*), extending into the submucosa (*sm*) without penetrating into the muscularis propria (*mp*) or adventitia (*ad*). **B** Corresponding endoscopic image of the ulcerative esophageal carcinoma

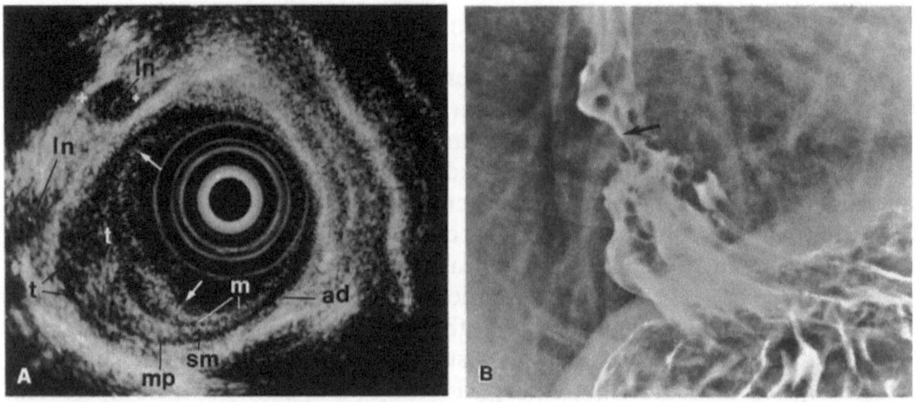

Fig. 3.7. A Endoscopic sonogram showing a semicircular hypoechoic tumor mass (*t*) penetrating through the adjacent muscularis propria (*mp*) into the adventitia (*ad*), with two sharply demarcated hypoechoic lymph nodes (*ln*) strongly suggestive of metastasis. Note the clear transition between normal and pathologic wall structure (*arrows*). *m*, mucosa; *sm*, submucosa. **B** Corresponding radiogram, showing polypoid stenosing tumor mass in the distal esophagus (*arrow*)

Staging by CT has proved unreliable because of the inability of CT to resolve the layers of the esophageal wall and document accurately the extent of mediastinal invasion [12]. In cases of extensive esophageal tumor penetration into the surrounding tissues, differentiation between intra- und extramural lesions may become difficult or even impossible, since a bronchus carcinoma immediately adjacent to the esophagus may have a similar echo pattern, especially if it penetrates into the esophageal wall. When it becomes possible to use the biopsy channel for endosonographically guided biopsy or even cytological puncture, the diagnosis may be firmly established.

Recently, we have been using the new (1987) TNM classification for endosonographic (ES) staging of esophageal carcinoma as follows [22]:

ES-T1: Hypoechoic tumor localized in the mucosa or submucosa or both with intact muscularis propria
ES-T2: Hypoechoic tumor in the mucosa and submucosa extending into the muscularis propria
ES-T3: Transmural hypoechoic tumor with penetration into the adventitia
ES-T4: Transmural hypoechoic tumor with penetration into adjacent structures, such as pericardium, descending aorta, tracheobronchial tree, diaphragm (crura diaphragmatica), or liver
ES-TX: Primary tumor cannot be assessed

Recently, a prospective study was performed with endosonography and CT in the preoperative TNM (1987) staging of esophageal carcinoma. Endosonography was superior to CT in the evaluation of the depth of tumor infiltration, especially in the early stages and in nonresectable carcinomas (overall accuracy: endosonography 89%, CT 89%), and in assessing regional lymph node metastases (overall accuracy: endosonography 80%, CT 51%). In cases of severe

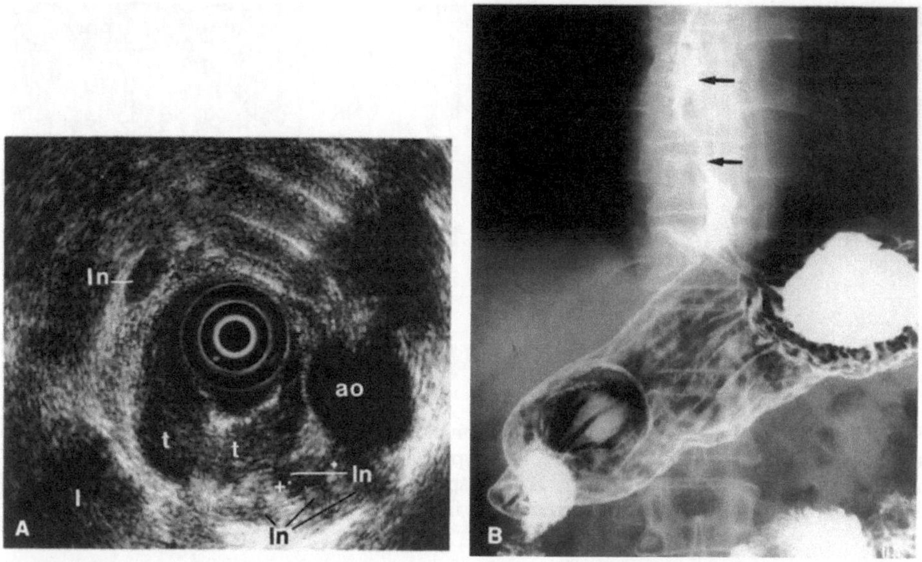

Fig. 3.8. A Endoscopic sonogram showing a hypoechoic polypoid transmural tumor (*t*) adjacent to the aorta (*ao*) with multiple lymph nodes (*ln*). Note a large, suspicious lymph node on the contralateral side of the aorta. *l*, liver. **B** Corresponding radiogram, showing the stenotic lesion in the distal esophagus (*arrows*)

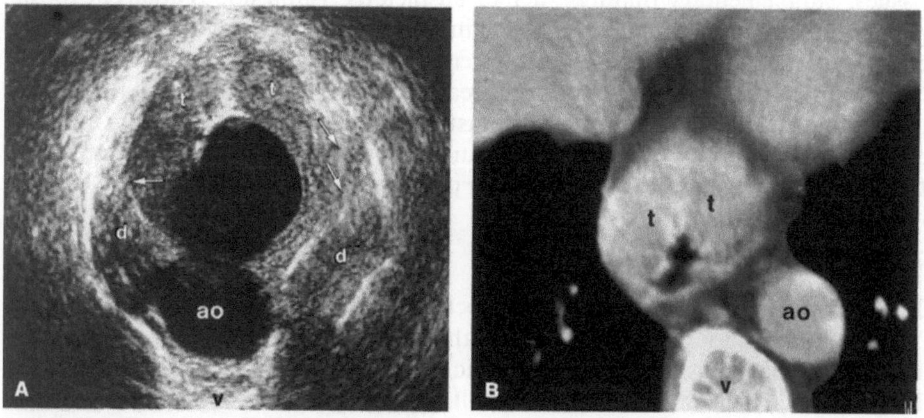

Fig. 3.9. A Endoscopic sonogram showing an extensive hypoechoic transmural tumor mass (*t*), with penetration into the surrounding tissues. Note the unclear demarcation into the surrounding tissues. Note the unclear demarcation of the tumor mass (*arrows*) and the diaphragm (*d*) bordering the aorta (*ao*). **B** Corresponding computerized tomography scan section, showing thickening of the esophageal wall (*t*). The penetration into the diaphragm is not visualized

stenosis, however, CT was superior to endosonography in diagnosing celiac lymph node metastases (distant metastases). The most important malignant submucosal tumor is leiomyosarcoma or -myoblastoma. It is usually visualized as an inhomogeneous tumor mass with sharply or bizarrely demarcated boundaries and is often associated with central ulceration or a fistula (Fig. 3.10). Differentia-

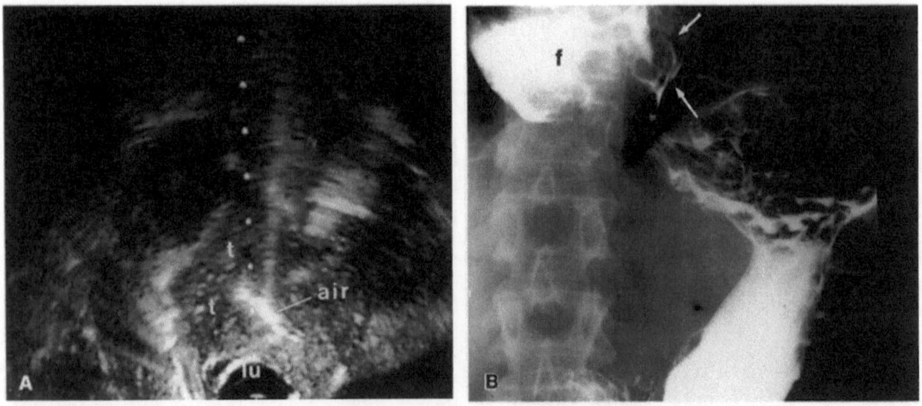

Fig. 3.10. A Endoscopic sonogram showing a semicircular hypoechoic tumor mass (*t*) penetrating deeply into the surrounding tissues. The hyperechoic structures within the mass are compatible with air in the fistula. *lu*, lumen. **B** Corresponding radiogram, showing a polypoid lesion (*arrows*) in the distal esophagus with an extensive fistula (*f*)

tion between an extensive leiomyoma and a -myosarcoma or -myoblastoma can sometimes be difficult because of the similarities in echo pattern. However, an extensive leiomyoma usually compresses but does not penetrate the surrounding tissues. Supplementary findings such as suspicious lymph nodes adjacent to the primary lesion may be helpful in ascertaining malignancy. A major advantage of endosonography is its capacity to differentiate a submucosal tumor from an extramural mass compressing the esophageal lumen, such as bronchus cancer, vascular abnormality, or lymph node metastasis. The diagnosis, however, must be confirmed by histology. In the near future endosonography may become essential in the detection of the optimal site for positive biopsy or cytology.

3.3.2 Gastric Lesions

Endosonography is accurate in the dectection and staging of gastric lesions. When a lesion is found endoscopically, the echo probe can be placed against the lesion, and the balloon and/or the gastric lumen filled with water to visualize the longitudinal extension and depth of infiltration, together with perigastric lymph node abnormalities. The water-filled stomach method allows clear visualization of any mucosal abnormalities because of the absence of compression by the water-filled balloon. The cardia and the pyloric region should be examined using both methods. Aspiration can be prevented by giving adequate sedation and by placing the patient in semivertical left lateral decubitus with meticulous constant pharyngeal aspiration of any secretions.

3.3.2.1 Benign Lesions

A gastric ulcer is visualized as a concave mucosal lesion covered with hyperechoic necrotic material, with an adjacent hypoechoic intramural structure. In cases of

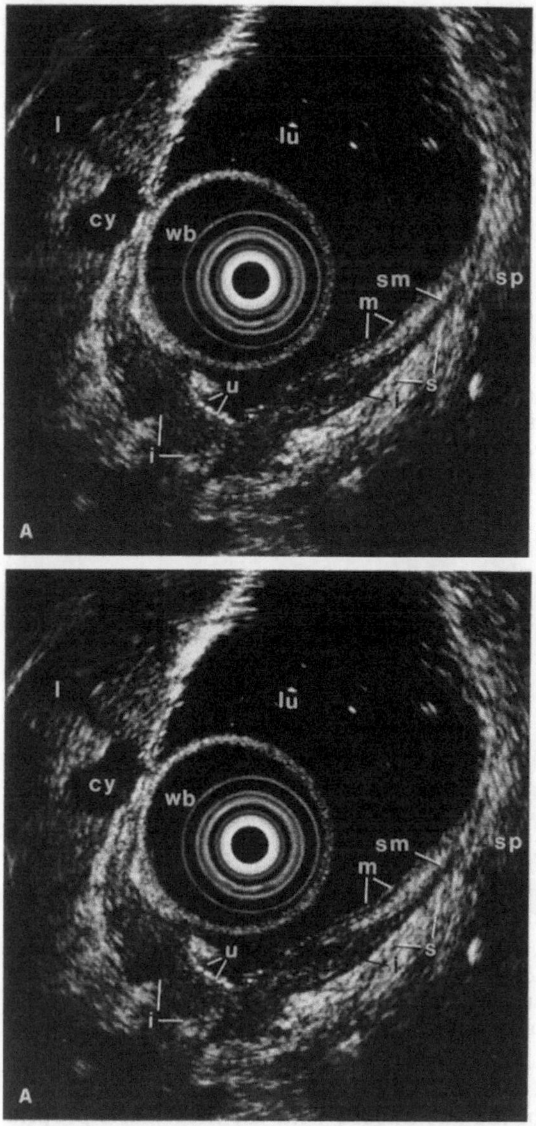

Fig. 3.11 A, B. Endoscopic sonograms. **A** Ulcerative lesion (*u*) with transmural infiltration (*i*) adjacent to the left liver lobe (*l*), proven to be benign by biopsies. *cy*, cystic lesion; *m*, mucosa; *sm*, submucosa; *sp*, spleen; *lu*, lumen. **B** Hypoechoic infiltration (*i*) penetrating into the muscularis propria (*mp*) adjacent to an extensive ulcer (*u*), proven to be non-Hodgkin lymphoma

extensive ulcers, deep penetration into the surrounding tissues can be visualized, usually associated with lymph node abnormalities. Differentiation between a benign and a malignant ulcer is impossible because of the similar echo patterns and the penetration of the hypoechoic abnormality through the muscularis propria (Fig. 3.11). Follow-up investigation may be very helpful in establishing the diagnosis. Disappearance of the hypoechoic echo pattern is highly indicative of a benign ulcer. In contrast, persistence of infiltration after the ulcer has healed strongly suggests a malignancy. In cases of extensive ulcers, endosonography may not be able to rule out a malignancy when follow-up investigation continues to show persistent intramural infiltration. Fundic or cardial varices are clearly imaged as bulging anechoic structures usually covered with normal mucosa,

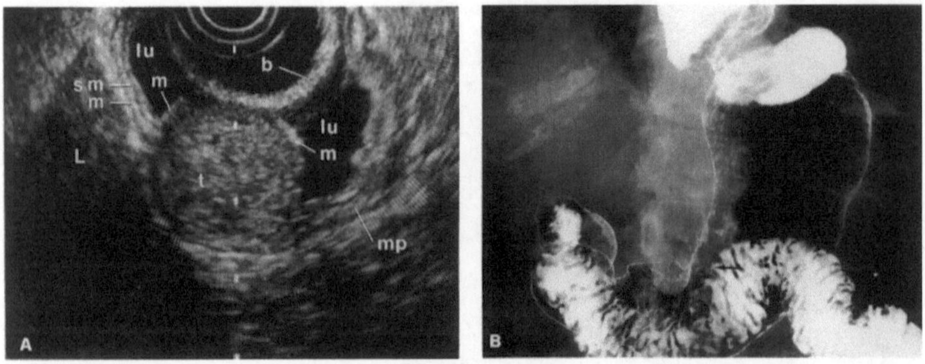

Fig. 3.12. A Endoscopic sonogram showing a round homogeneous hypoechoic echo pattern (*t*) protruding into the lumen (*lu*) covered with normal mucosa (*m*), which is strongly suggestive of leiomyoma. *L*, liver; *sm*, sub-mucosa; *mp*, muscularis propria; *b*, water-filled balloon. **B** Barium meal radiogram showing a smooth round double contour at the lesser curvature (*arrow*)

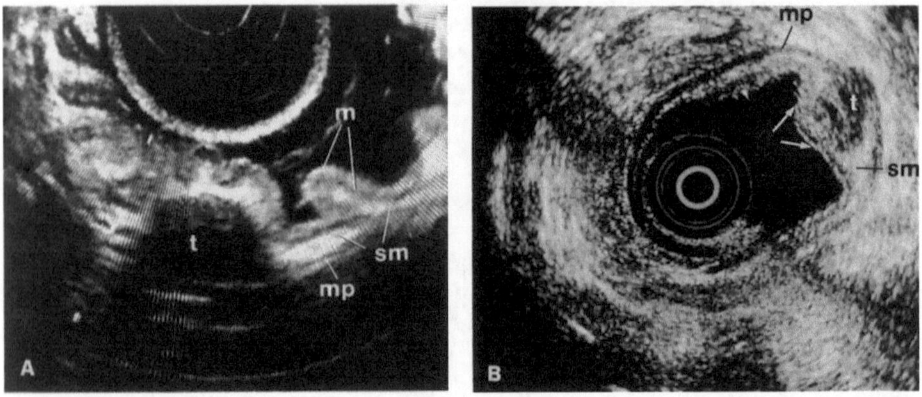

Fig. 3.13 A, B. Endoscopic sonograms. **A** Local thickening of the muscularis propria (*mp*), seen as a sharply demarcated hypoechoic structure (*t*) originating from the muscularis propria below normal mucosa (*m*). **B** A clearly demarcated hypoechoic echo pattern (*t*) in the submucosal layer (*sm*), with corresponding bulging of the mucosal layer (*arrows*)

localized in the mucosa or even in the submucosa with the muscularis propria remaining intact. Perigastric collateral veins directly adjacent to the varices are often visualized. In cases of extensive portal hypertension, ductular-like anechoic intramural varices, localized particularly in the fundus of the stomach, can often readily be seen. These are associated with a perigastric anechoic structure running towards the splenic hilum and with a dilated splenic vein. This is of the utmost importance because splenoportography may not be able to give such detailed information, which is essential for planning of surgical treatment.

Ectopic pancreas is mostly localized along the posterior wall of the antrum and is visualized as a small bulging lesion encircled by a hypoechoic rim. The latter contains a ductular-like hypoechoic structure communicating with the gastric lumen.

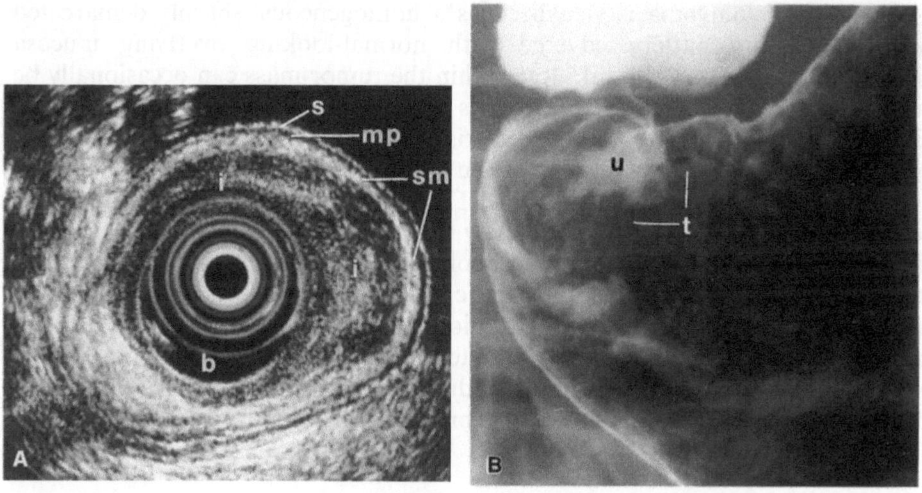

Fig. 3.14. A Endoscopic sonogram showing hypoechoic infiltration (*i*) into the submucosal layer (*sm*) without penetration into the muscularis propria (*mp*) and serosal layer (*s*). *b*, water-filled balloon. **B** Corresponding radiogram, showing a smooth round double contour (*t*) with a central ulcerative lesion (*u*)

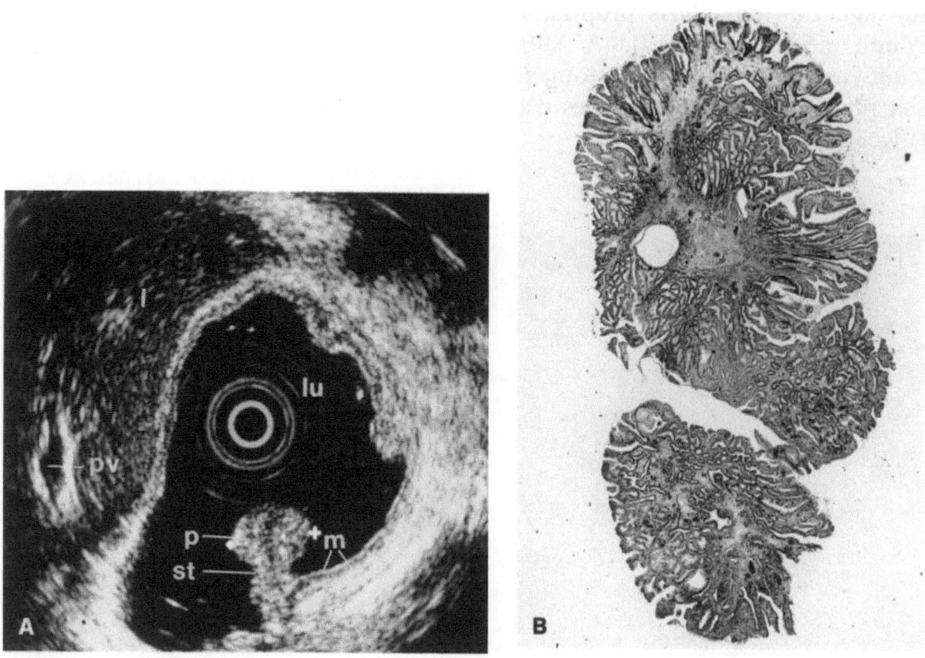

Fig. 3.15. A Endoscopic sonogram showing a polyp (*p*) containing some hypoechoic structures extending into the stalk (*st*) without penetrating into the adjacent gastric wall. *m*, mucosa; *lu*, lumen; *l*, liver; *pv*, portal vein. **B** Corresponding histological section, showing a hyperplastic polyp

A gastric leiomyoma is visualized as a homogeneous, sharply demarcated hypoechoic echo pattern covered with normal-looking overlying mucosa (Fig. 3.12). However, a central ulcer within the tumor mass can occasionally be seen. Local thickening of the muscularis propria can sometimes be recognized (Fig. 3.13); this appears to be characteristic of leiomyoma. An ulcer within a polypoid lesion protruding into the lumen may be taken for a leiomyoma because of the similar echo pattern (Fig. 3.14). The origin of a lesion bulging into the lumen which is found endoscopically or radiographically can readily be determined with endosonography. The commonest extramural lesions compressing the gastric lumen are pancreatic pseudocyst, distended gallbladder, hepatosplenomegaly, and distended colon. A submucosal tumor and an extramural lesion can readily be differentiated by endosonography. A gastric polyp is visualized as a polypoid lesion protruding into the lumen with no evidence of penetration into the adjacent muscularis propria of the gastric wall (Fig. 3.15).

3.3.2.2 Malignant Lesions

Early gastric cancer is visualized as a hypoechoic echo pattern limited to the mucosa and/or submucosa with no evidence of penetration into the muscularis propria; suspicious lymph nodes may or may not be present (Fig. 3.16). In contrast, advanced cancer is visualized as a hypoechoic area penetrating into or through the muscularis propria, usually associated with suspicious regional lymph nodes (Fig. 3.17). A submucosal smooth muscle tumor such as leiomyosarcoma or -myoblastoma is visualized as a hypoechoic tumor mass with sharply demarcated boundaries occasionally associated with central ulceration (Fig. 3.18).

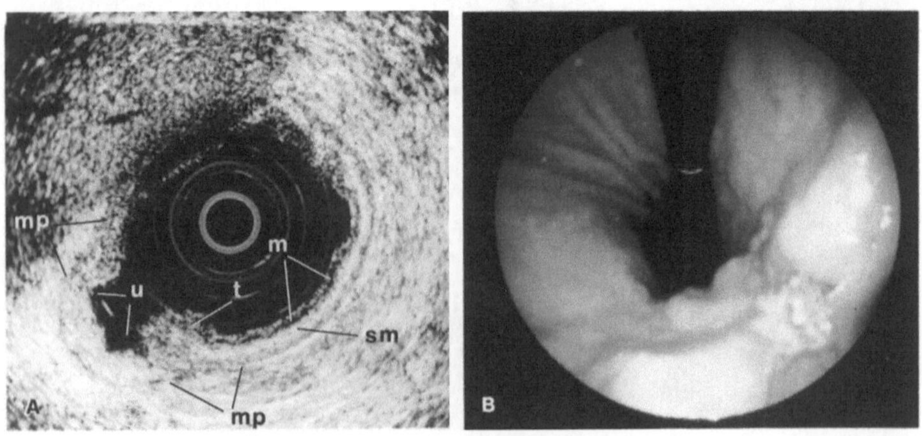

Fig. 3.16. A Endoscopic sonogram showing a circumscribed hypoechoic lesion in the mucosa and submucosa (*t*) adjacent to an ulcer (*u*), with no penetration into the muscularis propria (*mp*). *m*, mucosa; *sm*, submucosa. **B** Corresponding endoscopic image, showing the ulcerative lesion at the angulus, proven to be an early gastric cancer (type III)

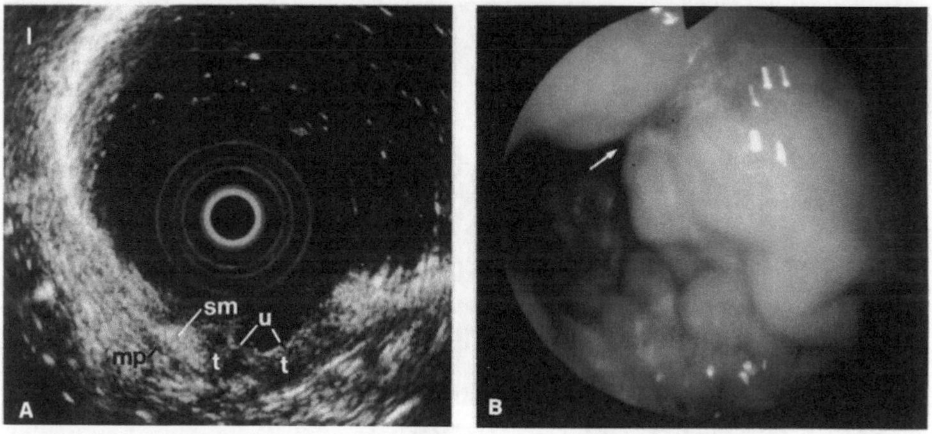

Fig. 3.17. A Endoscopic sonogram showing hypoechoic tumor (*t*) infiltration into the submucosal layer (*sm*), penetrating into the muscularis propria (*mp*) directly adjacent to the ulcer (*u*). *l*, liver. **B** Corresponding endoscopic image, showing the ulcer (*arrow*) with nodular margins

In assessing the resectability of gastric tumors we divided patients into three groups as follows:

Group I (local resection with curative intent): endosonography visualizes a clearly demarcated hypoechoic tumor with no penetration through the organ boundaries (muscularis propria); there may or may not be regional lymph node involvement (Figs. 3.19, 3.20).

Group II (palliative resection): endosonography visualizes a clearly delineated hypoechoic tumor mass penetrating deeply into the muscularis propria but with no evidence of deep penetration into the surrounding organs; there is distant lymph node involvement (Fig. 3.21).

Group III (nonresectable): endosonography visualizes a hypoechoic tumor mass penetrating deeply into the surrounding tissues (e.g., hepatoduodenal ligament, major blood vessels such as celiac trunk, portal vein, superior mesenteric artery, and aorta, with metastasis to the greater omentum and bursa omentalis) and/or organs (e.g., liver, pancreas, colon) (Fig. 3.22). In cases of diffuse signet ring cell carcinoma of the stomach (linitis plastica), resection is of no benefit to patients, because even when the carcinoma is locally resectable the prognosis is still very poor. Recently, we have been using the new (1987) TNM classification for staging [23]:

- ES-T1: Hypoechoic tumor localized in the mucosa or submucosa with intact muscularis propria
- ES-T2: Hypoechoic tumor localized in the submucosa with penetration into the muscularis propria and/or subserosa
- ES-T3: transmural hypoechoic tumor with penetration into the serosa, usually detected only by virtue of the presence of ascites
- ES-T4: transmural hypoechoic tumor with penetration into adjacent structures and organs
- ES-TX: Primary tumor cannot be assessed

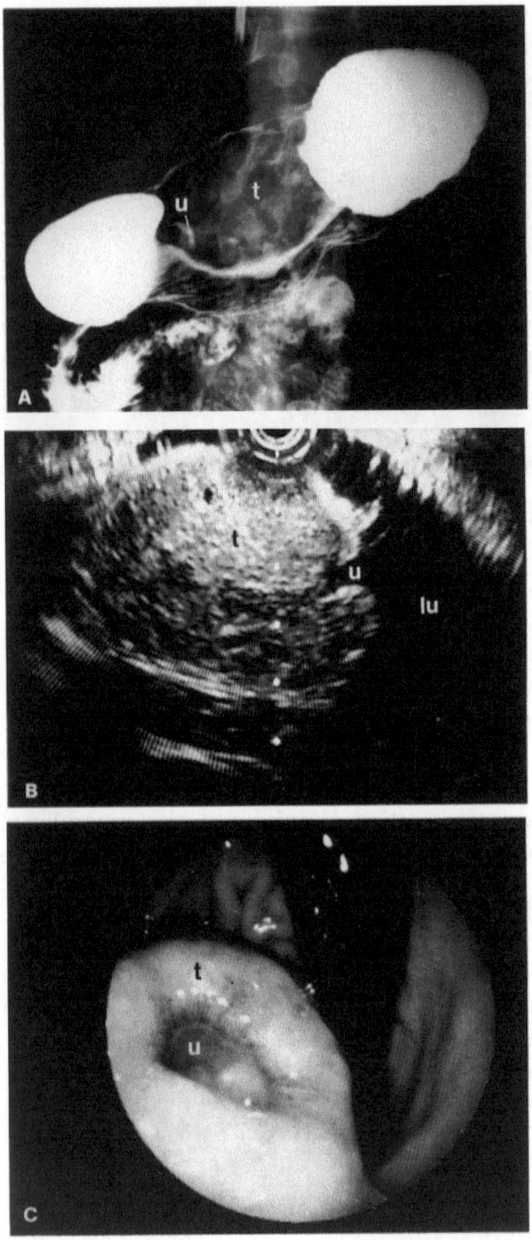

Fig. 3.18. A Radiogram showing an extensive bulging mass (*t*) with an ulcer (*u*). **B** Corresponding endoscopic sonogram, showing the extensive inhomogeneous hypoechoic tumor mass (*t*) protruding into the lumen (*lu*) with an ulcerative lesion (*u*). **C** Endoscopic image, showing the tumor mass (*t*) protruding into the lumen carrying an ulcer (*u*). **D** Corresponding histological section, revealing a leiomyosarcoma (*t*) with an ulcerative lesion (*u*). *m*, mucosa; *sm*, submucosa

Fig. 3.20. A Endoscopic sonogram showing a transmural hypoechoic tumor (*t*) adjacent to an ulcerative lesion (*u*). *lu*, lumen; *l*, liver. **B** Corresponding histological section, showing a tumor (*t*) penetrating into the muscularis propria (*mp; arrows*) with an ulcerative lesion (*u*)

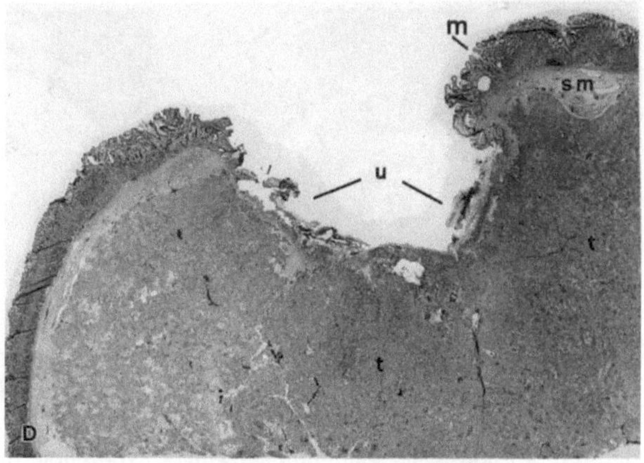

Fig. 3.18. D

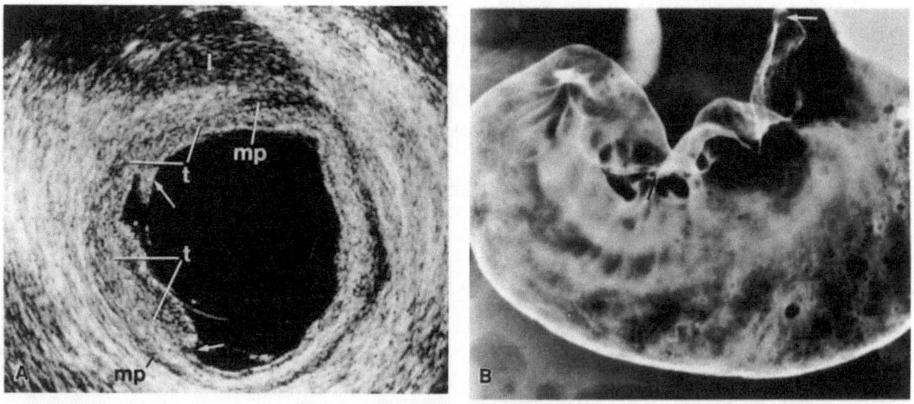

Fig. 3.19. A Endoscopic sonogram showing a clearly demarcated hypoechoic tumor (*t*) penetrating into the muscularis propria (*mp*), with some nodular margins (*arrows*) adjacent to the liver (*l*). **B** Corresponding radiogram showing a double contour (*arrows*) at the lesser curvature

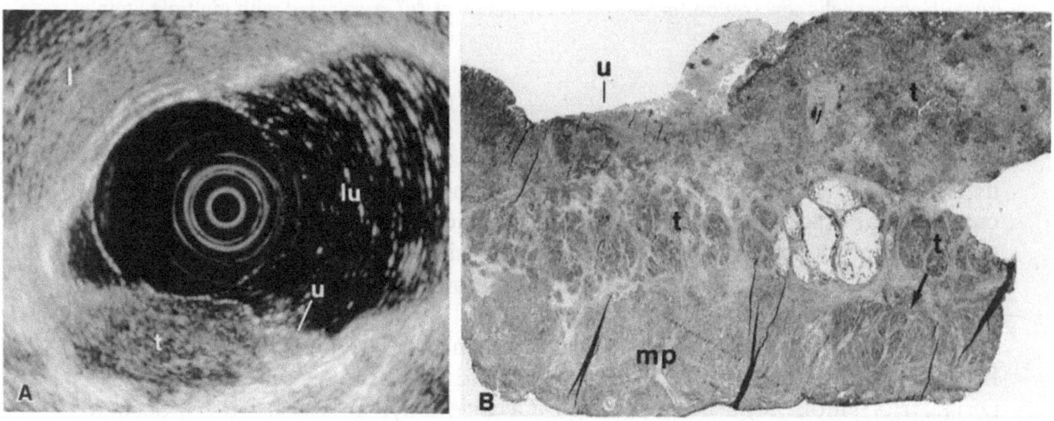

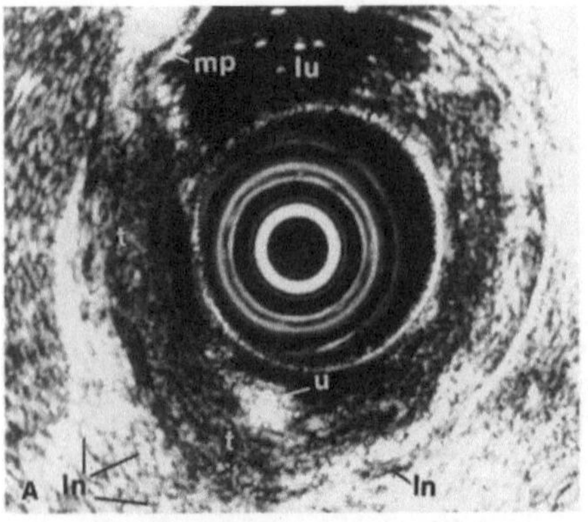

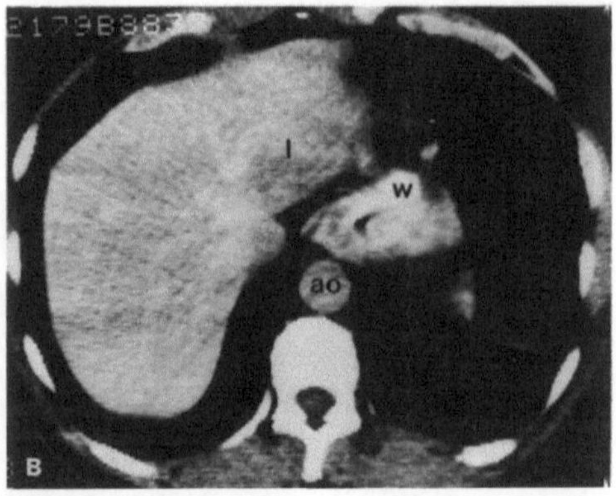

Fig. 3.21. A Endoscopic sonogram showing a hypoechoic tumor (*t*) penetrating into the muscularis propria (*mp*) adjacent to an ulcerative lesion (*u*), with some small adjacent lymph nodes (*ln*) not suggestive of malignancy. *l*, liver; *lu*, lumen. **B** Corresponding computerized tomography scan, showing thickening of the wall (*w*) adjacent to the liver (*l*) and aorta (*ao*)

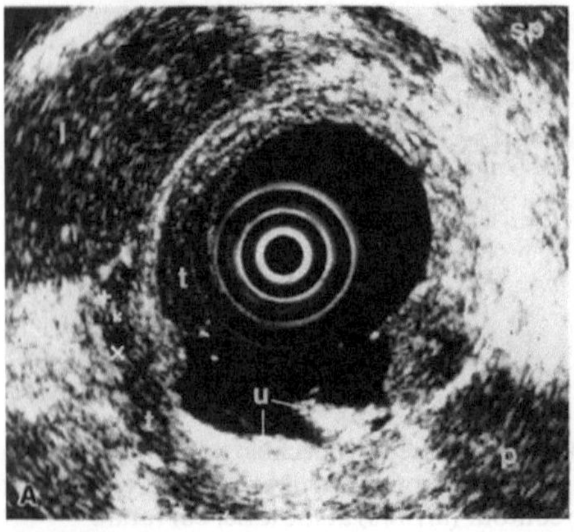

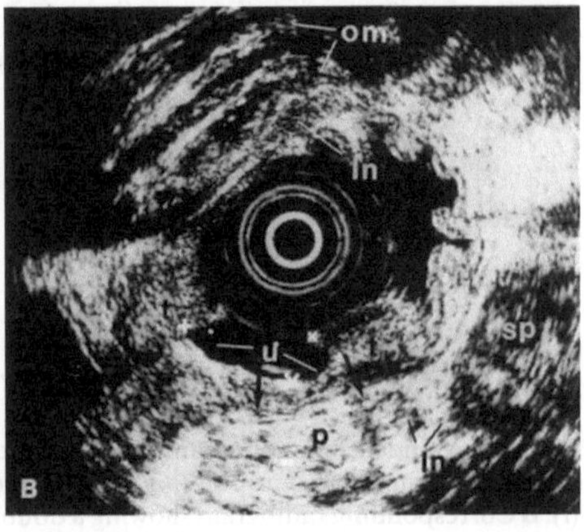

Fig. 3.22 A, B. Endoscopic sonograms. **A** Hypoechoic tumor (*t*) penetrating deeply into the pancreas (*p*) adjacent to an ulcerative lesion (*u*). *l*, liver; *sp*, spleen. **B** Tumor (*t*) adjacent to an ulcer (*u*) with some slight penetration (*arrows*) into the pancreas (*p*), associated with multiple lymph nodes (*ln*). *om*, omentum majus

Recently we have performed a prospective study in the preoperative TNM (1987) staging of gastric carcinoma. As in the case of esophageal carcinoma, the depth of infiltration has been used as a criterion, in preference to tumor size, circumferential involvement, and obstruction. Endosonography is accurate in the evaluation of the tumor category and in diagnosing regional lymph node involvement. In the evaluation of nonmetastatic lymph nodes and distant metastases, however, endosonography is less accurate.

Endosonography usually visualizes gastric non-Hodgkin's lymphoma as diffuse transmural and ulcerative infiltration and polypoid lesions, together with perigastric lymph node abnormalities. Occasionally, an extensive hypoechoic

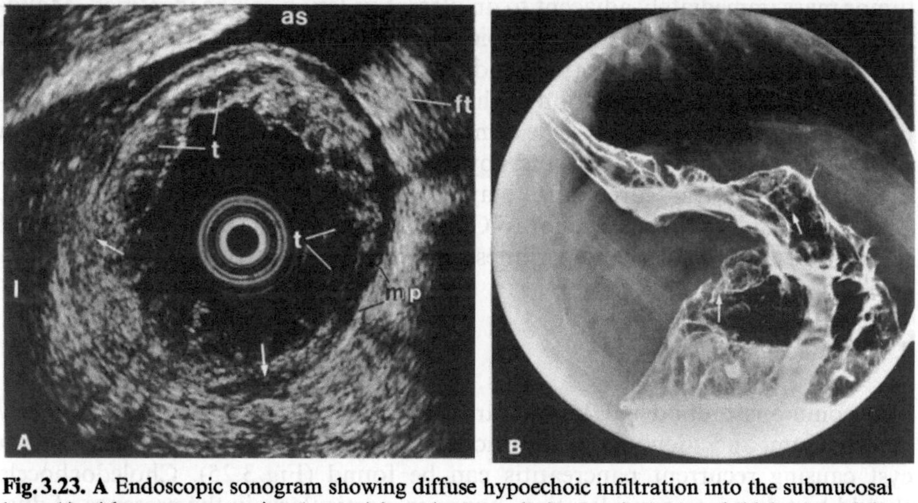

Fig. 3.23. **A** Endoscopic sonogram showing diffuse hypoechoic infiltration into the submucosal layer (*t*) with some penetration (*arrows*) into the muscularis propria (*mp*) and thickening of the gastric wall associated with ascites (*as*). *l*, liver; *ft*, fat tissue. **B** Corresponding radiogram, showing a double contour in the proximal stomach (*arrows*)

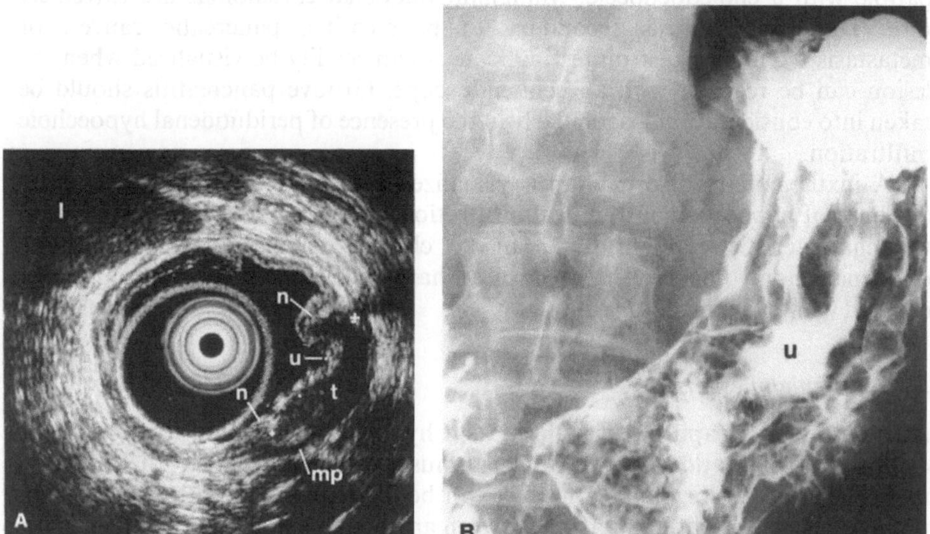

Fig. 3.24. **A** Endoscopic sonogram showing sharply demarcated hypoechoic tumor (*t*) penetrating into the muscularis propria (*mp*) directly adjacent to an ulcer (*u*) with nodular margins (*n*). *l*, left liver lobe. **B** Corresponding radiogram, showing the ulcer (*u*) localized at the greater curvature of the stomach

tumor mass immediately adjacent to an ulcerative lesion can be identified. Malignancies appear to be more hypoechoic than the surrounding tissues (Fig. 3.23). The transition between a normal and a pathologic wall structure can be seen clearly (Fig. 3.24). Determination of the longitudinal extent and depth of infiltration is also feasible, which is of the utmost importance in planning therapy and in follow-up after surgery, lasertherapy, chemotherapy, or radiotherapy. Occasionally a gastric carcinoma may be detected after radiotherapy [16]. Endosonography proved superior to CT because it permits clear visualization of both mural abnormalities and periintestinal lymph node involvement [20].

3.3.3 Duodenal Lesions

The commonest duodenal lesions are ulceration, peripapillary/juxtapapillary diverticulum, and adenoma of the duodenal papilla. Occasionally, a duplication cyst causing recurrent pancreatitis can be found (Fig. 3.25). Choledochocele should be taken into consideration, however, particularly in the presence of ductular structures within the intramural lesion. The absence of choledochus within the cystic lesion is strongly suggestive of a duplication cyst. In contrast, the presence of choledochus within or directly adjacent to the cystic lesion is compatible with a choledochocele. Malignant duodenal carcinomas are extremely rare. Duodenal stenosis secondary to pancreatitis, pancreatic cancer, or metastasis from extragastrointestinal cancer can readily be visualized when the lesion can be reached with an echoendoscope. Groove pancreatitis should be taken into consideration, particularly in the presence of periduodenal hypoechoic infiltration.

A juxtapapillary diverticulum is visualized as a limited excavation with no evidence of hypoechoic intramural infiltration. By filling the lesion with water, the characteristic configuration can be clearly visualized. Occasionally, a duodenal leiomyoma is visualized as a sharply delineated hypoechoic tumor covered with intact mucosa.

3.3.3.1 Benign Lesions

Adenoma of the papilla is visualized as a hypoechoic polypoid lesion with no evidence of penetration into the adjacent muscularis propria. The adjacent common bile duct and/or pancreatic duct can be dilated secondary to tumor compression. However, differentiation between an adenoma and a carcinoma can occasionally be difficult or even impossible if the adjacent muscularis propria cannot be seen. A juxtapapillary diverticulum is visualized as a concave lesion, usually with no evidence of abnormal hypoechoic intramural patterns unless inflammatory changes are present. The adjacent common bile duct and/or pancreatic duct may sometimes be dilated. A duodenal polyp is visualized as a hypoechoic polypoid lesion with a clearly delineated wall architecture; there is some hypoechoicity in the mucosa and/or submucosa with no evidence of penetration into the adjacent duodenal wall. A polyp with a long stalk can be visualized more clearly after rapidly filling the lumen with water. This water-

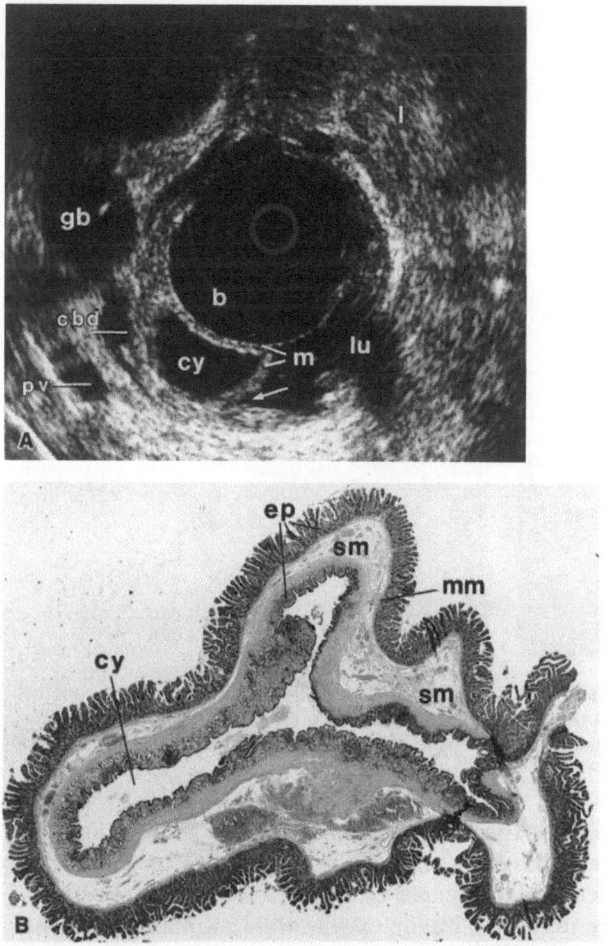

Fig. 3.25. A Endoscopic sonogram showing an anechoic cystic lesion (*cy*) directly adjacent to the mucosa (*m*), causing a bulging lesion (*arrow*). Note the anatomical relationship to the gallbladder (*gb*) and the common bile duct (*cbd*). *pv*, portal vein; *lu*, lumen; *b*, water-filled balloon. **B** Corresponding histological section, showing a duodenal duplication cyst (*cy*) covered with intact mucosa. *ep*, epithelium; *mm*, muscularis mucosae; *sm*, submucosa

filled lumen method is of the utmost importance for achieving clear visualization of the submucosal layer. Occasionally, villous adenoma adjacent to the papilla of Vater can be found, particularly in patients with polyposis coli. In such cases the water-filled method is the investigation of choice to clearly determine the presence or absence of focal invasion into deeper submucosal layers.

3.3.3.2 Malignant Lesions

Duodenal carcinoma is visualized as a hypoechoic intramural lesion, with or without penetration into the muscularis propria (Fig. 3.26). Extensive car-

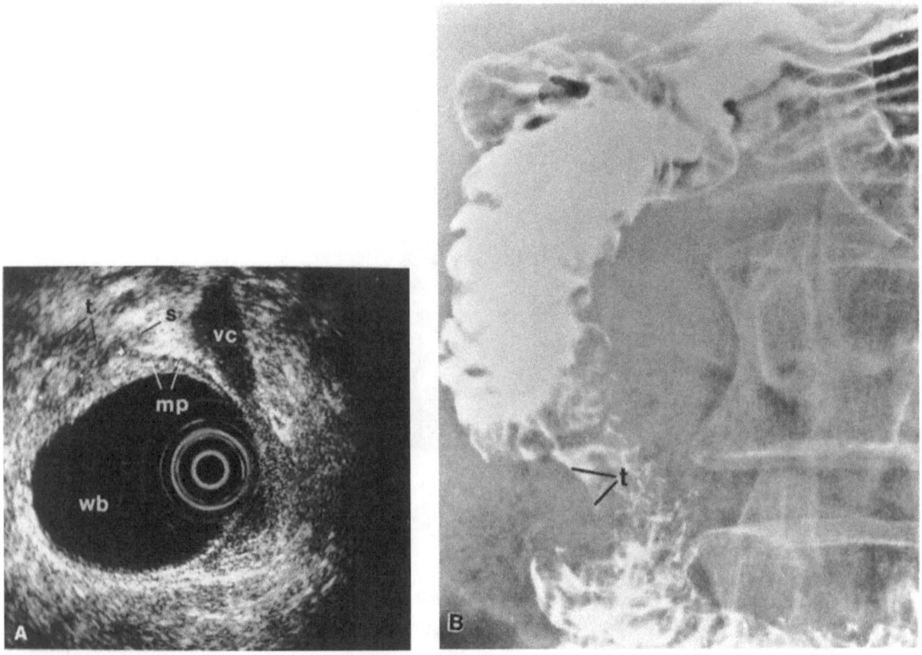

Fig. 3.26. A Endoscopic sonogram showing a clearly demarcated hypoechoic tumor (*t*) penetrating through the muscularis propria (*mp*) into the serosal layer (*s*) adjacent to the vena cava (*vc*). *wb*, water-filled balloon. **B** Corresponding radiogram, revealing a filling defect (*t*) on the lateral side of the descending duodenum

cinomas may cause obstruction of the lumen. Criteria for the TNM staging of duodenal carcinoma are comparable with those for gastric carcinoma (Sect. 3.3.2.2). However, the commonest cause of postbulbar duodenal obstruction is not primary duodenal carcinoma, but an extramural lesion, usually a pancreatic neoplasm. Groove pancreatitis is diagnosed when a diffuse hypoechoic area is seen, localized between the duodenal wall and the pancreas; there is no evidence of the abnormality extending into the pancreatic parenchyma, but it is usually associated with an obstruction of the pancreatic duct and/or the common bile duct. Pancreatic carcinoma localized in the head of the pancreas may infiltrate and obstruct the adjacent duodenum, showing up as a hypoechoic tumor mass penetrating directly into the duodenal wall. A hypoechoic tumor mass immediately adjacent to the duodenal wall compressing or bulging into the lumen is strongly suggestive of a metastatic lesion. The primary lesion is often of extragastroduodenal origin, such as ovary or breast cancer, Hodgkin's lymphoma, cholangiocarcinoma, or pancreatic cancer. Malignant duodenal polyps are extremely rare. The commonest peripapillary neoplasm is carcinoma of the duodenal papilla, which is visualized as a hypoechoic polypoid lesion, often penetrating into the common bile duct and/or pancreatic duct. Usually one can readily differentiate between an adenoma and a carcinoma prior to sphincterotomy. Penetration of a hypoechoic structure into the adjacent muscularis propria is strongly suggestive of malignancy. In contrast, the absence of such penetration is indicative of benignity. However, biopsies are necessary for definitive diagnosis.

3.3.4 Tumors in the Common Bile Duct and Proximal Biliary System

The distal part of the biliary system can be visualized by placing the echo probe in the second part of the duodenum. By gradually withdrawing the instrument, using the typical location of the distal bile duct adjacent to the duodenal lumen as a landmark, the common bile duct, the hepatic duct, and the region of bifurcation can readily be visualized [19].

However, exact topographic anatomical knowledge is necessary for correct positioning of the echo probe. The most important structure for topographic anatomical orientation is the portal vein, which is localized adjacent and parallel to the common duct. Occasionally, the hepatic artery can be identified between the common duct and the portal vein.

3.3.4.1 Distal Common Bile Duct Lesions

Benign Lesions. Benign tumors in the distal common bile duct are adenomas, which may originate from the peripapillary region and protrude into the lumen of the common duct. Impacted stones in the ampullary region may cause an obstruction and some times simulate malignant obstruction. By placing the echo probe directly against the lesion, malignancy can readily be ruled out if no evidence of a hypoechoic tumor mass is found. A concretion is visualized as a hyperechoic structure usually associated with dorsal shadowing. A bile duct tumor is visualized as a hypoechoic lesion localized in the common bile duct, usually with dilation of the latter. After biliary surgery or occasionally after cholecystectomy, a hyperechoic structure can be identified immediately adjacent to the ductular narrowing of the proximal part of the common bile duct, with prestenotic dilation; this is compatible with postsurgical changes. Moreover, metallic clips can be visualized as hyperechoic structures.

Malignant Lesions. Bile duct carcinoma is visualized as a polypoid tumor protruding into or obstructing the lumen of the bile duct. With adequate placing of the echo probe against the lesion, the origin of the latter can often be clearly identified (Fig. 3.27). In cases of extensive carcinoma penetrating into the adjacent pancreatic parenchyma, differentiation between bile duct carcinoma and pancreatic cancer can be difficult or even impossible, particularly if the pancreas is also infiltrated. Such an abnormality is similar to a double duct lesion seen on endoscopic retrograde cholangiopancreaticography (ERCP) (Fig. 3.28). A carcinoid lesion in the peripapillary region is visualized as a round or ellipsoid hypoechoic lesion compressing or penetrating into the pancreatic or common bile duct. After insertion of a biliary endoprosthesis, the site of the lesion can readily be identified, using the hyperechoic echo pattern of the endoprosthesis as a guide. In contrast, CT scan images are often interfered with by endoprostheses.

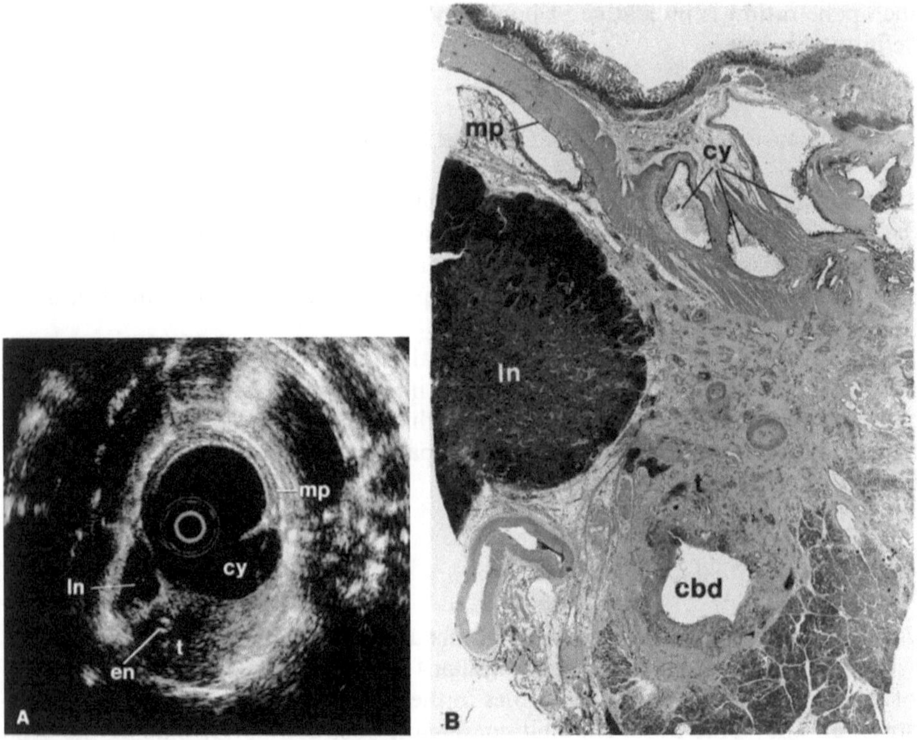

Fig. 3.27. A Endoscopic sonogram of resection specimen showing a round hypoechoic intraductal echo pattern (*t*) containing an endoprosthesis (*en*), with visualization of a cystic lesion (*cy*). An ellipsoid hypoechoic lymph node is seen on the contralateral side (*ln*), immediately adjacent to the main lesion. **B** Corresponding histological section, showing tumor infiltration (*t*) immediately adjacent to the common bile duct (*cbd*), with a cystic benign. *mp*, muscularis propria

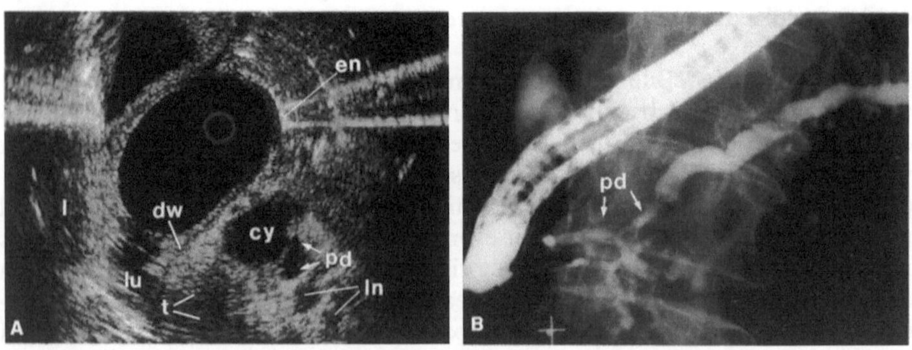

Fig. 3.28. A Endoscopic sonogram showing a hypoechoic tumor (*t*) adjacent to a cystic lesion (*cy*) and the pancreatic duct (*pd*), with a biliary endoprosthesis (*en*). *lu*, lumen; *ln*, lymph node; *l*, liver. **B** Endoscopic retrograde cholangiopancreatogram revealing circumscribed narrowing of the pancreatic duct (*pd*) in the periampullary region

Moreover, the real-time dynamic properties of endosonography allow more detailed information to be obtained on tumor penetration around or into the major blood vessels, which is of the utmost importance in assessing resectability. The most important blood vessels are the portal vein, the hepatic artery or the celiac trunk, and the mesenteric artery. Benign and malignant lesions can thus be readily distinguished.

Bifurcation Tumors. A bifurcation tumor of the bile duct (Klatskin tumor) is visualized as a hypoechoic tumor with polycyclic or roundly demarcated boundaries protruding into or compressing the adjacent bile duct, with prestenotic dilation of the intrahepatic biliary tree of the left and/or right system. Lymph nodes directly adjacent to the tumor can be identified, usually localized in the hilum of the liver or along the common bile duct and adjacent to the cystic duct. A tumor with sharply demarcated boundaries, and with no evidence of penetration into the liver parenchyma or lymph node involvement, is an indication for curative resection (Figs. 3.29, 3.30). A tumor penetrating into the adjacent liver parenchyma, usually associated with involved lymph nodes, strongly suggests a palliative procedure. Penetration of the tumor mass into the adjacent major blood vessels and deeply into the liver parenchyma suggests non-resectability (Fig. 3.31). In the case of an extensive mass, differentiation between a bifurcation tumor and a solitary liver metastasis may sometimes be difficult because of their similar echo patterns. Recently, we have been using the new TNM classification for staging extrahepatic bile duct carcinoma (Klatskin) [24]. Criteria for the staging of tumor categories are as follows:

T1: Hypoechoic intraductal tumor invades the mucosa or muscle layer
  T1 a: Hypoechoic tumor invades the mucosa
  T1 b: Hypoechoic tumor invades muscle layer (muscularis)
T2: Hypoechoic tumor invades hyperechoic perimuscular tissue
T3: Hypoechoic tumor invades adjacent structures: liver, gallbladder, portal vein, or hepatic artery

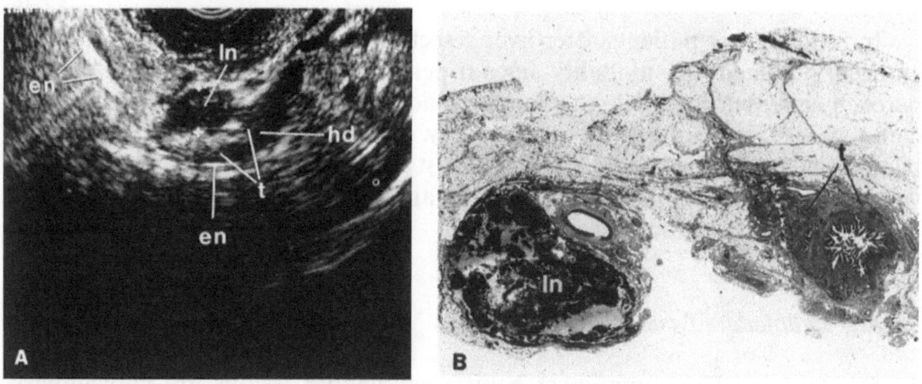

Fig. 3.29. A Endoscopic sonogram showing a hypoechoic intraductal tumor (*t*) with an endoprosthesis (*en*) and a sharply delineated hypoechoic lymph node (*ln*). *hd*, hepatic duct. **B** Corresponding histological section, revealing the intraductal carcinoma (*t*) with a metastatic lymph node (*ln*)

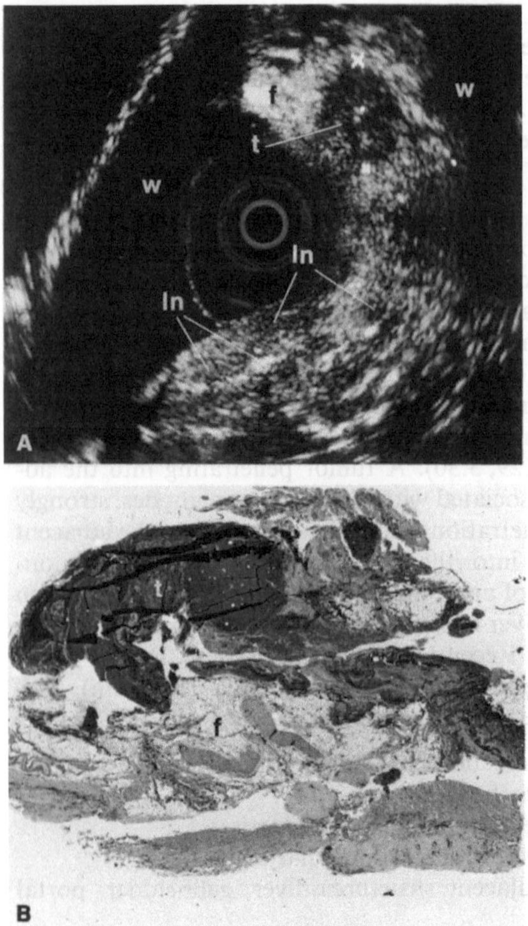

Fig. 3.30. A Endoscopic sonogram of a resection specimen showing a sharply demarcated hypoechoic tumor (*t*) with some adjacent fat tissue (*f*) and small, innocuous, hyperechoic lymph nodes (*ln*). **B** Corresponding histological section, showing a cholangiocarcinoma (*t*) with adjacent fat tissue (*f*)

In follow-up of patients after liver resection endosonography appears to be an accurate diagnostic modality since it permits imaging of both ductular and parenchymal abnormalities, together with adjacent lymph node involvement. In contrast, ERCP is unable to visualize any ductular abnormalities because the biliary system cannot be filled with contrast medium after biliary surgery. Conventional transcutaneous ultrasonography and CT are also inaccurate because of artifacts secondary to postsurgical changes.

3.3.4.2 Gallbladder Lesions

Benign Lesions. The commonest benign gallbladder lesions are cholelithiasis and/or cholecystitis. A solitary stone or multiple concretion can be seen as a round or ellipsoid hypoechoic structure with dorsal shadowing, which can usually be detected by conventional ultrasound. A small stone (even with a diameter of

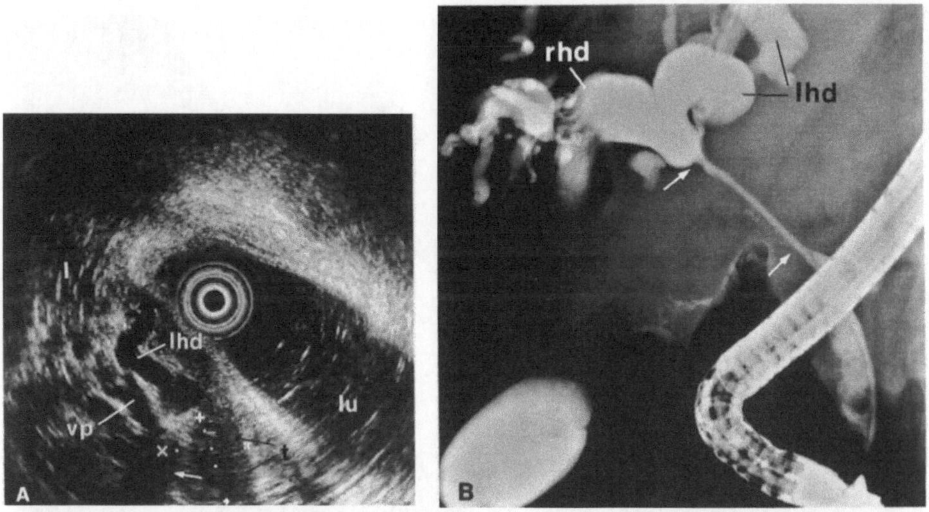

Fig. 3.31. A Endoscopic sonogram showing dilation of the left hepatic duct (*lhd*) due to a bifurcation tumor (*t*), with some suspicious penetration (*arrow*) into the adjacent portal vein (*vp*). *l*, liver; *lu*, lumen. **B** Corresponding endoscopic retrograde cholangiopancreatogram, revealing narrowing of the common hepatic duct (*arrows*), with dilation of the left (*lhd*) and right (*rhd*) hepatic ducts

less than 5 mm) can be clearly identified as a small round or ellipsoid hyperechoic structure. The commonest small concretion is a cholesterol stone, usually localized adjacent to the wall of the gallbladder, imaged as a small hyperechoicity and simulating a polyp. However, absence of a stalk (sessile or penduculated polyp) and displacement of the hyperechoicity when the patient's position is changed are more characteristic of cholesterol stones than of polyps.

Cholecystitis is visualized as thickening of the wall with no evidence of hypoechoic tumor masses protruding into the lumen of the gallbladder or penetration into the surrounding tissues. The thickening of the gallbladder is usually secondary to a hyperechoic echo pattern compatible with inflammatory changes.

Stones localized in the neck of the gallbladder or in the cystic duct may cause obstruction of the adjacent common hepatic duct, which may simulate malignant stenosis on ERCP (Mirrizzi syndrome). Endosonography may rule out malignancy because of its capacity to visualize the primary lesion as a hyperechoic lesion compressing the adjacent bile duct without any evidence of a tumor mass immediately adjacent to the stenotic area.

Malignant Lesions. Carcinoma of the gallbladder is visualized as a polypoid hypoechoic lesion originating from the wall and protruding into the lumen or penetrating into the surrounding tissues (Fig. 3.32). Gallbladder carcinoma penetrating deeply into the surrounding tissues and with no evidence of multiple distant lymph node involvement is an indication for curative resection. A carcinoma penetrating directly into the adjacent common bile duct or hepatic duct, usually associated with lymph node involvement, strongly suggests palliative

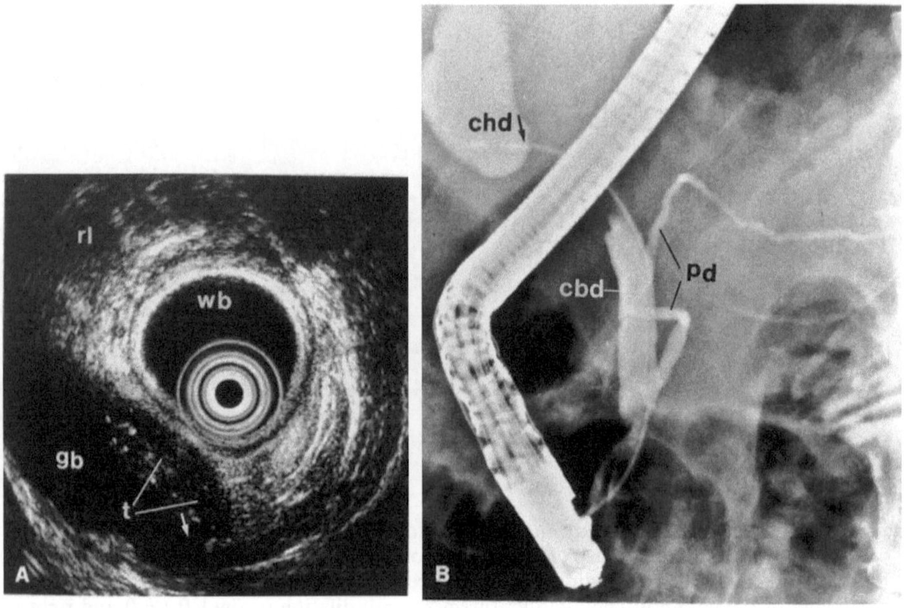

3.32

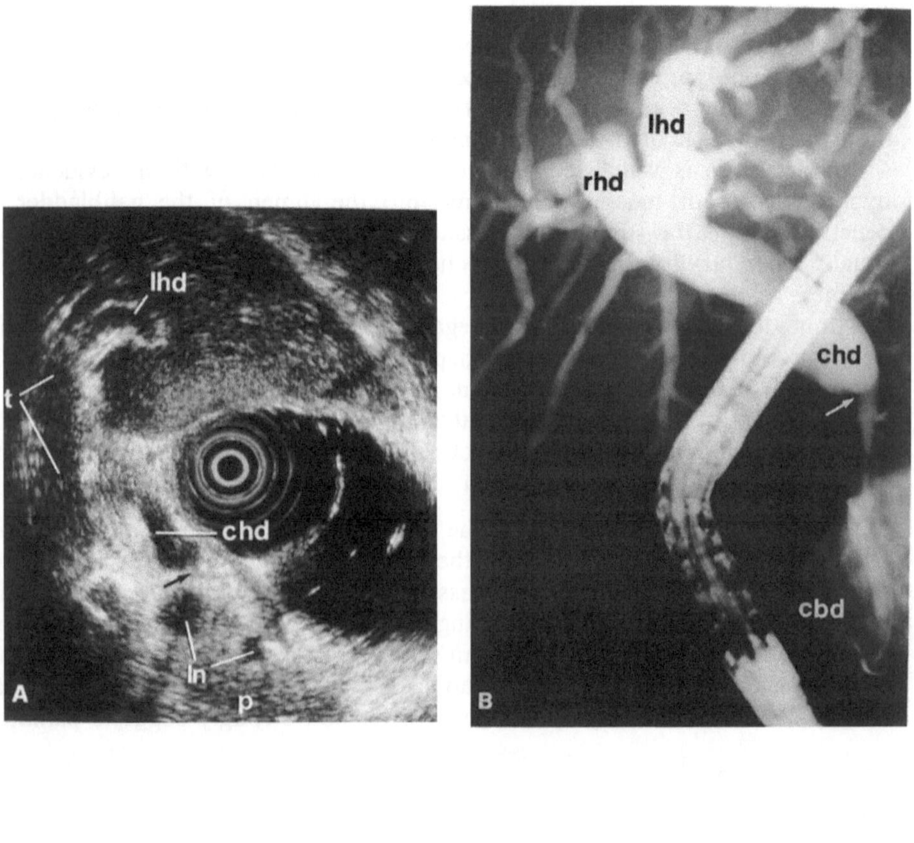

3.33

resection. Deep penetration of the carcinoma into the adjacent tissue, e.g., the gallbladder bed or the adjacent duodenum, is highly suggestive of non-resectability. Carcinoma of the gallbladder with continuous penetration into the proximal biliary system can sometimes be difficult to distinguish from a Klatskin tumor because of the similar echo pattern and intrahepatic ductular dilation (Fig. 3.33). A carcinoma penetrating into the adjacent distal bile duct and the pancreatic head may simulate pancreatic or common bile duct carcinoma on ERCP, or even simulate groove pancreatitis, which may readily be distinguished by endosonography. Occasionally, sludge phenomena of the gallbladder may simulate the presence of gallbladder malignancy because of some hypoechoic pattern immediately adjacent to the wall of the gallbladder. However, such a pseudotumorous lesion can be displaced by changing the position of the patient. Duodenal stenosis may often be multifactorial. The origin of such a lesion can readily be identified by placing the echo probe against or into the stenotic area.

3.4 Future Prospects

Endosonography allows clear visualization of intramural abnormalities together with the surrounding tissue, because target lesions are approached directly with a high-frequency ultrasound beam. Moreover, extramural lesions directly adjacent to the gastrointestinal tract can be clearly visualized. This is of the utmost importance because most gastrointestinal lesions can be reached endoscopically and therefore also endosonographically. Endosonography thus appears to be very helpful in detection, in staging, and in follow-up after treatment of intra- und extramural lesions. When a lesion is found endoscopically, endosonography can be performed to detect its origin and assess its extent. The possibility of using the biopsy channel for endosonographically guided puncture or biopsy may further enhance not only the diagnostic but also the therapeutic value of the procedure. Endosonographically guided cystogastrostomy and/or cystoduodenostomy may remove the necessity for extensive surgical procedures. Moreover, nodal or mural malignancy can readily be ruled out. There is no doubt that endosonography will become an important diagnostic and therapeutic procedure in gastroenterology.

Fig. 3.32. A Endoscopic sonogram showing a polypoid hypoechoic tumor (*t*) in the wall of the gallbladder (*gb*), with some penetration into the surrounding structures (*arrow*). *rl*, right liver lobe; *wb*, water-filled balloon. **B** Corresponding endoscopic retrograde cholangiopancreatogram, revealing narrowing of the distal common hepatic duct (*chd*), without visualization of the gallbladder and with a normal pancreatic duct (*pd*). *cbd*, common bile duct

Fig. 3.33. A Endoscopic sonogram showing dilation of the common hepatic duct (*chd*), with narrowing (*arrow*) directly adjacent to two suspicious lymph nodes (*ln*). An extensive hypoechoic tumor (*t*) is seen in the bifurcation of the bile duct, extending to the common hepatic duct. *p*, pancreas. **B** Corresponding endoscopic retrograde cholangiopancreatogram, revealing the narrowing (*arrow*) and dilation of extra- and intrahepatic duct. *rhd*, right hepatic duct; *lhd*, left hepatic duct

In the future, the possibility of performing ultrasonic procedures via the biopsy channel, particularly for assessing circumscribed intramural lesions (e.g., polyps or intramucosal submucosal carcinomas), may further enhance their diagnostic value. The combination of videoendoscopy with endosonography may result in an outstanding diagnostic procedure for teaching and for documentation of both endoscopic and ultrasonic images. The small diameter of the echo probe compared to the standard instrument enables easier passage of the probe through the pylorus or even through a stenosis. Improvement in endoscopic imaging and the smaller echo probe make for easier maneuvering of the instrument.

References

1. Baker HL, Good CA (1955) Smooth muscle tumors of the alimentary tract. Their roentgen manifestations. AJR 74:246–254
2. Caletti G, Bolondi L, Brocchi P et al. (1983) Staging of gastric cancer by means of endoscopic ultrasonography (Abstract). Gastroenterology 84:13866
3. Di Magno EP, Regan PT, Clain JE, James EM, Buxton JL (1982) Human endoscopic ultrasonography. Gastroenterology 83:824–829
4. Faivre J, Bory R, Moulinier B (1978) Benign tumors of oesophagus: value of endoscopy. Endoscopy 10:264–268
5. Fargenburg D, Farman J, Dallemand S et al. (1975) Leiomyoblastoma of the stomach. report of 9 cases. Radiology 117:297–300
6. Heyder N, Lutz H, Lux G (1983) Ultraschalldiagnostik via Gastroskop. Ultraschall Med 4:84–93
7. Kaneko E, Kumagai J, Honda N et al. (1983) Evaluation of the new giant-biopsy forceps in the diagnosis of mucosal and submucosal gastric lesions. Endoscopy 15:322–326
8. Lux G, Heyder N, Demling L (1982) Endoscopic ultrasonography – technique, orientation and diagnostic possibilities. Endoscopy 4:220–225
9. Nauert TC, Zornoza J, Ordonez N (1982) Gastric leiomyosarcomas. AJR 139:291–297
10. Papazian A, Gineston JL, Capron JP, Quenum C (1984) Leiomyoblastoma of the stomach: endoscopic treatment. Endoscopy 16:157–159
11. Phillips JC, Lindsay JW, Kendall JA (1970) Gastric leiomyosarcoma: roentgenologic and clinical findings. J Dig Dis 15:239–246
12. Quint LE, Glazer GM, Orringer B (1985) Esophageal carcinoma: CT findings. Radiology 155:171–175
13. Scand J Gastroenterol 19 (Suppl 94):1–106
14. Scand J Gastroenterol 19 (Suppl 102):5–37
15. Scand J Gastroenterol 21 (Suppl 123):1–169
16. Shani A, Schutt AJ, Weiland LH (1978) Primary gastric malignant lymphoma followed by gastric adenocarcinoma. Report of 4 cases and review of the literature. Cancer 42:2039–2044
17. Strohm WD, Classen M (1984) Endosonographie mit einem Gastrofiberskop. Ultraschall Med 5:84–93
18. Tio TL, Tytgat GNJ (1984) Endoscopic ultrasonography in the assessment of intra- and transmural infiltration of tumours in the oesophagus, stomach and papilla of Vater and in the detection of extraoesophageal lesions. Endoscopy 4:220–225
19. Tio TL, Tytgat GNJ (1986) Atlas of transintestinal ultrasonography. Mur Kostverloren, Aalsmeer
20. Tio TL, den Hartog Jager FCA, Tytgat GNJ (1986) Endoscopic ultrasonography of Non-Hodgkin lymphoma of the stomach. Gastroenterology 91:401–408
21. Tio TL, den Hartog Jager FCA, Tytgat GNJ (1986) The role of endoscopic ultrasonography in assessing local resectability of oesophagogastric malignancies. Scand J Gastroenterol 21 (Suppl 123):78–86

22. Tio TL, Cohen P, Coene PP, Udding J, den Hartog Jager FCA, Tytgat GNJ (1989) Endosonography and computed tomography of esophageal carcinoma. Gastroenterology 96:1478–1486
23. Tio TL, Coene PPLO, Schouwink MH, Tytgat GNJ (1989) Esophagogastric carcinoma: preoperative TNM classification with endosonography. Radiology 173:411–417
24. Tio TL, Wijers OB, Sars PRA, Tytgat GNJ (1990) Preoperative TNM classification of proximal extrahepatic bile duct carcinoma by endosonography. Sem Liver Dis (in press)
25. Welch JP (1975) Smooth muscle tumors of the stomach. Am J Surg 130:279–285

4 Endorectal Sonography

U. HILDEBRANDT, J. BEYNON, G. FEIFEL, and N. J. McC. MORTENSEN
With a contribution by P. LANGENSCHEIDT and B. KRAMANN

Extracorporeal ultrasonic scanners have always been considered unsatisfactory for imaging the gastrointestinal tract. The reasons are the presence of intestinal gas and the limited resolution of the low frequencies used. The rectum expecially, hidden as it is within the bony structures of the pelvis, is not accessible to extracorporeal ultrasound. However, as interest in the diagnostic imaging of rectal cancer has grown, refined sonographic techniques combining endoscopy and sonography have been introduced.

4.1 History

The first attempt at ultrasonic intraluminal scanning was made in the mid-1950s by Wild and Reid (Fig. 4.1). They used a rotating scanner in the rectum to detect echo pattern changes due to cancer, and found that "in general cancer tissue returned more sound than normal control tissue".

Having designed and produced three successful echo-endoprobes, Wild and Reid expressed the hope that their work would "inspire interest in the development of endoprobic ultrasonic techniques for the much needed detection of early, localized neoplastic foci in the mucosa of the lower bowel" [45]. The screening of an asymptomatic population for cancer using ultrasound was achieved by Watanabe [44], who used a specially designed chair for the detection of prostatic cancer by radial scanning of the prostate from the rectal lumen. Alzin [2] and Dragsted [11] reported on the imaging of rectal cancer using a scanner designed for urological use. Since then a considerable number of papers have reflected the growing interest in the new field of endosonographic imaging of rectal cancer imaging [13, 16, 21, 29, 32]. Based on our own experience with endorectal ultrasound since 1983 in Homburg, since 1984 in Bristol and since 1986 in Oxford [4–6], it is our aim to describe the technique, to interpret the results and to discuss the many controversies that have arisen.

4.2 Patient Preparation

We do not use either anaesthesia or sedation. The rectum has to be evacuated with an enema, so that it is completely clean. If preparation is unsatisfactory, faeces between the water balloon and the rectal wall will reflect the sound energy.

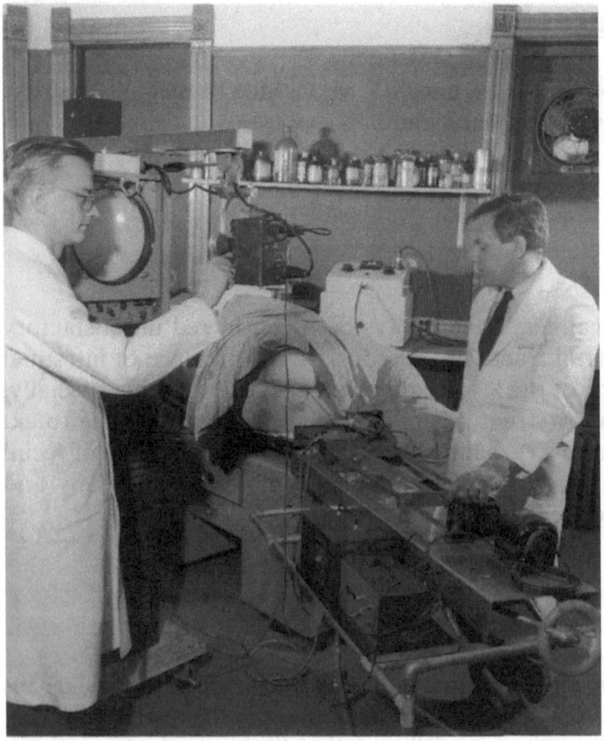

Fig. 4.1. Photograph from 1956 showing John Wild (*right*) and John Reid (*left*) with the first endoluminal real-time instrument. The extraction unit, adjustable for height, is shown next to Wild. Reid is seen supervising the real-time image on the display unit and the automatic display camera (Courtesy of John Wild)

This causes a "blind sonogram" with poor resolution beyond the faecal barrier. Faeces may also mimic a lesion where there is none. The patient is placed in one of three positions for examination: the left lateral, the supine or the lithotomy position. In Homburg we prefer the latter since we are accustomed to perform endoscopies with the rigid rectoscope in this technique. The advantage is that the visually determined tumour site within the 360° circumference coincides topographically with the sonographic evaluation of the tumor when the probe is handled in the proposed manner. A tumour extending from 12 to 3 o'clock is imaged on the sonogram in the right upper quarter of the rectal circumference. In Bristol and Oxford we prefer the left lateral position and have acceptable results.

4.3 Equipment

The first instrument we used was the prototype 9526 manufactured by Brüel and Kjaer (Naerum, Denmark). It was equipped with a 3.5-MHz radially scanning transducer. Since 1983 we have used the commercially available Brüel and Kjaer radial scanner type 1846.

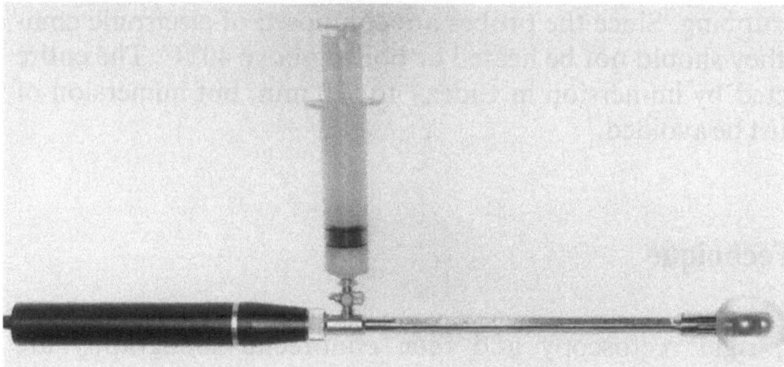

Fig. 4.2. Endorectal probe (Brüel and Kjaer, Naerum, Denmark)

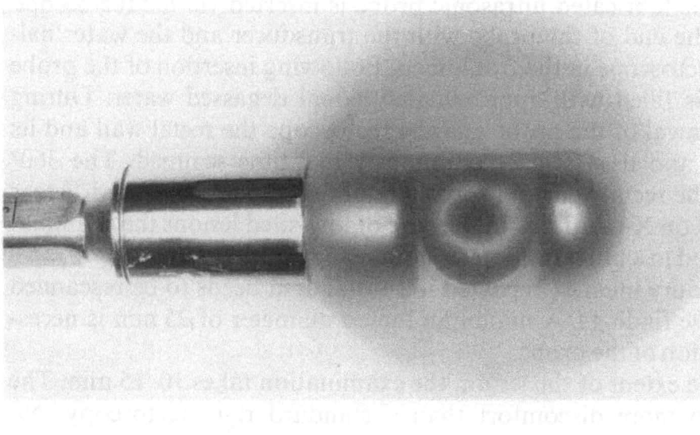

Fig. 4.3. A 7-MHz transducer surrounded by a water-filled balloon

The Brüel and Kjaer radial scanning probe is 24 cm long (Fig. 4.2). A transducer is fitted to the end of the rod and rotates mechanically at a rate of 4–6 cycles per second. The reflections of the transmitted ultrasonic waves are received at a 90° angle. Scanning radially to the axis of the rectal probe, a 360° display of the rectum and the surrounding tissues is provided. A thin rubber balloon is attached over the transducer (Fig. 4.3) and filled with degassed water, thus providing an acoustic path for the ultrasonic waves. To prevent transmission of infectious diseases (e.g. AIDS) all probes may be covered with a disposable latex sheath. Using the latter it is necessary to place water or gel between the transducer balloon and the latex sheath for proper acoustic interfacing. Gel is applied to the tip of the endoscopic probe before insertion into the rectum.

4.4 Cleaning and Disinfection

When a disposable latex sheath is used it is simply changed prior to examining the next patient. Normally the probe is washed with water and foreign matter is removed by gentle scrubbing. Since the probes are composed of electronic components and plastics they should not be heated or boiled above 40° C. The entire probe can be disinfected by immersion in Cidex® for 20 min, but immersion of the connector area must be avoided.

4.5 Examination Technique

Digital examination, rigid rectoscopy and then endorectal sonography are carried out in either the lithotomy or the left lateral position. We use a rectoscope of 20 cm length and 20 mm internal diameter which is introduced into the rectum as far as possible. The lubricated ultrasonic probe is inserted via the rectoscope (Fig. 4.4) such that the end of the probe with the transducer and the water balloon is beyond the rectoscope in the free lumen. Following insertion of the probe the rubber balloon is filled with approximately 60 ml degassed water. During simultaneous withdrawal of the probe and the rectoscope the rectal wall and its surrounding organs and tissues are continuously real-time scanned. The 360° transverse views of the rectal wall and surrounding tissues are monitored. Areas of interest are copied on X-ray films. In the case of low-sited lesions the examination may be performed in a blind fashion without using the rectoscope.

The whole procedure must be repeated if a distal area needs to be rescanned to clarify inconclusive findings. A minimum lumen diameter of 25 mm is necessary to achieve insertion of the probe.

Depending on the extent of the lesion, the examination takes 10–15 min. The procedure causes no more discomfort than a standard rigid rectoscopy. No major complications have been encountered.

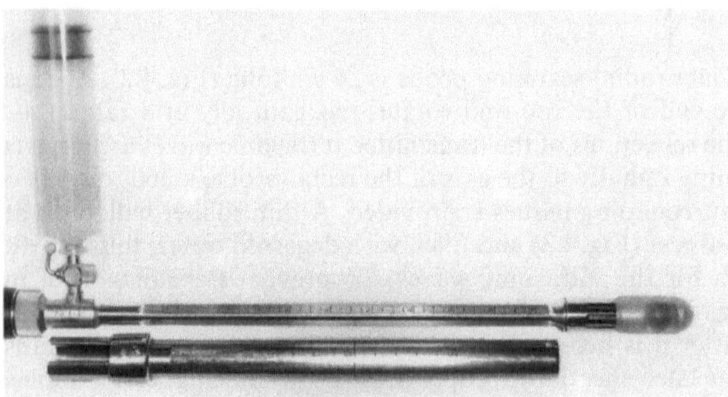

Fig. 4.4. The probe, 24 cm long and 19 mm in diameter at the thickest part, fits through the 20-cm rectoscope of 20 mm internal diameter (Karl Storz, Tuttlingen, FRG)

4.6 Sonographic Characteristics of the Rectal Wall

Sonographically the rectal wall is represented by three hyperechoic and two hypoechoic circles when a 7-MHz transducer is used (Figs. 4.5, 4.6). The inner hyperechoic (white) circle represents a combination of the rubber balloon and the interface of water and mucosa, the middle hyperechoic circle, the interface between mucosa and muscularis propria, the outer hyperechoic circle, the interface between muscularis and fat. The inner hypoechoic (dark) circle represents the mucosa. No differentiation can be made between mucosa and submucosa: probably the submucosa is overlaid by the middle hyperechoic circle or part of it. The outer hypoechoic circle represents the muscularis propria.

The sonographic appearance of the different layers of the rectal wall was first assessed by Boscaini and Montori [8, 9] who performed in vitro ultrasonographic studies on polyethylene membranes of different thickness and on surgical specimens from the rectal wall, using a 5-MHz linear scanner (PLB 505S, Toshiba).

We reached similar conclusions using a 7-MHz radial scanner (Brüel and Kjaer). In vitro studies of the excised rectum in a water bath revealed that the balloon alone, when filled with water, was imaged as a white circle. On scanning the rectal wall without using a balloon, the inner white circle was shown to represent the interface which arose when part of the wave was reflected at the surface of the mucosa. When a balloon was used the reflection of the balloon merged with this interface to give one hyperechoic circle. On injection of saline into the submucosa we were able to demonstrate that the resulting thickened plane belonged to the inner hyperechoic circle representing the mucosa. After removal of the mucosa and submucosa disruption of the inner hypoechoic circle was observed while the outer hypoechoic circle remained unchanged.

4.5
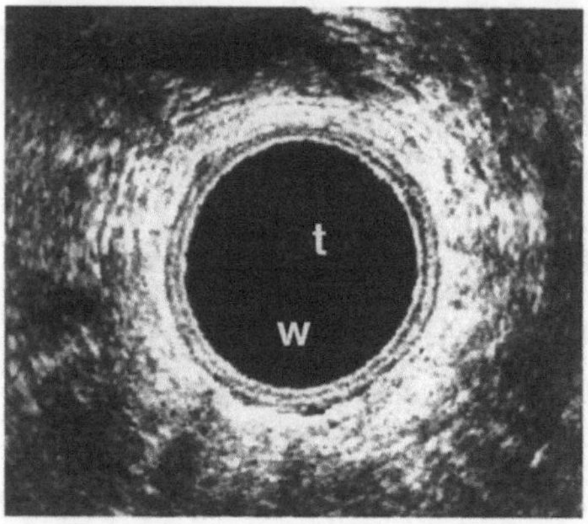

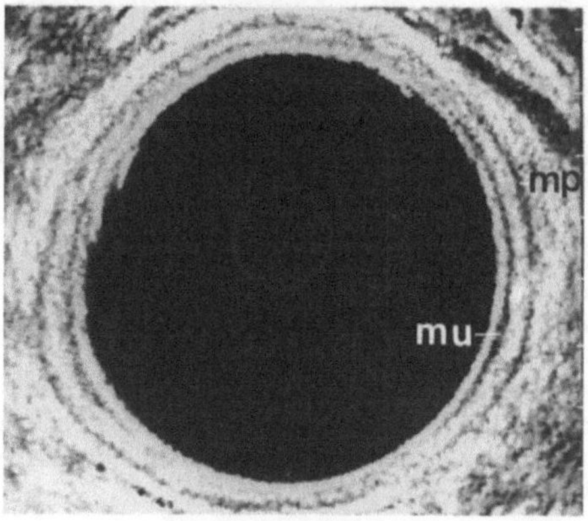

4.6

Fig. 4.5. Sonogram of the intact rectal wall. *t*, transducer; *w*, water-filled balloon. The three hyperechoic circles represent interfaces. The inner hypoechoic circle corresponds to the mucosa, the outer hypoechoic circle to the muscularis propria

Fig. 4.6. Magnification of the sonographic appearance of the rectal wall showing the hypoechoic mucosa (*mu*) and muscularis propria (*mp*) and the three hyperechoic interfaces

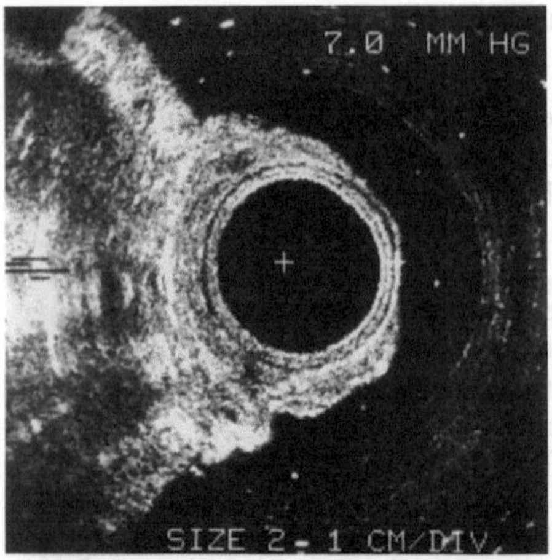

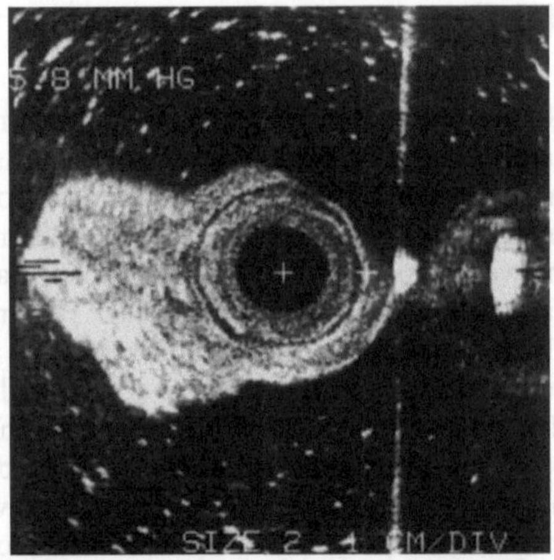

4.9

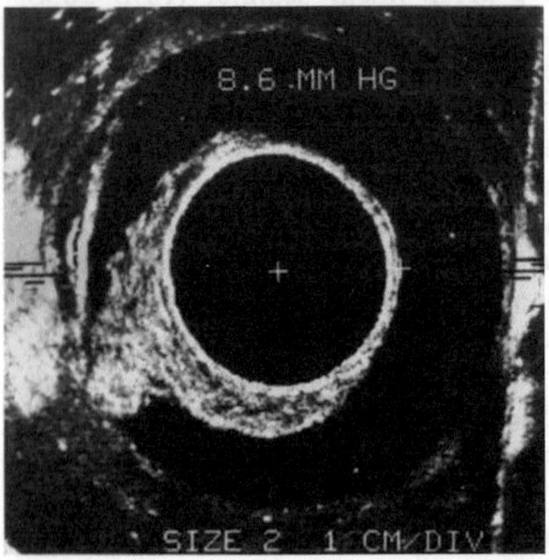

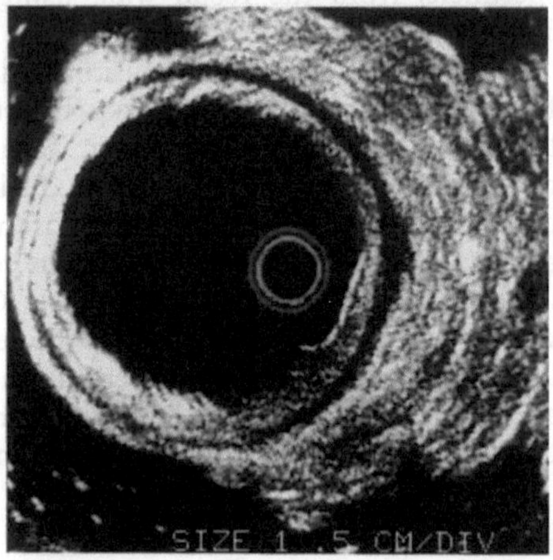

4.10

Fig. 4.7. Water-bath study of the rectal wall. The ideal distance of the transducer from the rectal wall (2.3 cm) provides imaging of the individual rectal layers on the right side of the circumference. Transducer position within water balloon marked by *cross*. Intraluminal pressure of rectum in vitro: 7.0 mm Hg

Fig. 4.8. Water-bath study of the rectal wall. The distance between transducer and rectal wall is less than 2 cm. The inner and middle interface are not sharply delineated. Due to the lesser extension the rectal wall appears thicker. Intraluminal pressure of rectum in vitro: 5.8 mm Hg

Fig. 4.9. In vitro examination. Extensive filling of the water balloon results in maximum distension of the rectal wall with compression of the layers and poor differentiation of mucosa and muscularis propria. Transducer distance from rectal wall 2.4 cm. Intraluminal pressure: 8.6 mm Hg

Fig. 4.10. In vitro study. The transducer is not at 90° to the rectal wall. As a result the wall is represented on the right by two interfaces and one layer and on the left *semicircle* by four interfaces and three layers

Three technical factors determine the sonographic appearance of the rectal wall:

1. The focal range of the transducer. The 7-MHz transducer has a focal range of 2–5 cm. Hence the individual rectal wall layers are best imaged when the transducer is positioned 2–5 cm away from the rectal wall (Figs. 4.7, 4.8).
2. The distension of the water balloon. When the balloon is filled with a high volume of liquid at high pressure, the rectal wall is distended and the mucosa is squeezed against the muscularis propria, resulting in a decrease in wall thickness. Even if the transducer is within the focal range the rectal wall may not be imaged as expected (Fig. 4.9).
3. The angle of the transducer with respect to the rectal wall. Sound waves from a transducer which deviate more than 2° from the ideal 90° position hit the rectal wall tangentially. As a result the sonographic appearance is changed (Fig. 4.10).

The sonographic appearance of the rectal wall is explained as follows. A single anatomic layer has two interfaces which appear on the sonogram as white lines. The imaging of an anatomic layer is only possible if the axial resolution is high enough to distinguish between the transmitted and the reflected ultrasound beam of the layer. Thus the layer has to have a minimum thickness depending on the frequency used. When a second anatomic layer which is also confined by two interfaces is added, and the second layer has a common interface with the first, then there will be three interfaces, i.e. three circles on the sonogram. The anatomic layers will appear as dark lines between the interfaces (Fig. 4.11). To generalize, if n layers have $n+1$ interfaces, then they will be represented by $n+1$ white circles. In the rectum, the two dark layers of mucosa and muscularis are accompanied by three white circles [4, 18].

Rifkin [29–31], who used amongst other equipment a 3.5-MHz and a 6.7-MHz radial scanner, described two layers, a hyperechoic inner layer that probably represented a combination of echoes from the balloon and the mucosa, and a hypoechoic layer representing the submucosa and muscularis. Konishi [21] analysed the structure of the rectal wall in vivo with a 7.5-MHz transducer and found six different layers. In vitro he used a 3.5-MHz radial and a 5.0-MHz linear array. With both scanners the normal rectal wall was visualized as having three layers. The inner hyperechoic layer was said to correspond to mucosa and sub-

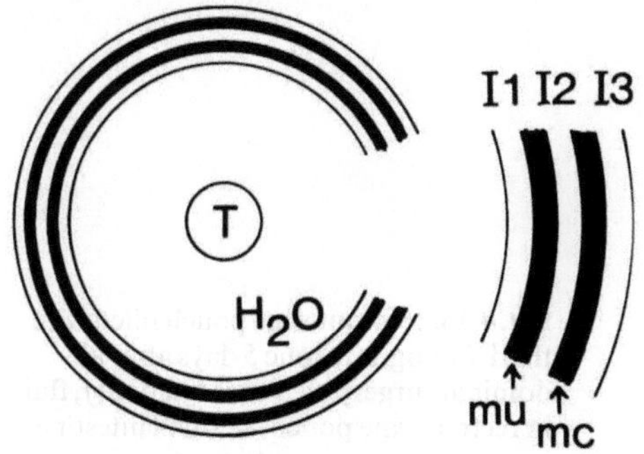

Fig. 4.11. Schematic interpretation of the sonographic appearance of the rectal wall. *T*, transducer; *I1*, *I2*, *I3*, inner, middle and outer interface; *mu*, mucosa, *mc*, muscularis propria

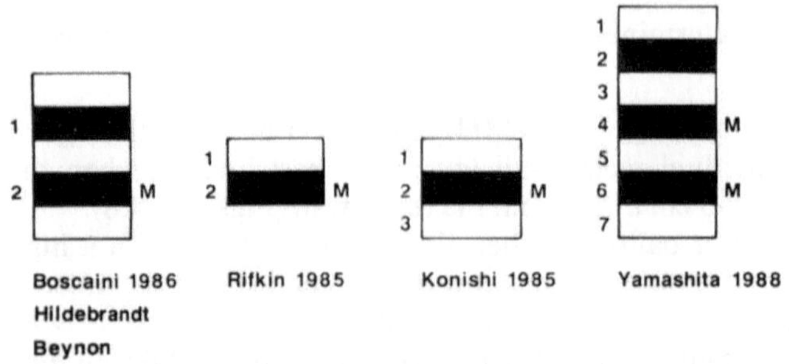

Fig. 4.12. Sonographic interpretation of the rectal wall. Boscaini and Montori [8], Hildebrandt et al. [18] and Beynon et al. [4] describe two hypoechoic lines as real anatomic layers: *1* mucosa, *2* muscularis. Rifkin and Marks [29] interpret a hyperechoic line as mucosa (*1*) and a hypoechoic line as muscularis (*2*). Konishi et al. [21] see two hyperechoic (*1, 3*) and one hypoechoic (*2*) anatomic layer. Yamashita et al. [46] describe four hyperechoic and three hypoechoic layers. All agree that the outermost hypoechoic layer corresponds to the muscularis (*M*)

mucosa, the middle hypoechoic layer, the muscularis propria. Yamashita [46] at times found a seven-layer structure of the normal rectal wall. Despite the different interpretations there is agreement on one point: the outer [35] hypoechoic layer is considered by all ultrasonographers to be the muscle layer (Fig. 4.12) [6, 7].

The peritoneum covers the upper third of the rectum in the front and at the sides and the middle third in the front only. The lower third of the rectum has no peritoneal covering. As there is no sonographic difference between the superior and the inferior rectum, we suggest that the serosa is not visible sonographically. This interpretation is not shared by others [21], who take the outer interface to be the serosa.

In the male the peritoneum is reflected from the rectum to the posterior wall of the bladder, where it forms the floor of the rectovesical pouch. In the female the peritoneum is reflected to the posterior fornix of the vagina, where it forms

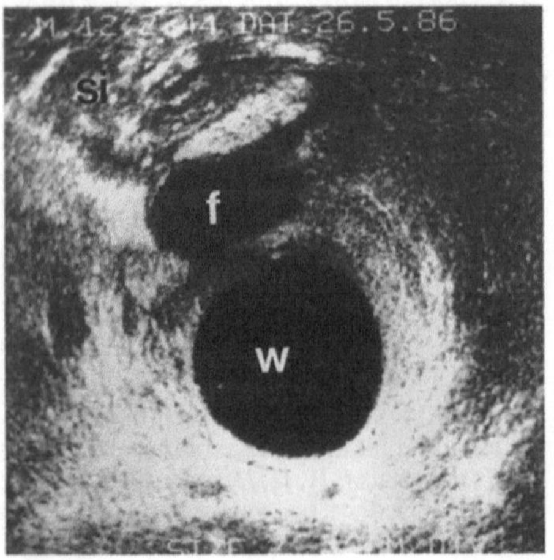

Fig. 4.13. Rectouterine pouch filled with fluid. Sonogram done 5 days after abdominal surgery. *w*, water balloon; *f*, fluid in rectouterine pouch; *si*, small intestine

the floor of the rectouterine pouch. When filled with fluid, in appendicitis for example, the pouch becomes visible on ultrasound in both males and females (Fig. 4.13).

Generally, no sonographic differentiation of the intra- and extraperitoneal part of the rectum can be achieved.

Neither is it possible to visualize the internal transverse rectal folds: when the balloon is filled with water, these folds, which consist of mucous membranes and circular muscles, are flattened. In the case of distension of the rectal ampulla, about double the amount of water is necessary to establish contact between the balloon and the rectal wall.

4.7 Sonographic Characteristics of the Pelvic Floor

The pelvic diaphragm, comprising the levator ani and coccygeal muscles, forms the pelvic floor. When the probe has been inserted into the anal canal, it can be demonstrated by ultrasound that this muscle sheet stretches between the pubis anteriorly and the coccyx posteriorly (Fig. 4.14). It is attached along the side walls of the pelvis to the obturator fascia. The internal obturator muscle is seen as a hypoechoic band in front of the hyperechoic reflection which represents the pubic ramus (Figs. 4.15, 4.16). The puborectal muscle forms a sling at the junction of the rectum and the anal canal. The junctional area is sonographically characterized by a thickening of the wall (Fig. 4.17).

14
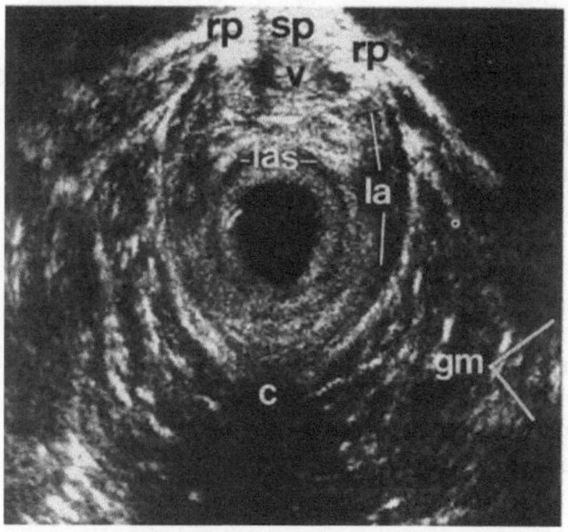

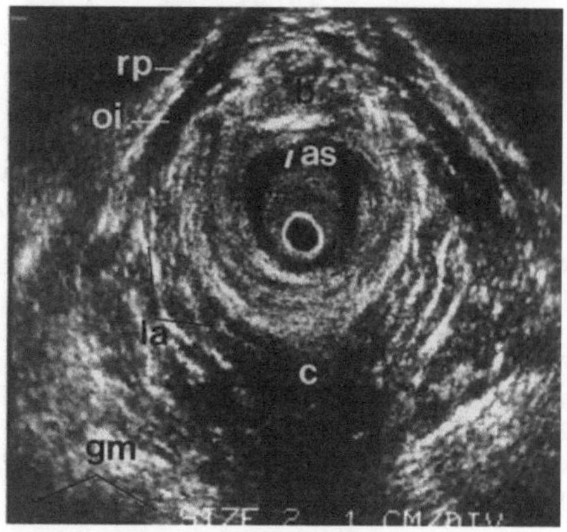

4.15

Fig. 4.14. Female pelvic floor. The levator ani muscle (*la*) stretches between the ramus pubis (*rp*) and the coccyx (*c*). *sp*, symphysis pubis; *v*, vagina; *ias*, internal anal sphincter; *gm*, gluteus maximus

Fig. 4.15. Male pelvic floor. The internal obturator muscle (*oi*) is seen as a hypoechoic band in front of the hyperechoic reflection which represents the ramus pubis (*rp*). *b*, bulb of penis; *ias*, internal anal sphincter; *la*, levator ani muscle; *c*, coccyx; *gm*, gluteus maximus

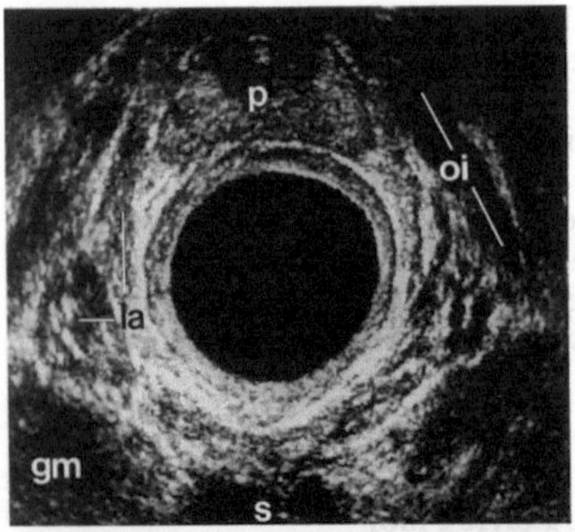

4.16

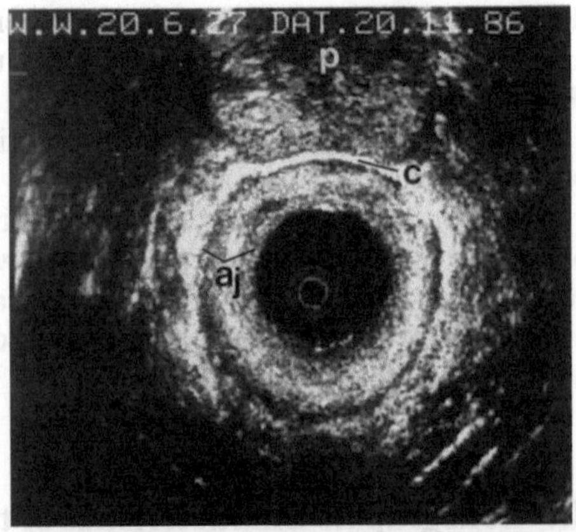

4.17

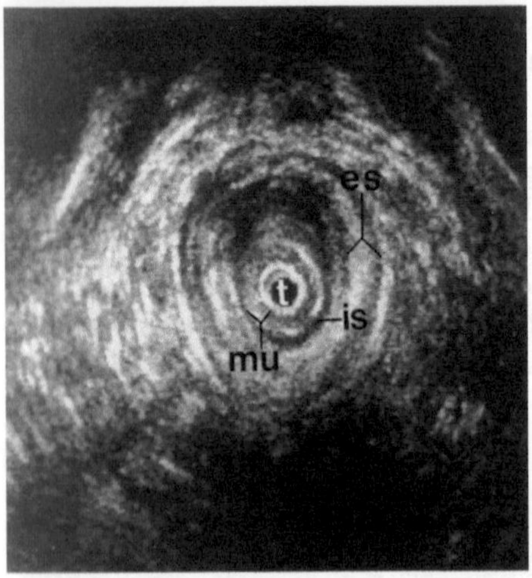

4.18

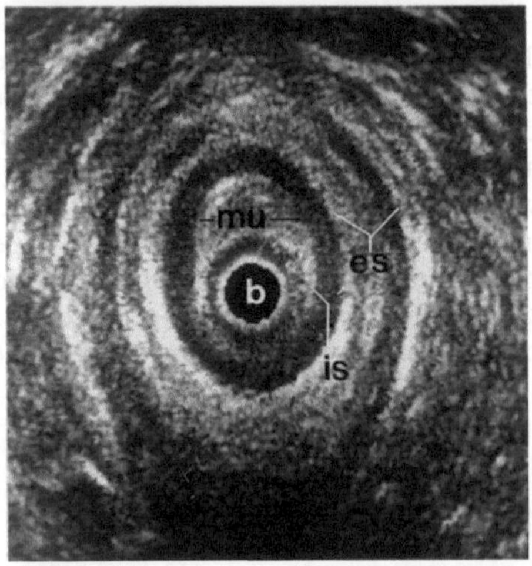

4.19

Fig. 4.16. Male pelvic floor. Sonogram beyond the anal canal with visualization of the levator ani muscle (*la*) and the prostate (*p*). The hyperechoic band behind the internal obturator muscle (*oi*) represents the ramus pubis. *s*, lower sacrum; *gm*, gluteus maximus

Fig. 4.17. The puborectal muscle is sonographically visualized as a thickening of the rectal wall at the anorectal junction (*aj*). *p*, prostate; *c*, cleavage plane between prostate and rectal wall

Fig. 4.18. Sonogram of the anal canal. The transducer (*t*) is surrounded by a small amount of water. The inner hyperechoic circle represents the mucosa (*mu*). Due to the transducer position the thickness of the mucosa appears variable. The next, hypoechoic layer corresponds to the internal sphincter (*is*). The subsequent hyperechoic and hypoechoic layers represent the external sphincter (*es*)

Fig. 4.19. Magnification of the anal canal. Innermost circle: balloon (*b*). Variably thick hyperechoic structure: mucosa (*mu*). In the rectum the mucosa is supposedly hypoechoic. Hypoechoic circle: internal sphincter (*is*). The next, hyperechoic and relatively hypoechoic structures are the external sphincter (*es*) together with the conjoined longitudinal muscle

20 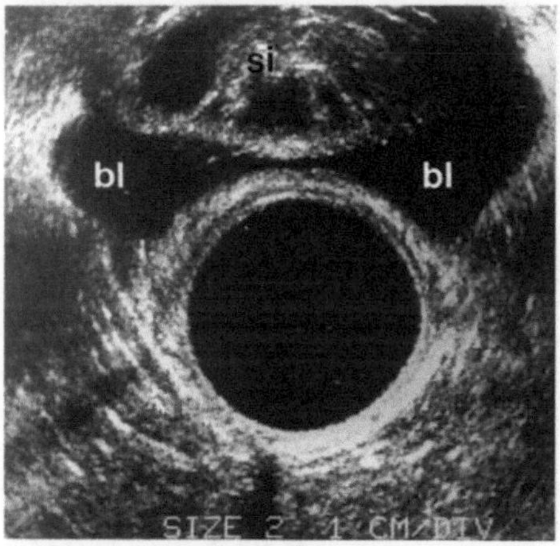

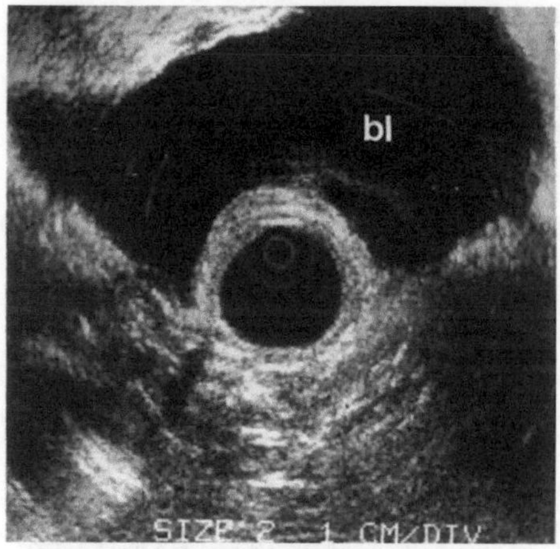 4.21

Fig. 4.20. Sonogram of the bladder (*bl*), partially filled with urine. The bladder wall is distorted by a loop of small intestine (*si*)

Fig. 4.21. Full distension of the bladder (*bl*). Transvaginal view after abdominoperineal excision

Within the anal canal the balloon cannot be inflated enough for the sphincter muscles to lie within the focal range. Despite this deficiency the internal sphincter appears more hypoechoic than the external sphincter. The mucosa is visualized as a hyperechoic structure (Figs. 4.18, 4.19).

4.8 Sonographic Relations of the Rectum

Posteriorly the rectum rests on the inferior three sacral vertebrae and the coccyx. Anteriorly, in the male it is related to the base of the bladder, the seminal vesicles and the prostate. The sonographic appearance of the bladder depends on how full it is (Figs. 4.20, 4.21). The emptied bladder shows a plicated wall structure. The prostate has a sharp outer margin and a homogeneous hypoechoic appearance. The rectovesical septum, which is closely associated with the prostate, represents a potential cleavage plane between the rectum and the prostate (Fig. 4.22). This fact is of clinical importance when a rectal cancer growing on the anterior wall has to be assessed for penetration into the prostate. Another landmark is the seminal vesicles, which extend to both sides of the prostate. They vary in size but are constantly hypoechoic (Fig. 4.23).

In the female, the vagina is anterior to the rectum. The rectum is separated from the cervix of the uterus and the posterior fornix of the vagina by the rectouterine pouch. Inferior to this pouch the rectovaginal septum separates the vagina and the rectum (Figs. 4.24, 4.25). Tumours penetrating into the septum or the posterior wall of the vagina are clearly visualized. Like the prostate in males, the uterus in females is sharply separated from neighbouring structures (Fig. 4.26). The ovaries and the uterine tubes are inconstantly visible, varying with the age of the patient (Figs. 4.27–4.29).

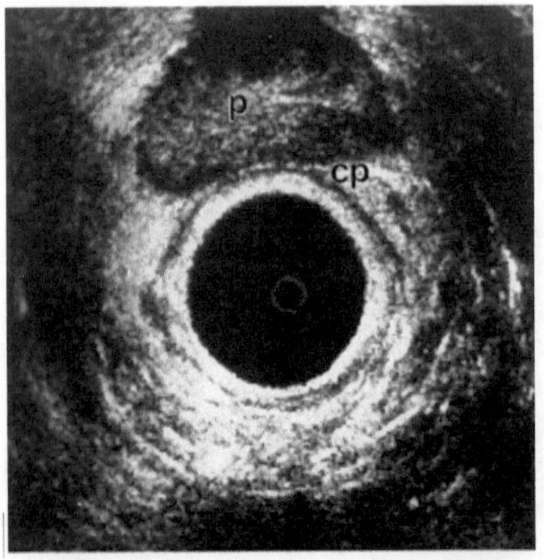

4.22

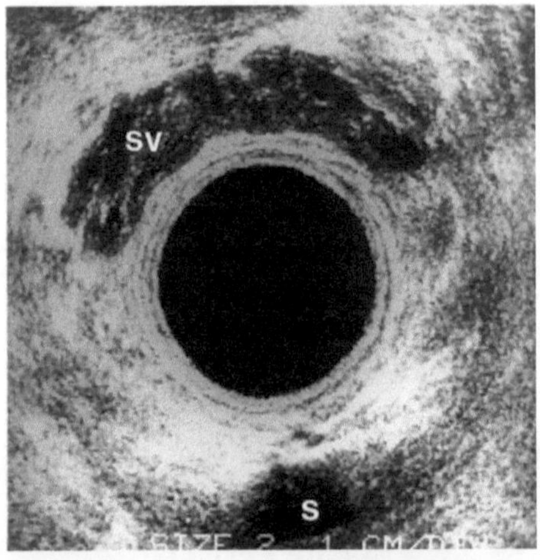

4.23

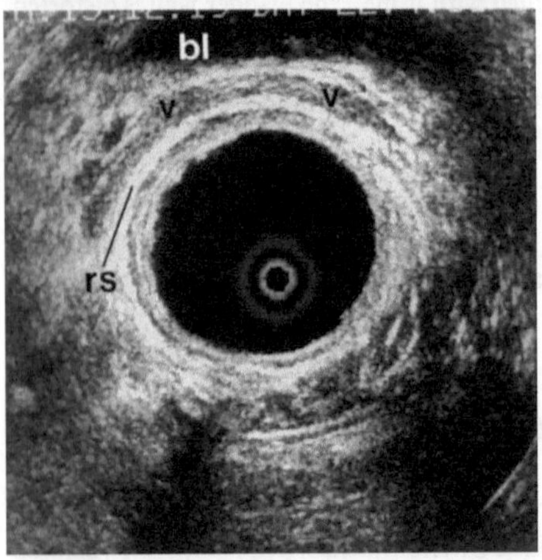

4.24

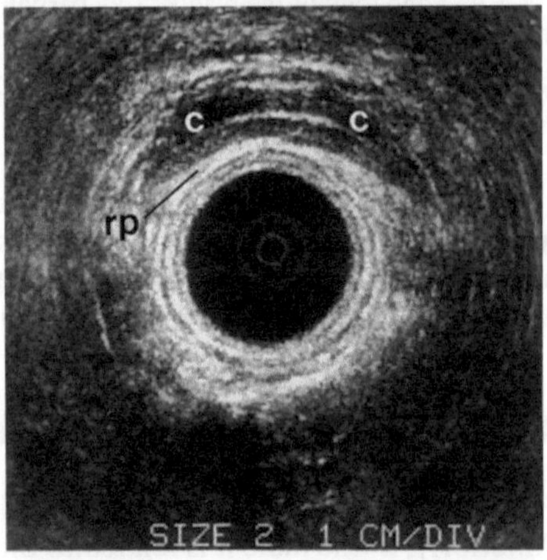

4.25

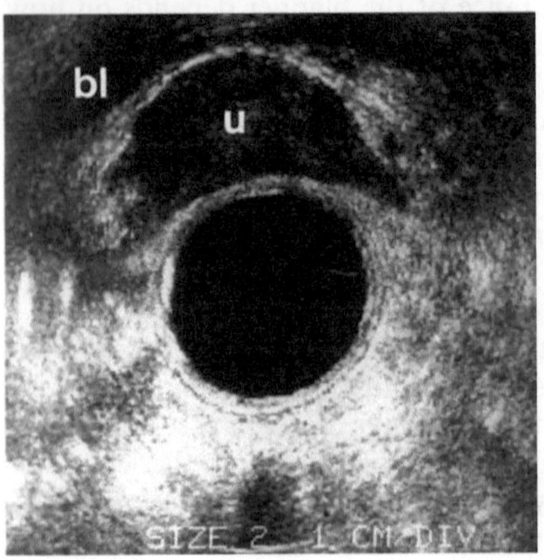

4.26

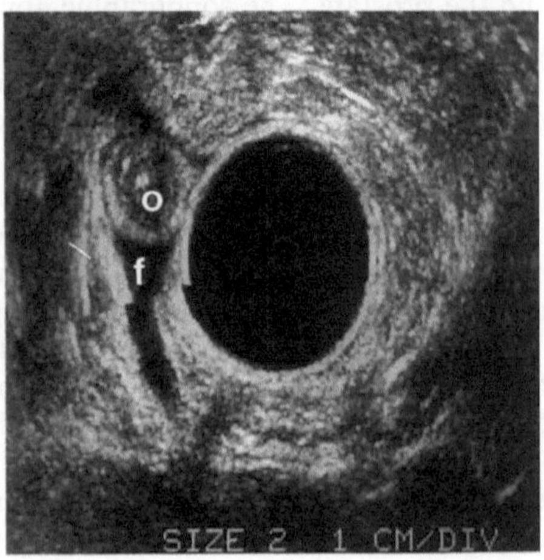

4.27

28 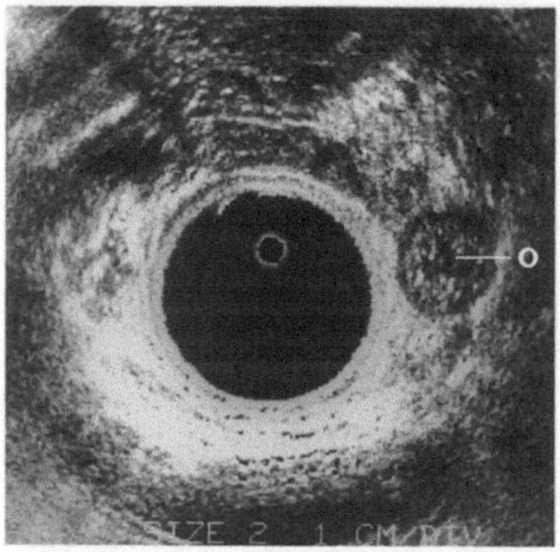

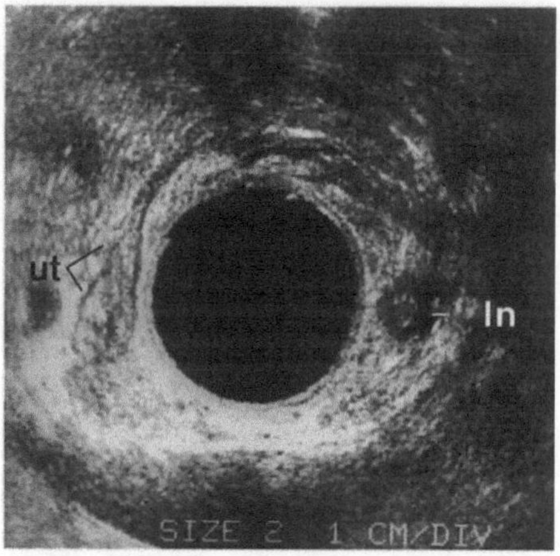 4.29

Fig. 4.28. Sonogram of the left ovary (*o*) in a 50-year-old patient. Diameter of ovary: 2 cm

Fig. 4.29. Sonogram demonstrating the right uterine tube (*ut*). At the opposite side of the rectal wall, a lymph node (*ln*) is seen

4.9 Sonographic Characteristics of Blood Vessels

There are five rectal arteries which anastomose freely with each other. The superior rectal artery (Fig. 4.30), a continuation of the inferior mesenteric artery, divides at the level of S3 into two branches which descend one on each side of the rectum (Fig. 4.31). The two middle rectal arteries are branches of the internal iliac arteries, and the two inferior rectal arteries are branches of the internal pudendal arteries. The venous drainage of the rectum is via the superior, middle and inferior rectal veins. There is rich anastomosis among all three (Fig. 4.32).

Blood vessels are hypoechoic. Most display a typical bright reflection of the echo (Fig. 4.33). Veins can often be differentiated from arteries from the fact that

Fig. 4.22. Sonogram showing cleavage plane (*cp*) between anterior rectal wall and prostate (*p*)

Fig. 4.23. Sonogram of seminal vesicles. Intact rectal wall, hypoechoic seminal vesicles (*sv*), hypoechoic structure behind the posterior rectal wall representing sacrum (*s*)

Fig. 4.24. Sonogram of the vagina (*v*), visualized as an elliptical hypoechoic structure separated from the anterior rectal wall by the rectovaginal septum (*rs*). *bl*, base of bladder

Fig. 4.25. The cervix (*c*) of the uterus is separated from the rectal wall by the rectouterine pouch (*rp*)

Fig. 4.26. Sonogram of uterus (*u*), showing wall of evacuated bladder (*bl*)

Fig. 4.27. Sonogram of the right ovary (*o*) in a patient with ileitis. The hypoechoic area corresponds to fluid (*f*) in the pelvis

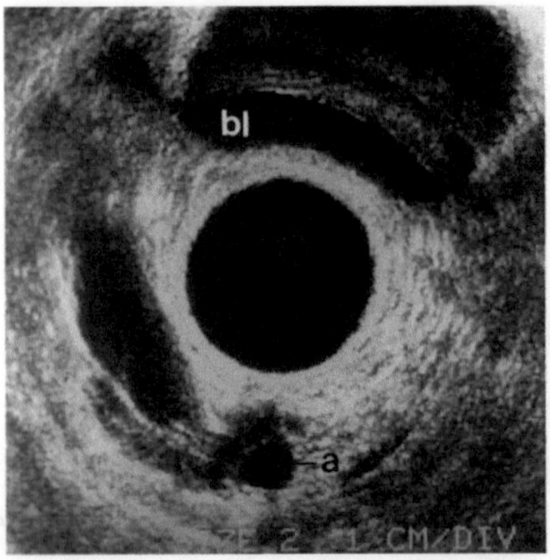

4.30

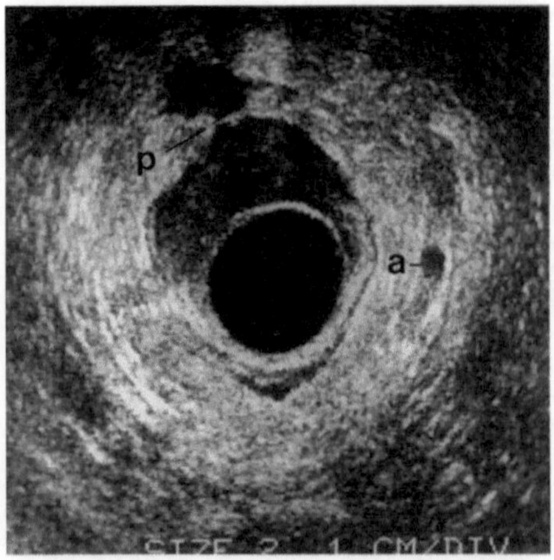

4.31

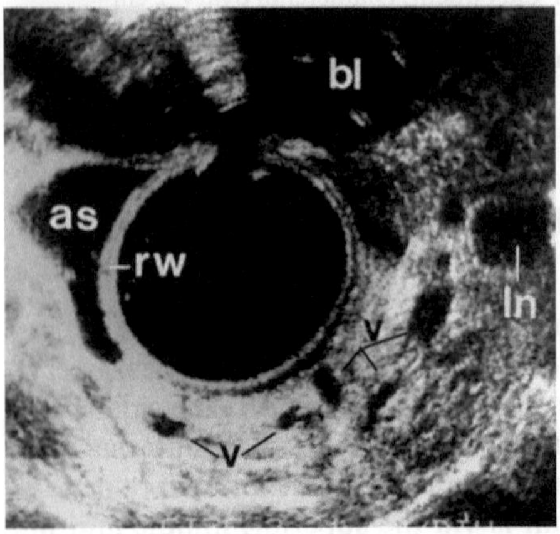

4.32

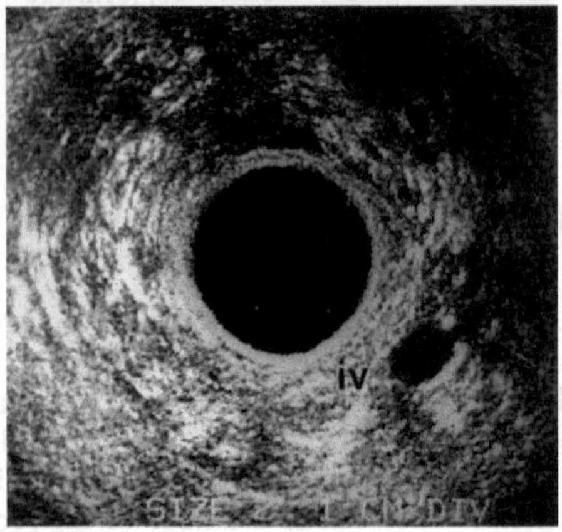

4.33

Fig. 4.30. Sonogram demonstrating the superior rectal artery (*a*). *bl*, bladder

Fig. 4.31. Rectal cancer with penetration (*p*) into the perirectal fat. On the right side of the sonogram, the left rectal artery (*a*) shows the typical bright reflection at the lateral border of the vessel

Fig. 4.32. Sonogram demonstrating perirectal veins (*v*) cut in different longitudinal and transverse planes. *bl*, bladder; *rw*, rectal wall; *ln*, lymph node; *as*, ascites

Fig. 4.33. Iliac vessel (*iv*) on the right side of the sonogram. The typical hyperechoic reflection is seen on the lateral border of the vessel

they run in different planes, whereas arteries run parallel to the longitudinal axis of the rectum and are mostly cut transversely by ultrasound. When veins and arteries run in parallel they cannot be differentiated from each other (Fig. 4.34).

Depending on the depth of insertion of the probe, it may be possible to follow the iliac vessels up to the bifurcation (Fig. 4.35, 4.36). The sonographic continuity of hypoechoic vessels is the criterion used to differentiate them from hypoechoic lymph nodes.

34 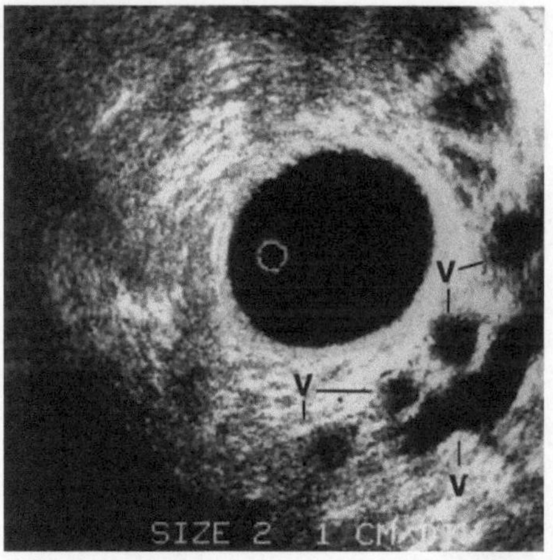

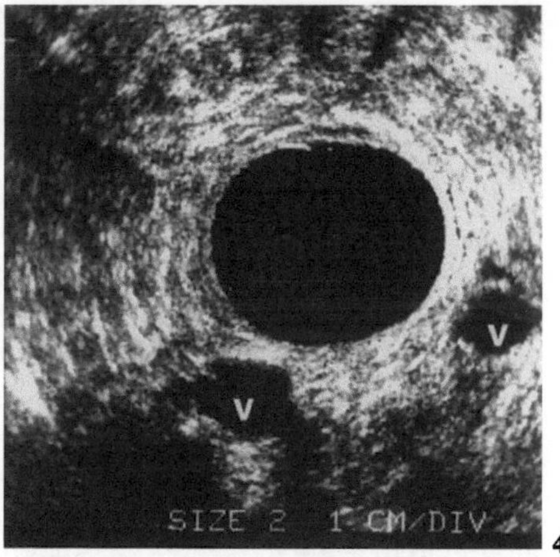 4.35

36 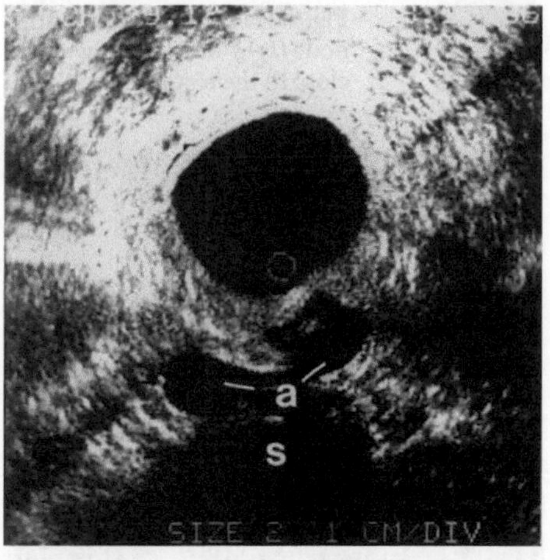

Fig. 4.34. Sonogram of external and internal iliac veins and arteries, which cannot be identified individually by ultrasound. *v*, vessel

Fig. 4.35. Iliac vessels (*v*) at the posterior wall of the rectum

Fig. 4.36. Iliac arteries (*a*) at the bifurcation. The hypoechoic area inferior to the vessels corresponds to the sacrum (*s*)

4.10 Sonographic Characteristics of Lymph Nodes

The lymph vessels from the part of the anal canal superior to the pectinate line drain into the internal iliac lymph nodes and through them into the common iliac and aortic lymph nodes. The lymph vessels inferior to the pectinate line drain into the superficial inguinal lymph nodes.

In a normal rectum the lymph nodes are generally not more than 3 mm in diameter. The number of perirectal nodes ranges between 8 and 20.

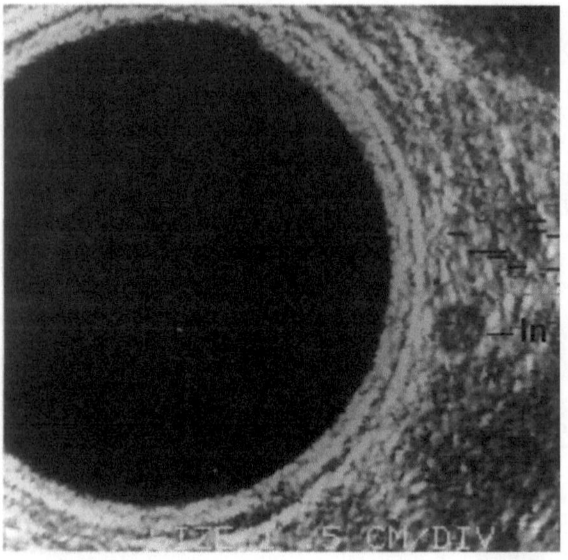

Fig. 4.37. Hyperechoic lymph node (*ln*) 4 mm in diameter close to the rectal wall

4.38

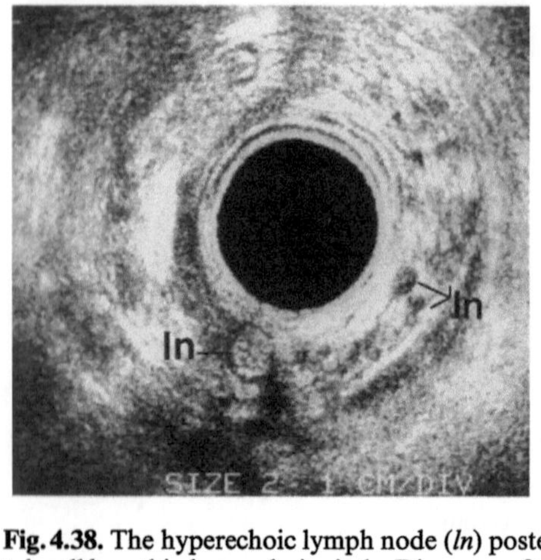

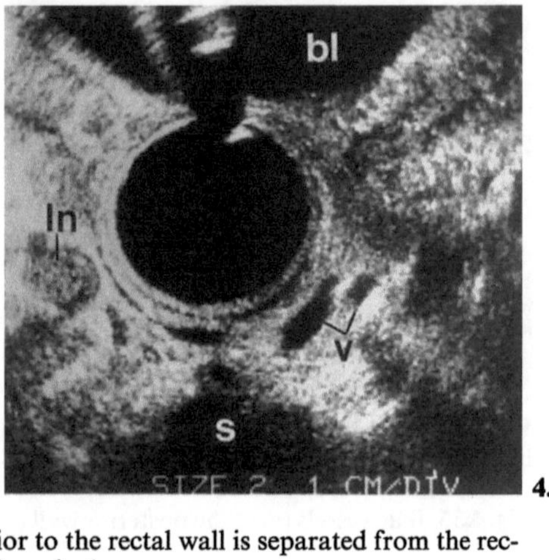

4.39

Fig. 4.38. The hyperechoic lymph node (*ln*) posterior to the rectal wall is separated from the rectal wall by a thin hypoechoic circle. Diameter of this node: 1 cm

Fig. 4.39. Sonogram of the perirectal area cephalad from a rectal cancer. On left side of sonogram: hyperechoic lymph node (*ln*) of 12 mm diameter surrounded by a hypoechoic circle. *bl*, bladder; *s*, sacrum; *v*, vein

With the use of the 7.0-MHz transducer, lymph nodes are visible on ultrasound. They appear in different echo patterns. Due to their fat-like echogenicity normal lymph nodes may not be visualized within the perirectal fat.

In Homburg the experience with the visualization and assessment of pararectal lymph nodes is based on 113 primary rectal cancers that were evaluated for lymph node metastases. As a result of our study we determined the following sonographic characteristics to differentiate lymph nodes.

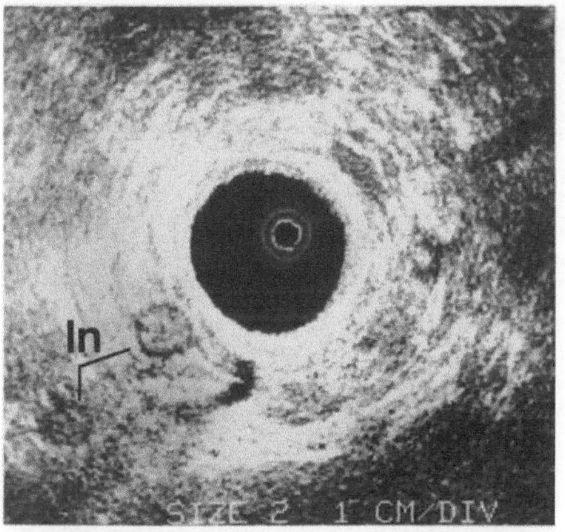

4.40

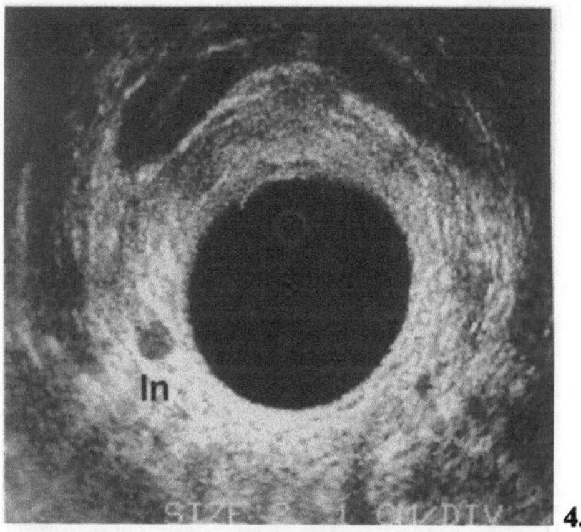

4.41

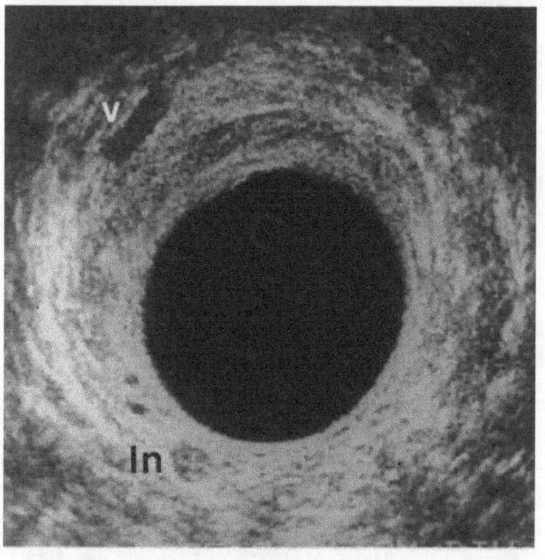

4.42

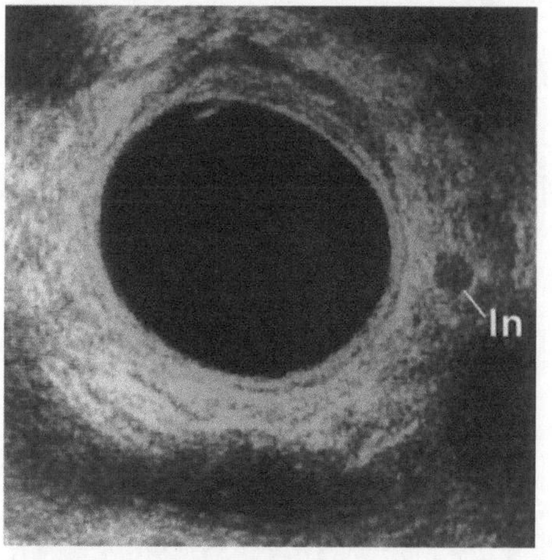

4.43

Fig. 4.40. The two hyperechoic lymph nodes (*ln*) in the lower left quadrant of the sonogram are demarcated from the perirectal fat by a hypoechoic circle

Fig. 4.41. Sonogram proximal to a rectal cancer. Due to the non-specific inflammation caused by tumour destruction of the mucosa a hyperechoic lymph node (*ln*: size 6 mm) is visible on the left side of the sonogram

Fig. 4.42. Hyperechoic lymph node (*ln*: size 5 mm) characteristic for non-specific inflammation at the posterior rectal wall. *v*, vein

Fig. 4.43. Hyperechoic lymph node (*ln*) of 5 mm diameter at the right side of the sonogram

1) *Normal lymph nodes* are not larger than 3 mm. Due to their fat-like echogenicity they are not visualized by ultrasound.

2) *Inflamed lymph nodes:* Lymph nodes which are enlarged due to non-specific inflammation are visualized by ultrasound from 4 mm diameter upward (Fig. 4.37). Normally they are hyperechoic. Hyperechoic lymph nodes are occasionally separated from the perirectal fat by a thin hypoechoic circle (Figs. 4.38–4.40), but mostly they are characterized by a homogeneous pattern

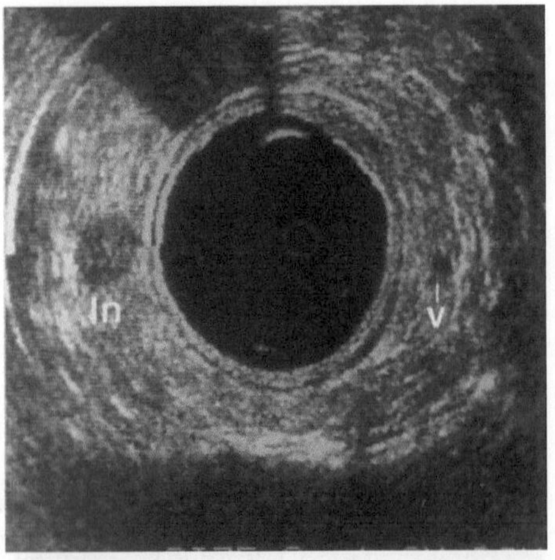

4.44

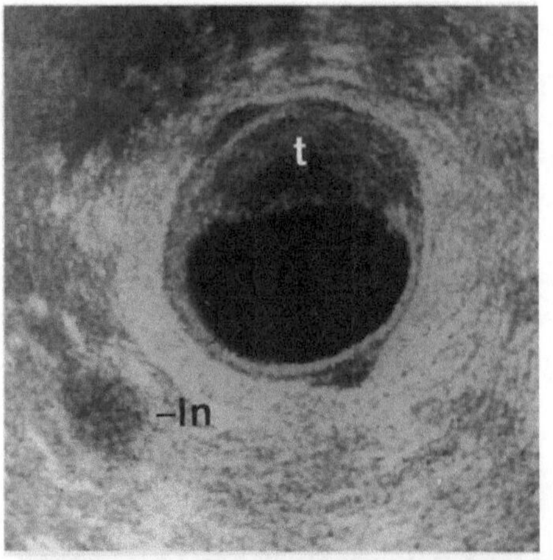

4.45

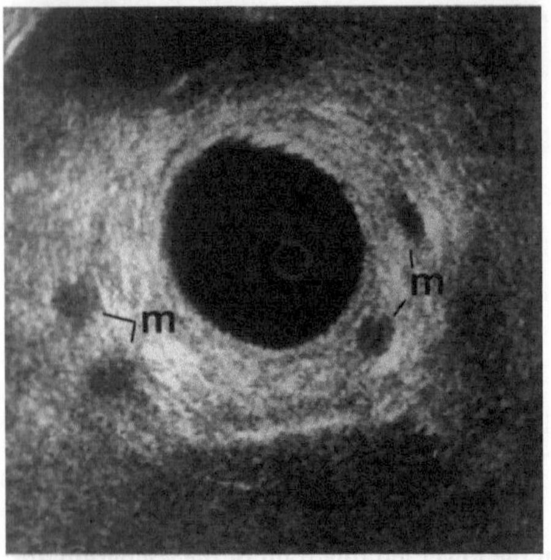

4.46

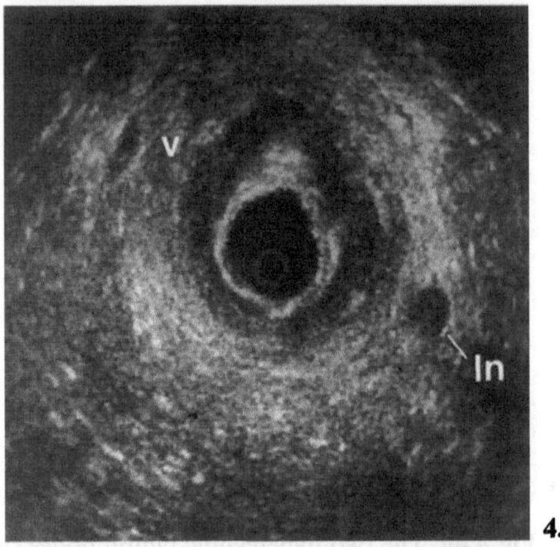

4.47

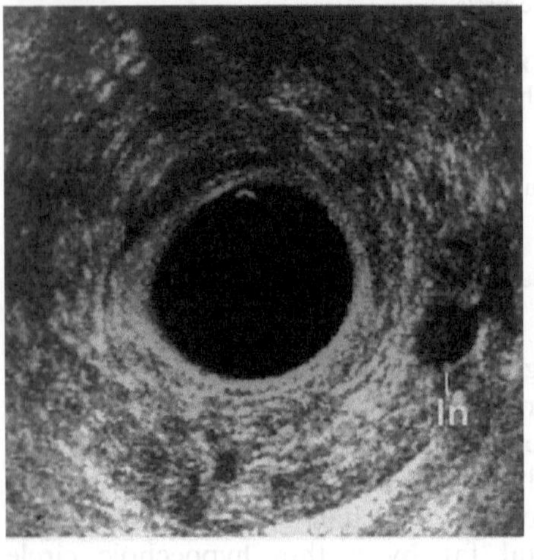

4.48

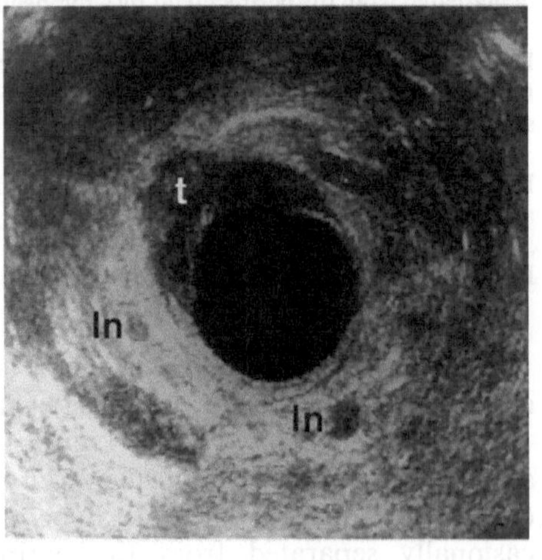

4.49

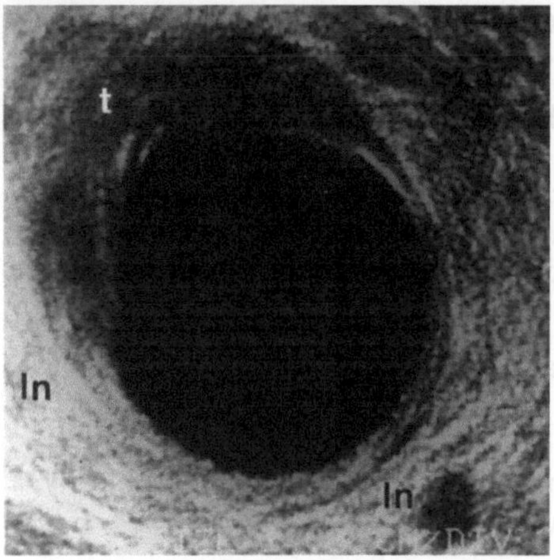

4.50

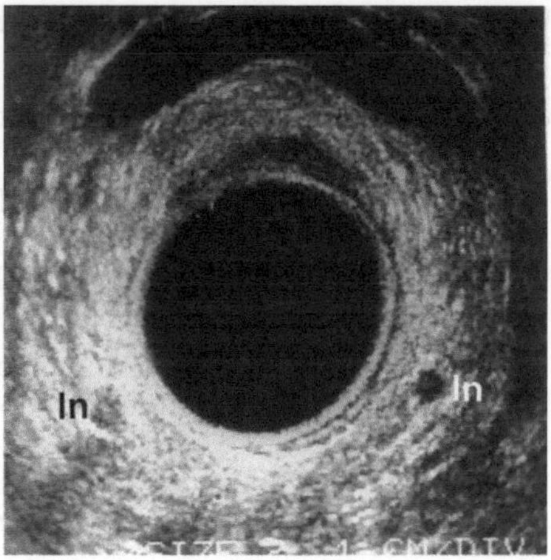

4.51

Fig. 4.44. Hyperechoic lymph node (*ln*) of 11 mm diameter at the left side of the sonogram. Blood vessel (*v*) of 2 mm size at the right side

Fig. 4.45. Rectal tumour (*t*) confined to the wall with a hyperechoic perirectal lymph node (*ln*) of 15 mm diameter. The enlargement of the node is caused by non-specific inflammation

Fig. 4.46. Sonogram proximal from a rectal tumour, demonstrating four hypoechoic lymph node metastases (*m*), size 6–8 mm

Fig. 4.47. Hypoechoic lymph node (*ln*) at the proximal part of the anal canal, close to a tumour which penetrates the anal sphincter. *v*, vein

Fig. 4.48. Hypoechoic lymph node (*ln*) of 9 mm diameter at the right side of the sonogram

Fig. 4.49. Sonogram of a rectal tumour (*t*) penetrating into the perirectal fat. The 3-mm hyperechoic lymph node (*ln*) on the left side of the image proved to be inflammatory. The hypoechoic node of 5 mm size at the posterior wall was histologically confirmed as involved node

Fig. 4.50. Magnification of Fig. 4.49

Fig. 4.51. In this case, both lymph nodes, the hyperechoic on the left and the hypoechoic on the right of the sonogram had been identified as non-specifically inflamed lymph nodes

which is less echogenic than the surrounding perirectal fat and does not exhibit the hypoechoic circle (Figs. 4.41–4.45).

3) *Involved lymph nodes:* Lymph nodes which are involved by tumour cells are characterized by a hypoechoic appearance (Figs. 4.46–4.48). Since non-specifically inflamed nodes may also have a hypoechoic pattern, the differentiation of involved and inflammatory nodes is not always possible (Figs. 4.49–4.51). The clinical impact of the evaluation of lymph nodes will be discussed later in this chapter.

4.11 Endosonographic Staging of Rectal Cancer

4.11.1 Assessment of Tumour Penetration Depth

In Homburg in 163 patients both preoperative staging by endorectal ultrasound and postoperative histopathological staging of the excised specimens were carried out. Based on the TNM system proposed by the UICC [37] we defined the tumours as follows:

uT1: Tumour confined to mucosa and submucosa (Figs. 4.52, 4.53). Sonographically, a uT1 tumour does not interrupt the middle interface (Figs. 4.54, 4.55).

uT2: Tumour confined to the rectal wall (Figs. 4.56, 4.57). Sonographically, a uT2 tumour does not interrupt the outer interface (Figs. 4.58–4.61).

uT1/pT1

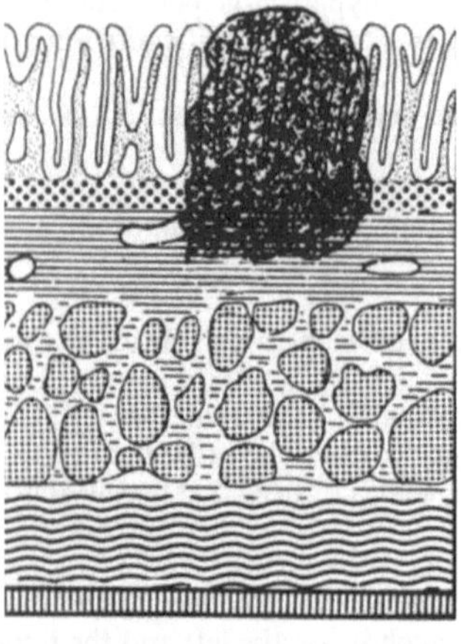

4.52

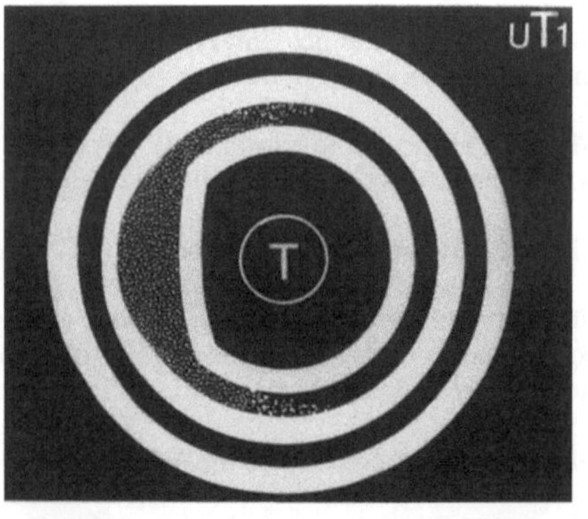

4.53

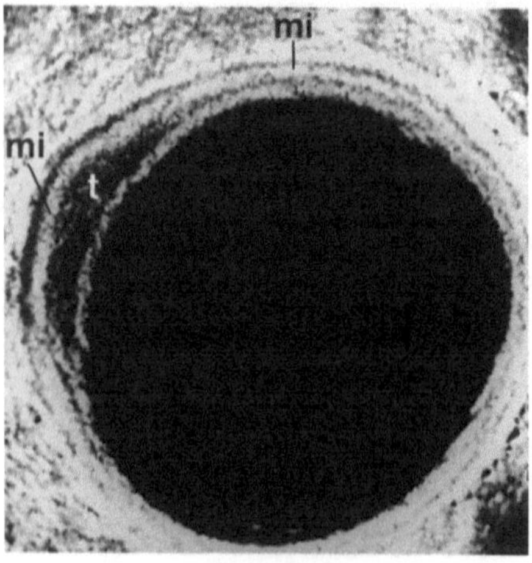

4.54

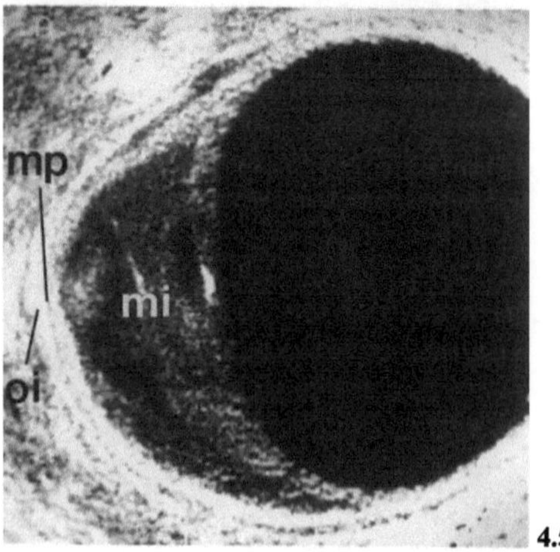

4.55

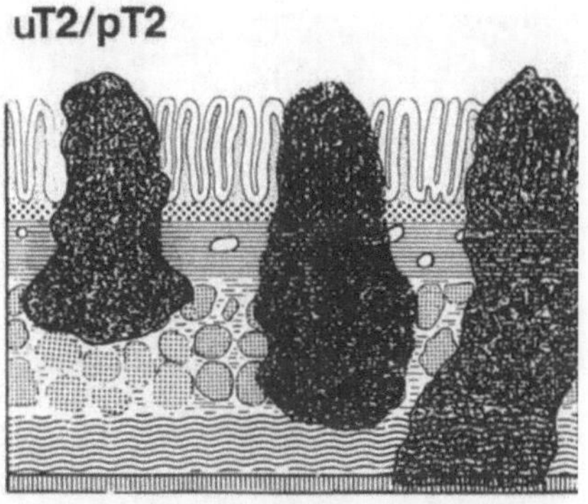

56

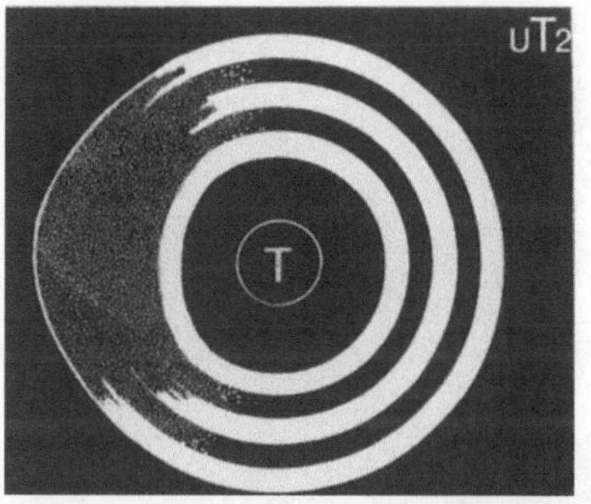

4.57

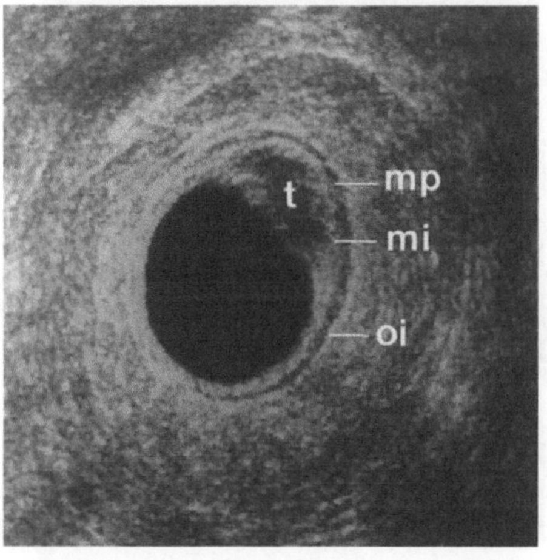

58

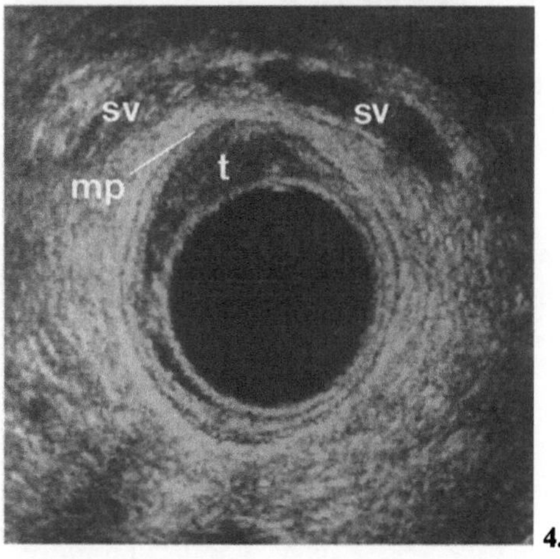

4.59

Fig. 4.52. Schematic illustration of the ultrasonic (u) tumour stage uT1, corresponding to the pathohistological (p) stage pT1. Tumour does not penetrate muscularis propria. (From [37])

Fig. 4.53. Schematic illustration of the ultrasonic tumour stage uT1. The middle interface, representing the borderline between submucosa and muscularis propria, is not interrupted

Fig. 4.54. Sonogram of a tumour stage uT1 on the left side. The middle interface (*mi*) is identified in the intact section of the rectal wall (*top*). In the tumour-bearing section of the wall the middle interface is not interrupted. Hence the tumour (*t*) is confined to the submucosal plane

Fig. 4.55. The thin hypoechoic line between the middle (*mi*) and outer (*oi*) interface represents the intact muscularis propria (*mp*). By definition the tumour stage is uT1

Fig. 4.56. Schematic illustration of tumour stage uT2, corresponding to pT2. Tumour must not penetrate through the rectal wall (From [37])

Fig. 4.57. Schematic illustration of the sonographic tumour stage uT2. The middle interface is interrupted, whereas the outer interface, representing the borderline with the perirectal fat, is intact

Fig. 4.58. Sonogram of tumour stage uT2. The middle interface (*mi*) is not sharply depicted. The tumour (*t*) penetrates but does not perforate the muscularis propria (*mp*). *oi*, outer interface

Fig. 4.59. Sonogram of tumour stage uT2. On the lateral rectal wall the middle interface is visible. Between 11 o'clock and 1 o'clock the tumour (*t*) has penetrated the muscle layer but is still confined to the wall. *sv*, seminal vesicles; *mp*, muscularis propria

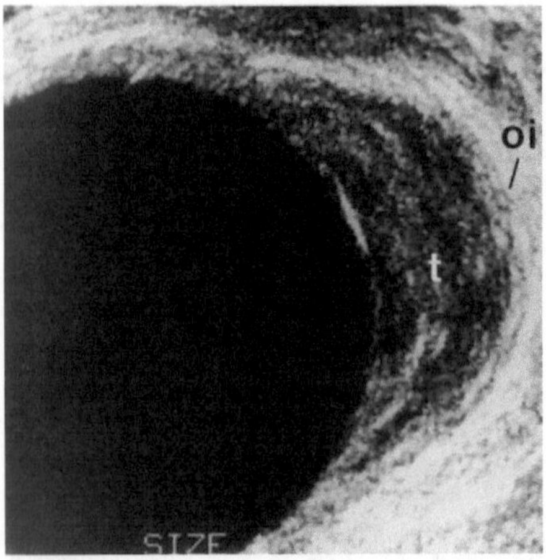

4.60

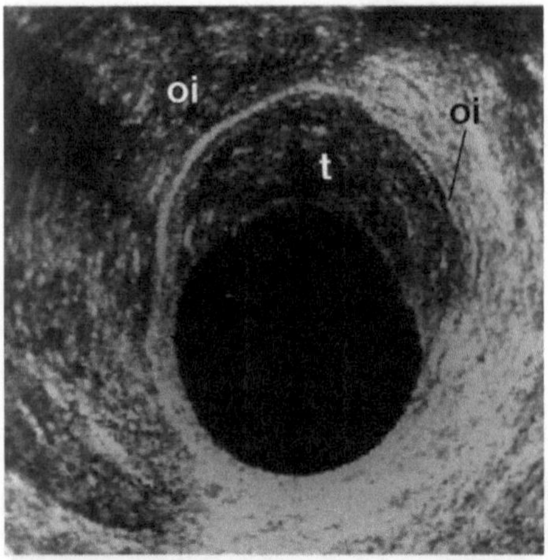

4.61

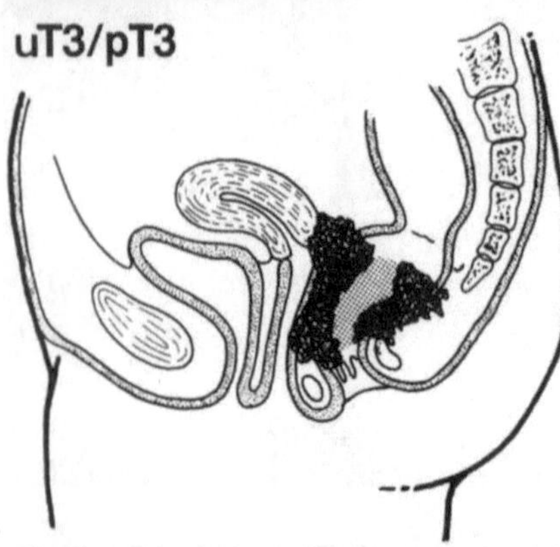

4.62

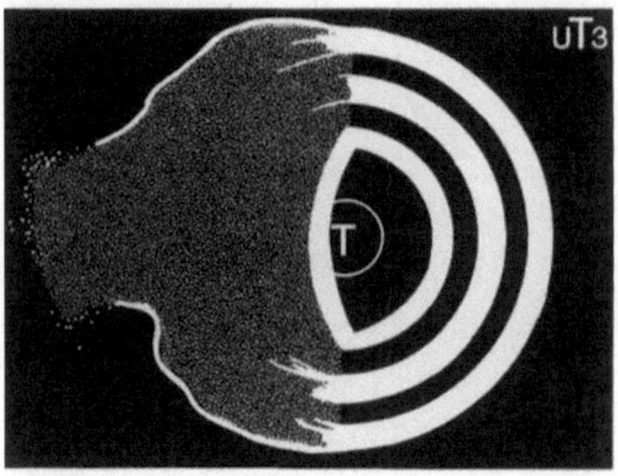

4.63

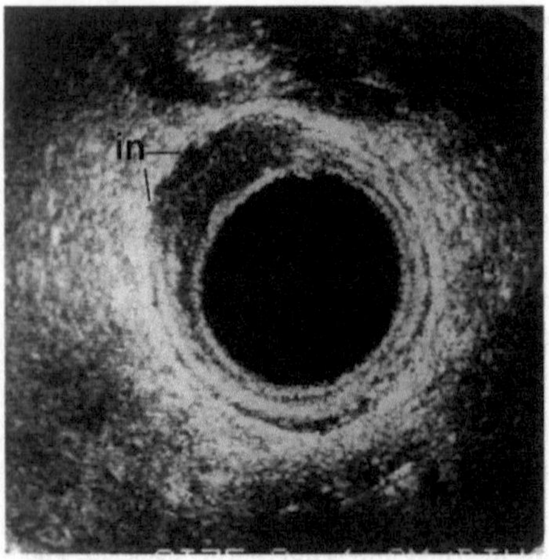

4.64

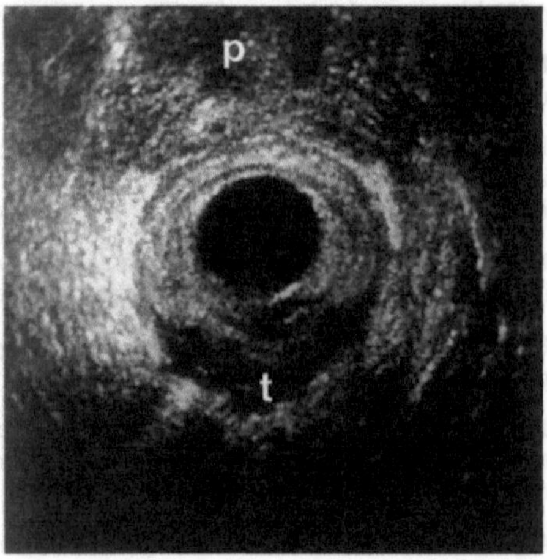

4.65

66
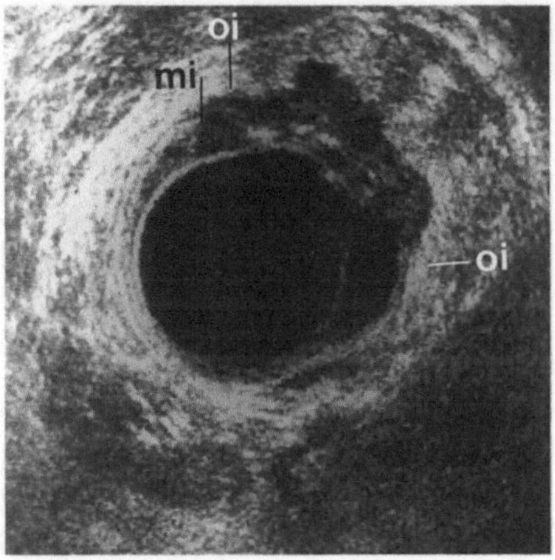

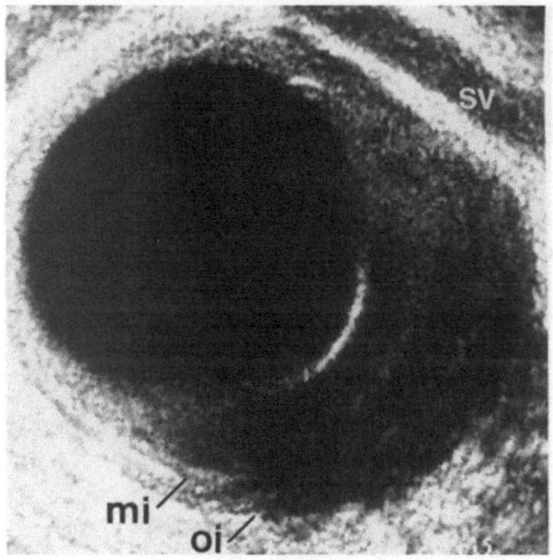

4.67

Fig. 4.60. Tumour stage uT2. The outer interface (*oi*) is not interrupted. The hypoechoic area at the *top* corresponds to the left seminal vesicle

Fig. 4.61. Tumour stage uT2. No interruption of the outer interface (*oi*) at the anterior rectal wall. *t*, tumour

Fig. 4.62. Schematic illustration of tumour stage uT3, corresponding to pT3. Tumour penetrates into the perirectal area or into neighbouring organs. (From [37])

Fig. 4.63. Schematic illustration of the sonographic tumour stage uT3. The outer interface has been disrupted by the penetrating tumour

Fig. 4.64. Tumour stage uT3. Minimal interruption (*in*) of the outer interface manifested by the jagged line. The depth of penetration of the tumour is about 2 mm

Fig. 4.65. Sonogram of a tumour stage uT3 at the anorectal junction. The jagged line shows the slight penetration into the perirectal fat. The tumour (*t*) is hypoechoic. p, prostate

Fig. 4.66. Tumour stage uT3. Normal layers of rectal wall seen on left side of the sonogram. The middle (*mi*) and outer (*oi*) interfaces are interrupted. Penetration depth about 5 mm

Fig. 4.67. Tumour stage uT3. Interruption of middle interface (*mi*) and outer interface (*oi*). Deepest penetration about 5 mm at 4 o'clock. *sv*, seminal vesicle

uT3: Tumour penetrating through the rectal wall into the perirectal fat or into neighbouring organs (Figs. 4.62, 4.63). Sonographically, stage uT3 is characterized by interruption of the outer interface (Figs. 4.64–4.68).

The organs which may be infiltrated by rectal cancer are the vagina, uterus, bladder and prostate. The cleavage plane between the penetrating tumour at the anterior rectal wall and the base of the prostate has not been invaded when the hyperechoic line is still intact (Fig. 4.69). Penetration into the prostate can be predicted when there is interruption of the hyperechoic line (Fig. 4.70). The uterus can be evaluated for tumour penetration in a similar way (Fig. 4.71). The rare cases of tumour perforation with perirectal abscess are visualized as areas of low echogenicity, similar to water (Fig. 4.72).

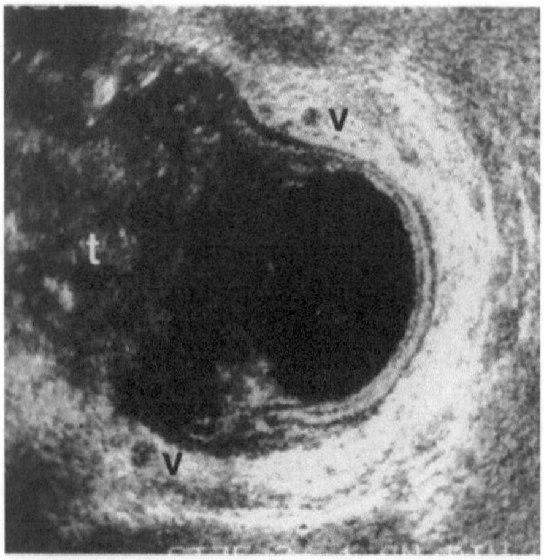

4.68

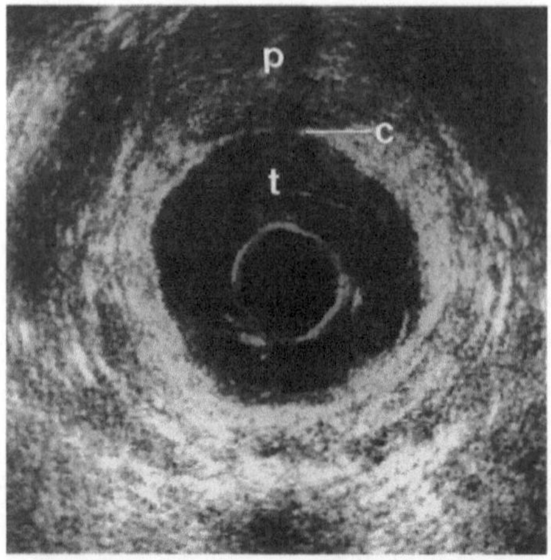

4.69

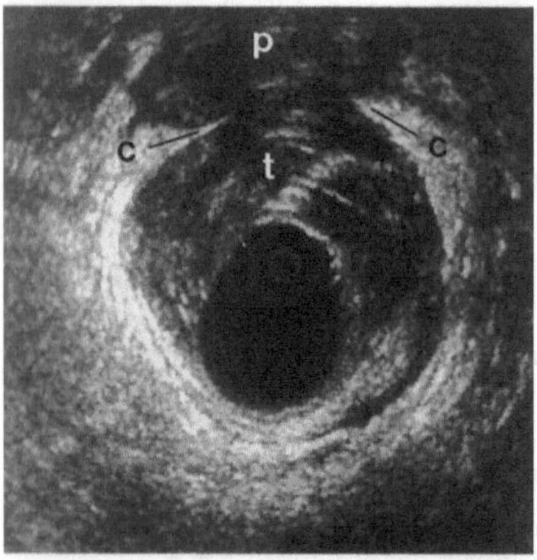

4.70

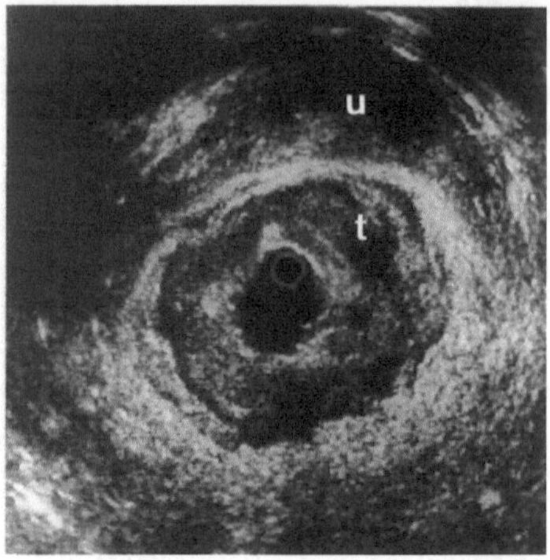

4.71

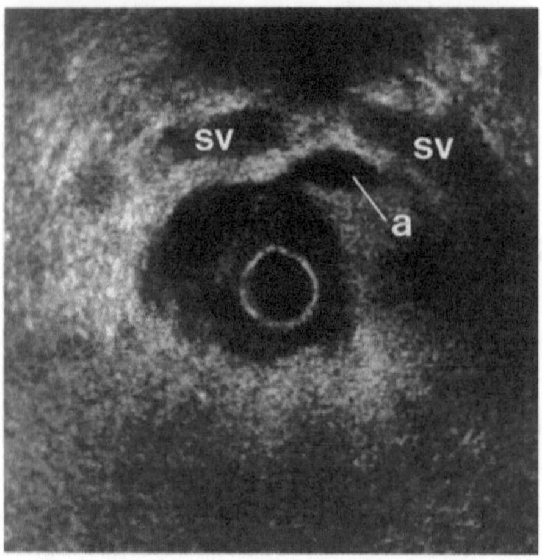

4.72

Table 4.1. Assessment of tumour penetration depth by endosonography (uT) compared to the pathohistological stage (pT)

uT1	10
pT1	9
Understaged	1
uT2	43
pT2	38
Overstaged	4
Understaged	1
uT3	110
pT3	93
Overstaged	17

4.11.1.1 Results

Ten tumours were sonographically assessed as stage uT1. In nine cases this was confirmed by histology. One case was understaged histologic examination revealed infiltration of the muscularis. Forty-three tumours were sonographically assessed as uT2, in 38 cases correctly. One tumour was understaged and four were overstaged. Of the 110 tumours assigned to uT3 on sonography, 17 were overstaged – histologically the tumours were confined to the rectal wall. The remaining 93 were staged correctly (Table 4.1).

Statistical analysis includes sensitivity, specificity, positive predictive value (PPV), negative predictive value (NPV) and accuracy. These were calculated as follows:

$$\text{Sensitivity} = \frac{tp}{tp+fn}$$

$$\text{Specificity} = \frac{tp}{tp+fn}$$

$$\text{PPV} = \frac{tp}{tp+fp}$$

$$\text{NPV} = \frac{tn}{tn+fn}$$

$$\text{Accuracy} = \frac{tp+tn}{tp+tn+fp+fn}$$

tp: true positive; *tn:* true negative; *fp:* false positive; *fn:* false negative.

The sensitivity, which expresses the potential of endosonography to assess the tumour stage T3, is 98% in this group of patients. The specificity, which means the potential of endosonography to predict stage uT2, including uT1, is 84%.

Fig. 4.68. Deep penetration of a tumour stage uT3 at the left side of the sonogram. On the right side, layers of the intact rectal wall. *v*, two blood vessels

Fig. 4.69. Circular rectal cancer. The hyperechoic cleavage plane (*c*) between tumour (*t*) and prostate (*p*) is not interrupted

Fig. 4.70. Rectal cancer stage uT3 at the anterior wall with penetration into the prostate. The cleavage plane (*c*) between tumour (*t*) and base of prostate (p) has been interrupted

Fig. 4.71. Circular tumour stage uT3 with destruction of the muscle layer, manifested by the characteristic jagged outer border. The plane between tumour (*t*) and uterus (*u*) is not interrupted

Fig. 4.72. Circular rectal cancer with narrow lumen and poor acoustic interfacing due to the low amount of water in the balloon (hyperechoic circle). The black area with no internal structure outside the tumour but within the perirectal fat corresponds to an abscess (*a*), confirmed by pathohistological examination of the excised specimen. *sv*, seminal vesicles

The PPV defines how many tumours staged T3 by ultrasound actually penetrate the rectal wall, and is 84%. The NPV defines how many tumours that are sonographically confined to the rectal wall are confirmed as stage T2 by histological examination, and is 98%. The accuracy is defined as the potential for endosonography to assess both stage T2 and stage T3, and is 87%.

4.11.1.2 Discussion

Why were two tumours sonographically understaged and 21 overstaged? One reason is the different frequencies used. Since case number 50 we have used the 7-MHz transducer. The preceding cases were staged with 3.5-MHz and 4.0-MHz transducers. Due to the poorer resolution of these low frequencies the different layers are imaged indistinctly, thus not enabling a sharp visualization of the margins of the tumour.

A second reason is the strictness of the criteria which were applied to evaluate ultrasonography in assessing rectal cancer. Tumour growth of merely 2–3 mm within or beyond the muscle-fat borderline cannot be assessed with the limited resolving power of ultrasonography. The high number of cases overstaged as uT3 reflects the tendency to overstage rather than understage the lesion. This is of clinical importance, since overstaging would not cause undertreatment.

The third reason for mis-staging by ultrasound is technical and anatomic.

If the region of interest does not lie within the focal length of the 7-MHz transducer, which ranges from 2 to 5 cm, or if the rectal wall is not hit at a 90° angle, distortion may occur. Especially in the lower third of the rectum, where the rectal ampulla narrows towards the anal canal, the ideal 90° position of the transducer is rarely achieved. The resulting tangential scanning plane causes sonographic overestimation of pT2 tumours.

4.11.2 Evaluation of Lymph Nodes

With the use of the 7.0-MHz transducer lymph nodes become visible by ultrasound. Preliminary experience suggests that hyperechoic nodes correspond histologically to nonspecifically inflamed nodes whereas hypoechoic nodes correspond histologically to lymph node metastases.

On the basis of the different echo patterns a prospective study was established. A total of 113 patients, i.e. those of the 163 mentioned above who were scanned with a 7.0-MHz transducer, entered the study. Hyperechoic nodes were defined as nonmetastatic, hypoechoic nodes were assumed to represent lymph node metastases. The number, site, size and echo pattern of the lymph nodes were recorded, and representative findings were photographed.

The 113 resected and fixed specimens were cut into serial transverse sections for purposes of comparison with the ultrasonic findings. The number and size of involved and noninvolved nodes was determined. The sonographic assessment of uN1 was based on the appearance of one single hypoechoic lymph node, because it was anticipated that not each individual lymph node would be detected sonographically prior to operation.

4.11.2.1 Results

Only about 50% of the total number of involved or nonsignificantly enlarged lymph nodes which were found by the pathologist in the resected specimens were seen preoperatively by ultrasound.

In 46 of the 113 patients we saw only hyperechoic lymph nodes on sonography and thus classified these 46 cases as N0. In 12 patients classified as N1 due to the presence of hypoechoic lymph nodes pathohistological examination revealed no lymph node metastases. Hence the specificity, the potential of endosonography to correctly identify nonmetastasized nodes, is 79%.

In 31 patients we correctly predicted lymph node metastases based on the visualization of hypoechoic lymph nodes. We did not predict lymph node metastases in 12 patients in whom the pathologist subsequently found at least one metastasized lymph node. The sensitivity, the potential of endosonography to predict lymph node metastases, is thus 72%. The accuracy, the rate of correct assessment of both involved and noninvolved nodes, is 76%.

4.11.2.2 Discussion

In the prospective study, lymph nodes were classified according to their echo patterns. Hypoechoic nodes were taken as metastasized, hyperechoic nodes as nonspecifically inflamed. It was demonstrated histologically, however, that hypoechoic nodes may be either metastatic or simply inflamed. The fact that both hypo- and hyperechoic nodes can be inflamed might be explained by different histological reactions in inflammatory nodes, such as follicular hyperplasia and sinus histiocytosis. On the basis of this study our present criteria for sonographic evaluation of lymph nodes are as follows:

1) Normal lymph nodes are not visualized due to their size and fat-like echogenicity. If lymph nodes are visible sonographically in a patient with rectal cancer the probability of lymph node metastasis is very low.
2) Hyperechoic lymph nodes are not metastasic. They are visualized by ultrasound due to nonspecific inflammatory changes.
3) Hypoechoic lymph nodes are probably metastatic, but nonspecific inflammation is possible.

Tio [40, 41] studied the sonographic echo pattern of pararectal lymph nodes and of nodes along the upper gastrointestinal tract. He found that irregularly hypoechoic nodes similar to or more hypoechoic than the primary lesion, together with sharply demarcated borders, were highly suggestive of malignancy. Lymph nodes with a homogeneous echo pattern more hyperechoic than the primary lesion and with blurred boundaries suggested benign inflammatory changes.

Precise differentiation between a benign and a malignant process in lymph nodes was not achieved by Aibe [1]. In his patient population the ultrasonic visualization rate of lymph nodes surrounding the esophagus was 33.7% in total and 43.4% for lymph node metastases. He concluded that endoscopic ultrasonography is useful for the detection of enlarged lymph nodes, but stated no clear sonographic criteria for differentiating benign and malignant lymph nodes.

4.11.3 Comparison Between Endorectal Sonography and Computed Tomography

P. Langenscheidt and B. Kramann

Endosonography and computed tomography (CT) were compared in 49 patients with rectal cancer. The staging was carried out in accordance with the classification suggested by the UICC. In 34 patients, alterations of the pelvic lymph nodes were also deliberately sought. In all cases, there was histological examination of the surgical specimen including the perirectal fat tissue.

The CT investigation was carried out with a Siemens DR 2 scanner. The slice thickness was 8 mm. Intravenous injections of contrast medium were carried out only in individual cases. The rectum and the sigmoid colon were filled with dilute contrast medium in only five patients. In the other patients, the rectum was contrasted by air insufflation after intramuscular injection of Buscopan (*N*-butyl scopolamine bromide). The CT investigations were performed by various staff members, but the scans were assessed by one of the authors who did not know the histological and endosonographic findings.

The CT criteria for the depth of infiltration were as follows:

Stages T1 and T2 were regarded as not primarily differentiable. Where there was a distinct regular delineation of the intestinal wall from the pararectal tissue or from the subserosal fat, stage T2 was assumed. The intraluminal extent of the tumours was not considered.

Stage T3 was assumed where there were discrete irregularities of the border between the outer circumference of the intestinal wall and the adjacent tissue. Furthermore, process-like dense structures projecting from the outer intestinal wall into the pericolic or perirectal tissue were also regarded as evidence of transmural spread.

Stage T4 was assumed where there were signs of infiltration of the tumour into adjacent organs.

Lymph nodes of the true pelvis with a diameter of more than 1 cm by CT, as well as grouped lymph nodes in the mesorectum even with a diameter of less than 1 cm by CT, are regarded as suggestive of metastases.

4.11.3.1 Results

Assessment of Tumour Penetration Depth. In 46 of 49 patients investigated (93.9%), direct agreement was found between the endosonographically and histologically determined depth of penetration. Three T2 tumours were classified sonographically as T3, i.e. wall penetration was inferred on the basis of the endosonogram but could not be verified histologically (Table 4.2).

CT diagnosis of the depth of penetration was correct in 37 cases (80.4%). Wall penetration was wrongly suspected in eight T2 tumours, and existing wall

Table 4.2. The results of endosonographic assessment of the depth of tumour penetration (uT) in comparison with the histological findings (pT) ($n=49$)

uT	pT			
	1 ($n=0$)	2 ($n=12$)	3 ($n=36$)	4 ($n=1$)
1	–	–	–	–
2	–	9	–	–
3	–	3	36	–
4	–	–	–	1

Table 4.3. The results of assessment of the depth of tumour penetration by computed tomography (ctT) in comparison with the histological findings (pT) ($n=49$)

ctT	pT			
	1 ($n=0$)	2 ($n=12$)	3 ($n=36$)	4 ($n=1$)
1	–	–	–	–
2	–	4	3	–
3	–	8	32	–
4	–	–	1	1

Table 4.4. The assessment of lymph node involvement by computed tomography (ctN) in comparison to the histological findings (pN) ($n=34$)

ctN	pN	
	Negative ($n=18$)	Positive ($n=16$)
Negative	9	4
Positive	9	12

penetration was not detected in three T3 tumours. In one case, infiltration of the tumour into an adjacent organ was suspected on the basis of CT but could not be confirmed (Table 4.3).

Among the 34 patients whose perirectal lymph nodes were evaluated, the pathologist found metastatic changes in 16 cases. Endosonography and CT identified these metastases in 13 and 12 cases respectively (Table 4.4).

Among the remaining 18 patients without histologically verifiable lymph node metastases, such metastases were diagnosed four times on endosonography and nine times on CT (Table 4.4). Altogether, then, the perirectal lymph nodes

Table 4.5. The accuracy of endorectal sonography (ES) and computed tomography (CT) in assessing rectal wall penetration ($n=49$)

	Sensitive	Specificity	PPV	NPV
ES	100%	75%	92.5%	100%
CT	91.9%	33.3%	80.9%	57.1%

Table 4.6. Accuracy of endorectal sonography (ES) and computed tomography (CT) in the assessment of lymph node involvement in the true pelvis ($n=34$)

	Sensitivity	Specificity	PPV	NPV
ES	81.3	77.8	76.5	82.4
CT	75	50	52.2	63.6

All data are percentages.

Table 4.7. Accuracy of the assessment of rectal wall penetration by endorectal sonography (ES) and computed tomography (CT)

Principal investigator	Year	*n*	Sensitivity (%)	Specificity (%)	PPV	NPV
ES						
Beynon [5]	1986	42	94	87	97	78
Rifkin [30]	1986	81	83	84	76	90
Romano [32]	1985	23	86.7	100	100	80
CT						
Beynon [5]	1986	42	86	62	91	50
Rifkin [30]	1986	81	55	79	64	50
Romano [32]	1985	23	86.7	100	100	80

All data are percentages.

were correctly evaluated in 27 of 34 cases by endosonography and in 21 of 34 patients by CT. With regard to the therapeutic consequences, the differentiation between stages T1/T2 and stages T3/T4, i.e. whether the tumour has penetrated the wall or not, is of special importance (Table 4.5). Table 4.6 displays statistical data on the detection of lymph node metastases in the true pelvis. The present study indicates that both endosonography and CT are suitable for determining the depth of tumour penetration, but comparison with the results of histological investigation of the surgical preparations indicates a superiority of endorectal sonography. Beynon [5], Rifkin [30] and Romano [32], arrived at similar results (Table 4.7).

4.11.3.2 Discussion

Depth of Penetration: The high accuracy of endorectal sonography in determining the depth of tumour penetration rests on the imaging of the wall layers as well as the interfaces regarded as boundary lines between the layers. Their status – intact or interrupted – serves to indicate the extent of tumour infiltration. Three tumours described as T2 on histological investigation were overstaged endosonographically, i.e. small interruptions of the outer interface were regarded as indicators of possible infiltration of the perirectal fat tissue. This reflects the tendency of the investigator to assume a more advanced tumour stage in borderline cases, with a view to therapeutic safety.

The good resolution of CT and its reliable discrimination of the rectal wall from the perirectal fat tissue make it a relatively good method for preoperative tumour staging. Since CT does not allow differentiation of the wall layers [10, 14, 20, 38], however, the UICC classification should not be applied. The objective of CT assessment is simply to ascertain whether there is wall penetration or infiltration into adjacent organs. Thoeni [38] based his assessment of the CT imaging of rectal carcinomas on the criteria of wall thickness and spread in the true pelvis and suggested a classification into stages I to IV. The high rate of agreement with Dukes' pathohistological classification, 95%, is surprising, since besides local penetration, Dukes' classification also considers lymph node involvement.

Eight of ten stage T2 tumours were overstaged on CT, i.e. wall penetration was wrongly suspected, and three tumours from the T3 group were understaged. Thus it seems on the one hand that tumours which have not penetrated the rectal wall can lead to an irregular appearance of its outer surface, while on the other hand infiltration of the perirectal fat can yield a smooth border on CT.

According to our observations, the degree of wall thickening, which has been specified by various authors [33, 38, 42] as a criterion of the depth of penetration, does not allow reliable differentiation between stages T2 and T3. Without bolus injection of contrast medium, differentiation between tumour and healthy rectal wall is not possible. The difficulty in detecting penetration of the outer intestinal wall layers in borderline cases results from this. However, the visualization of the perirectal fascia, which is prerectally thickened in pathological lesions, and its significance for the assessment of the extent of tumour infiltration is reported by Grabbe [14]: In our opinion, the relevance of the recognition of this fascia lies more in the distinction between early and advanced stage T3 than in the detection of wall penetration.

Evaluation of Lymph Nodes: In vitro investigations of reactively enlarged and metastatically infiltrated lymph nodes indicated differences in echogenicity depending on histology. This observation led to the use of the criterion echogenicity in the evaluation of lymph nodes by endosonography.

In four of 18 cases without histologically demonstrated lymph node metastases, involvement of lymph nodes was suspected on the basis of endosonography. Thirteen of 16 metastatically altered lymph nodes were correctly diagnosed as such. Two of the three misinterpreted cases involved carcinomas of the upper third of the rectum, of which the cranial lymph drainage area is not accessible to endosonography owing to the latter's limited range. In the third case, hyperechoic lymph nodes were observed in the perirectal fat and described as reactively altered. Both reactively enlarged and metastatically involved lymph nodes were then found in the histological preparation.

So far, there are few studies on the endosonographic staging of lymph nodes. The criterion of echogenicity was applied by Tio [41] for evaluation of paragastric lymphomas in endosonographic investigations of the stomach.

Rifkin [30] suggested regarding all endosonographically discernible lymph nodes as potentially malignant. In doing so, he attained a surprisingly high specificity of 91%, with only six false-positive diagnoses amongst 66 patients without lymph node metastases ($n=81$). These results cannot be reproduced in our patient population. Dispensing with the criterion of echogenicity for differentiation of malignant from reactively enlarged lymph nodes would have led to a major rise in the rate of false-positive findings, i.e. to a marked loss of specificity of the method with no appreciable increase in sensitivity (Table 4.8). For this reason, it appears sensible to retain this criterion, even if further in vitro and in vivo studies are necessary.

The results attained by CT in the assessment of lymph node involvement showed an adequate sensitivity of 75%. Twelve of 16 positive cases were correctly diagnosed, but the specificity, at only 50%, was inadequate. Routine intravenous injection of contrast medium probably would have led to greater specificity in labeling of vessels in the perirectal space. This applies in particular to tumours with inflammatory alterations, in the vicinity of which vessels which can simulate lymph nodes when imaged in a certain plane are not uncommonly visualized more readily on CT.

In the studies of Dixon [10], Grabbe [14] and Rifkin [30], lymph node diameters of more than 1 cm or more than 1.5 cm were the sole criterion of metastatic involvement, whereas we rated the increased occurrence of small lymph nodes as an indication of possible metastatic spread, by analogy with our experience in the mediastinum. Evaluation of the diameter of imaged lymph nodes alone appears to be of dubious value, since reactive changes can also lead to an appreciable increase in size, while seven of 16 of the lymph node metastases demonstrated histologically in our patients were less than 10 mm in size. This uncertainty of the size criterion is reflected in the published results (Dixon: specificity 96%, sensitivity 39%; Grabbe: specificity 91.5%, sensitivity 34.4%;

Table 4.8. Results of lymph node staging with and without applying the criterion of echogenicity for the detection of malignancy ($n=34$)

	True negative	False negative	True positive	False positive	Sensitivity	Specificity
Simple sonographic detectability [30]	9	9	14	2	87.5%	50%
Differentiation of echogenicity (Feifel/Hildebrandt)	14	4	13	3	81.3%	77.8%

Table 4.9. Assessment of tumour penetration depth by computed tomography. (From [39])

Principal investigator	Year	*n*	Accuracy (%)
Dixon [10]	1981	47	77
Thoeni [38]	1981	39	92
Zaunbauer [47]	1981	11	100
Van Waes [42]	1983	21	81
Grabbe [14]	1985	155	79
Thompson [39]	1986	25	79
		472	77.1

Table 4.10. Assessment of lymph node metastases by computed tomography. (From [39])

Principal investigator	Year	*n*	Sensitivity (%)	Specificity (%)
Dixon [10]	1981	47	36	96
Zaunbauer [47]	1981	11	100	100
Grabbe [14]	1985	154	34	92
Thompson [39]	1986	25	22	75

Rifkin: specificity 100%, sensitivity 23%), which are similar to one another with regard to their high proportion of false-negative findings. The detection of early tumour invasion constitutes a problem, which indicates the limitations of preoperative diagnosis by means of imaging methods. We attribute the poorer results in the evaluation of lymph nodes, despite the good resolution of CT, primarily to the lack of a "tissue parameter" such as echogenicity in endorectal sonography. However, CT is superior in the assessment of lymph nodes nearer to the origin of the inferior mesenteric artery, which may be especially important in higher-located tumours.

With regard to the clinical application of the methods compared here, endorectal sonography in the hands of an experienced investigator appears to be superior to CT for determination of the depth of tumour infiltration, and is hence adequate as the sole method supplementing conventional diagnostic measures. It also appears to be superior in the assessment of perirectal lymph nodes (Tables 4.9, 4.10). Supplementary CT is indicated in tumours of the upper third of the rectum with potential metastatic spread via the mesenteric, para-iliac and para-aortic efferent lymphatics, and in stenosing carcinomas which cannot be passed by the rectoscope or the ultrasound probe. CT may also be indicated in some circumstances to verify or exclude infiltration of adjacent organs by advanced tumours.

4.12 Endosonography and Palliative Treatment of Rectal Cancer

High-risk patients can be treated palliatively by laser therapy, cryosurgery, infrared coagulation or transanal resection. The aim of these procedures in patients with inoperable rectal cancer is to control bleeding, to relieve obstruction and to

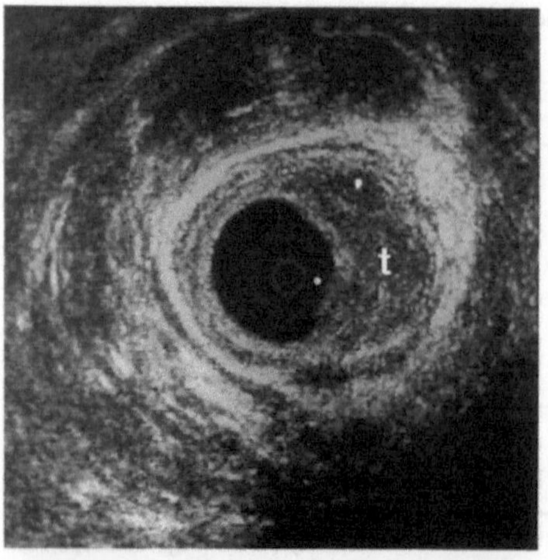

4.73

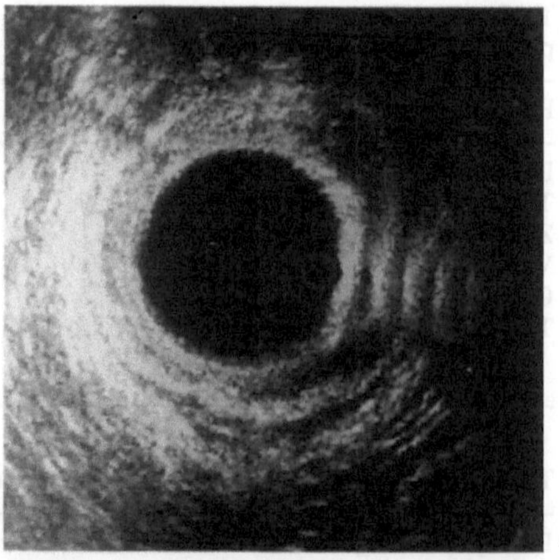

4.74

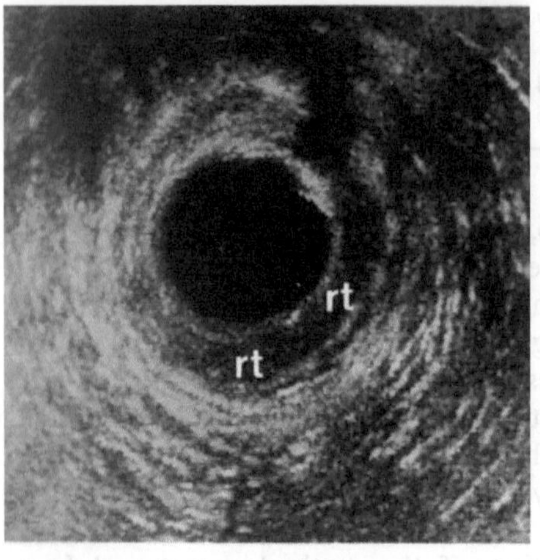

4.75

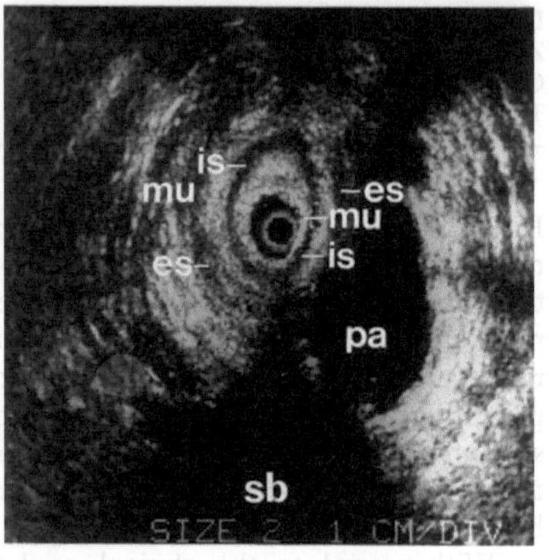

4.76

Fig. 4.73. Supra-anal rectal cancer in a poor-risk patient. The semicircular tumour (*t*) on the right side of the sonogram does not penetrate into the perirectal fat

Fig. 4.74. Sonogram of the tumour shown in Fig. 4.73 immediately after palliative infrared coagulation. Due to the tissue changes resulting from coagulation the sound waves are reflected at the coagulation site

Fig. 4.75. Sonogram in the same case 4 weeks later. The hypoechoic thickening of the right circumference of the rectal wall represents the residual tumor (*rt*)

Fig. 4.76. Sonogram of perianal abscess. The transducer is placed within the anal canal. On the left side of the image, mucosa (*mu*), internal sphincter (*is*) and external sphincter (*es*) are clearly demonstrated. On the right side, mucosa (*mu*) and internal sphincter are intact. The external sphincter is inflamed from the outside by the perianal abscess (*pa*). Hypoechoic area at bottom of sonogram: space between buttocks (*sb*)

avoid colostomy. Endosonography is a useful tool for monitoring tumour growth between treatment sessions and for evaluating tumour thickness during the treatment procedure in order to avoid perforation (Figs. 4.73–4.75).

4.13 Endosonography of Anorectal Abscesses

Five types of anorectal abscesses can be discerned: perianal, ischiorectal, submucosal, intersphincteric and supralevator. It is important to distinguish the different types because their treatment differs.

4.13.1 Perianal Abscess

The perianal abscess, the commonest of the five types, is situated superficially lateral to the anal verge. Clinically it presents as an area of erythema, induration or fluctuance. Proctoscopy may be difficult to perform because of pain, but when it is possible blind endoanal sonography can be performed as well. When only erythema is found clinically, with no apparent mass, endosonography may help to establish an early diagnosis. Despite the absence of fluctuance or significant induration an abscess may already be present (Fig. 4.76).

4.13.2 Ischiorectal Abscess

Ischiorectal abscess mostly presents as a large erythematous induration of the buttock. Proctoscopy is usually deferred because of severe pain. In our series we have no case documented by endosonography. Whether the evaluation of the extension of the abscess cavity by endosonography may affect the choice of incision remains to be seen.

4.13.3 Submucosal Abscess

A submucosal abscess arises from an infected crypt in the anal canal. The infection develops cephalad and presents as a mass within the lower part of the rectum or upper anal canal. The sonographic appearance of a submucosal abscess is characteristic: Due to the inflammatory reaction the mucosa is thickened. The hypoechoic muscularis propria and the hypoechoic abscess form an integrated whole. As at intact sites, the outer interface provides sharp delineation of the rectal wall from the perirectal fat (Figs. 4.77, 4,78).

4.13.4 Intersphincteric Abscess

An intersphincteric abscess occurs between the internal and external sphincters of the anus. The patient often feels a sense of fullness in the rectum. Pus discharge

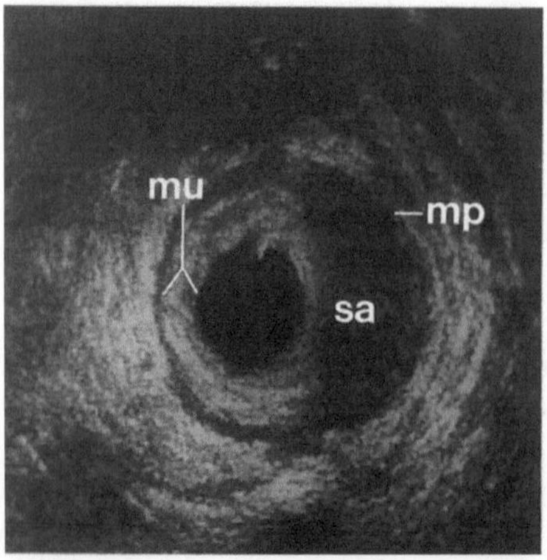

4.77

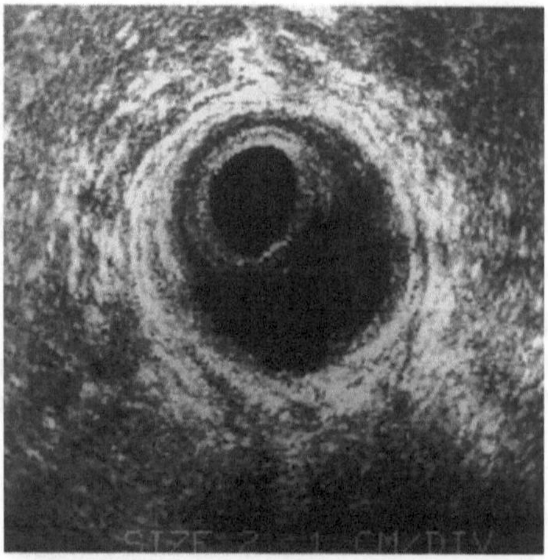

4.78

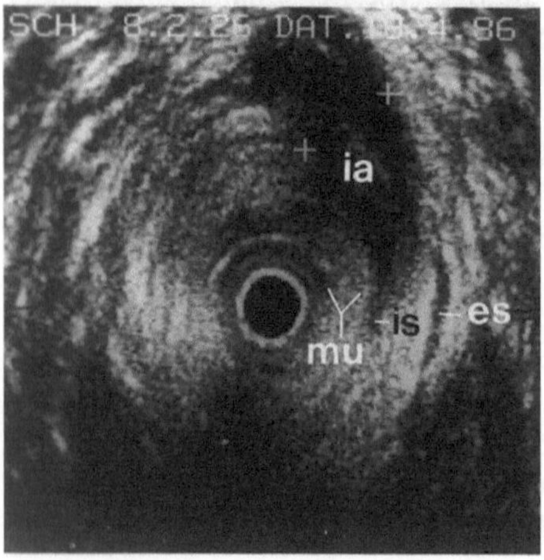

4.79

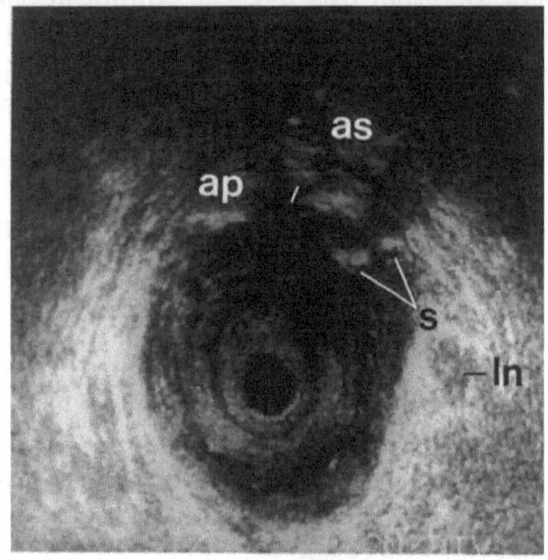

4.80

Fig. 4.77. Sonogram of submucosal abscess. The mucosa (*mu*) on the left side of the image appears thickened due to inflammation. The halfmoon-shaped hypoechoic area on the right side represents the submucosal abscess (*sa*) together with the muscularis propria (*mp*)

Fig. 4.78. Sonogram of submucosal abscess. Mucosa, submucosa and muscularis propria form a hypoechoic unity: the outer hyperechoic interface represents the intact borderline with the perirectal fat

Fig. 4.79. Sonogram of intersphincteric abscess. Mucosa (*mu*), internal sphincter (*is*) and external sphincter (*es*) are discernible on the right side of the image. The internal and external sphincter merge with the intersphincteric abscess (*ia*)

Fig. 4.80. Sonogram of necrotizing perineal infection. The structures of the anal sphincter are blurred in the anterior perineum (*ap*). Hyperechoic spots (*s*) with acoustic shadow (*as*) represent gas. (*ln*) lymph node

may be noted. Digital examination reveals a tender submucosal mass. On proctoscopy the mucosa appears oedematous. Ultrasound examination demonstrates the intact mucosa and the abscess between the two sphincters. The two sphincter muscles and the abscess appear hypoechoic on ultrasound and form an integrated whole (Fig. 4.79).

4.13.5 Supralevator Abscess

Supralevator abscess is rare and has not been documented by ultrasound in our series. Perianal and buttock pain are the presenting complaints. Two types can be seen. In one the abscess arises from pelvic sepsis, and transrectal drainage is the correct treatment. The other is an abscess secondary to a transsphincteric fistula. External drainage is then the appropriate treatment. Whether endosonography might help to decide between external and transrectal drainage could be worth investigating.

4.14 Necrotizing Perineal Infection

A relatively rare condition is spontaneous necrotizing infection of the perineum. One patient presented with a short history of discrete circumscribed perianal pain, tenderness and swelling. Immediately after hospitalization an endorectal sonographic examination was performed (Fig. 4.80). In comparison to the normal anal canal anatomy the different structures appeared to merge one into another. The anterior area of the perineum had a distinctive homogeneous hypoechoic appearance due to inflammation. Some hyperechoic spots with acoustic shadow represented gas in the necrotic tissue. The clinical feature of a rapid onset of perineal infection and the endosonographic detection of gas indicated that the underlying infection was a necrotizing process rather than a simple abscess. During preparation for operation the infection rapidly disseminated to the external genitalia. Wide surgical debridement with removal of all necrotic tissue was performed.

Adenomas by definition are benign. Due to their relationship with the subsequent development of cancer, their sonographic imaging is of some interest.

Rectal adenomas can be classified into three morphological types: polypoid, villous and mixed. They may be as small as 1 mm or larger than 7 cm, pedunculated or sessile.

Macroscopically the surface may be relatively smooth or nodular. Rectal bleeding is the commonest presenting complaint, but in patients with a large villous adenoma a change in bowel habit and mucous discharge are commonly observed.

It is not usually possible to determine the benign or malignant nature of polyps by inspection during sigmoidoscopy. Despite the generalizations about surface morphology, size, and presence or absence of a pedicle, the only certain means of establishing the diagnosis is histologic examination. Transanal excision is the preferred method of removing rectal adenomas. Large lesions can be removed via a posterior excision or an anterior rectal resection with or without restoration of intestinal continuity.

The aim of preoperative endosonography of adenomas is to evaluate whether carcinoma in adenomas are visible on ultrasound. Generally, the larger the lesion, the greater the likelihood of malignant change. Polypoid adenomas under 1 cm in diameter have been shown to have a 1% incidence of malignant change, while villous adenomas have a 10% risk of malignancy. Among adenomas larger than 2 cm, malignant change occurs in 35% of polypoid lesions and in 50% of villous adenomas.

Based on our experience with endosonography of more than 30 rectal adenomas we can state the following:

1) With the transducer in the ideal 90° position the two borderlines of the muscularis propria, e.g. the middle and outer interfaces, are visible on ultrasound (Figs. 4.81, 4.82).
2) Flat villous adenomas are sonographically characterized by a circumscribed thickening of the inner hypoechoic layer representing the mucosa.
3) The surface of polypoid adenomas is broken by clefts into multiple nodules. The water-filled balloon presses the adenoma against the rectal wall, and the resulting sonographic picture resembles that of a lobular or cystic tumour (Fig. 4.83).

4.81
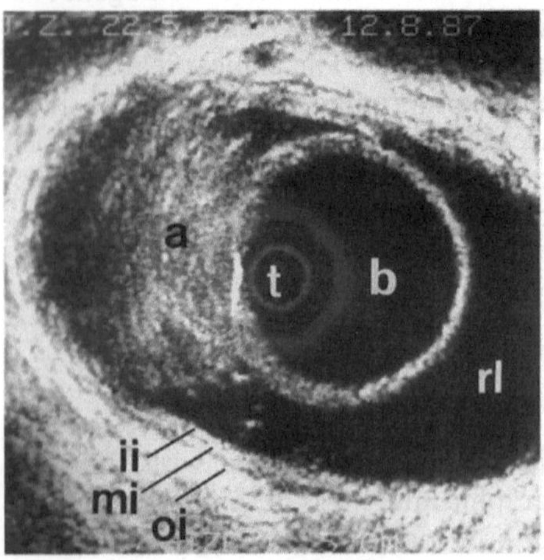

4.82
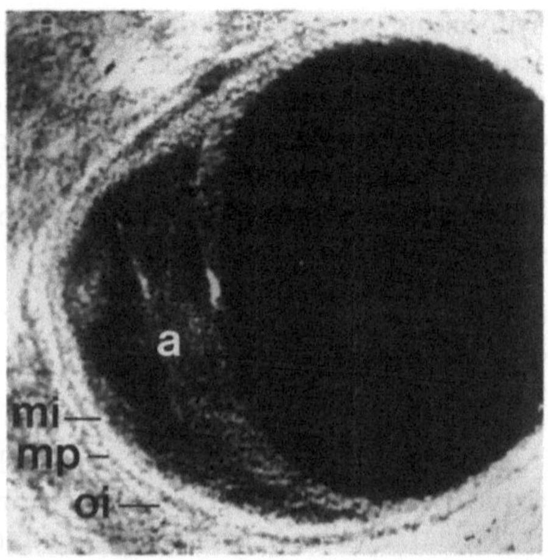

Fig. 4.81. Sonogram of adenoma (*a*). The rectal lumen (*rl*) is filled with water. The balloon (*b*) which surrounds the transducer (*t*) swims in the rectum. The three interfaces (*ii, mi, oi*) and the muscularis propria are visualized. The adenoma appears homogeneous, with sound amplification close to the transducer

Fig. 4.82. Sonogram of adenoma (*a*). The muscularis propria (*mp*) is demonstrated between the middle (*mi*) and outer (*oi*) interfaces

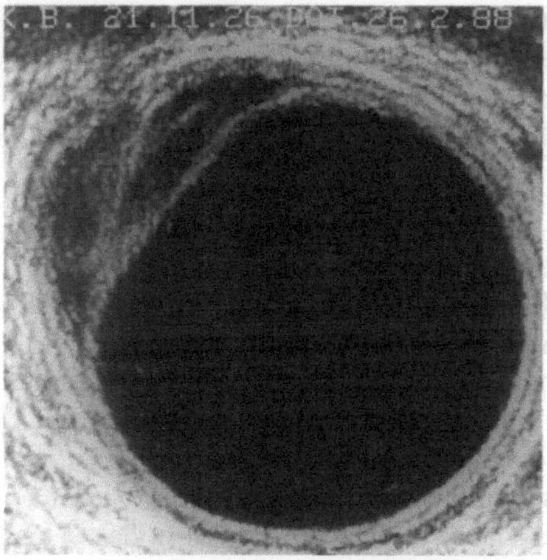

4.83

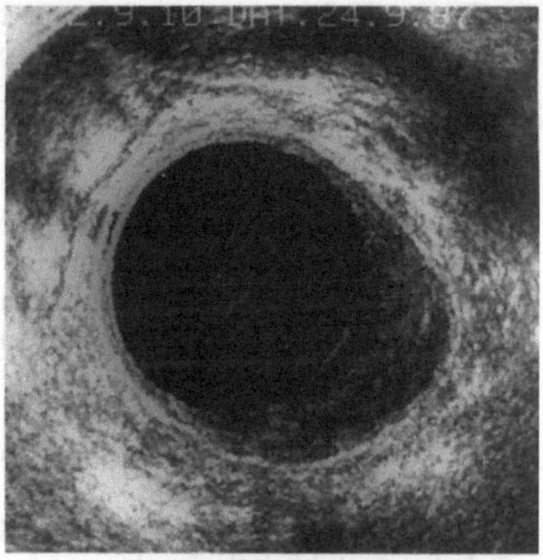

4.84

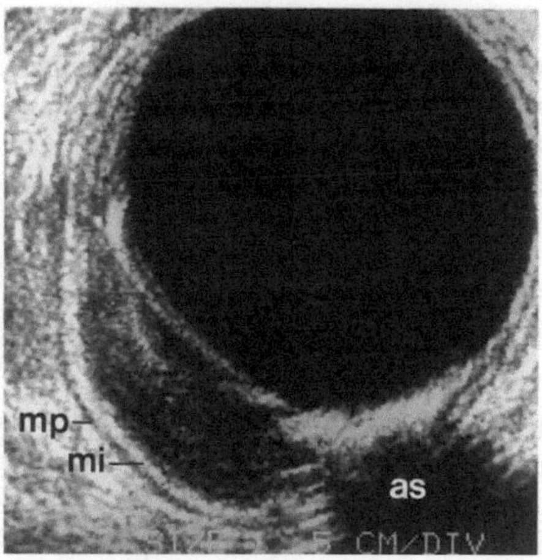

4.85

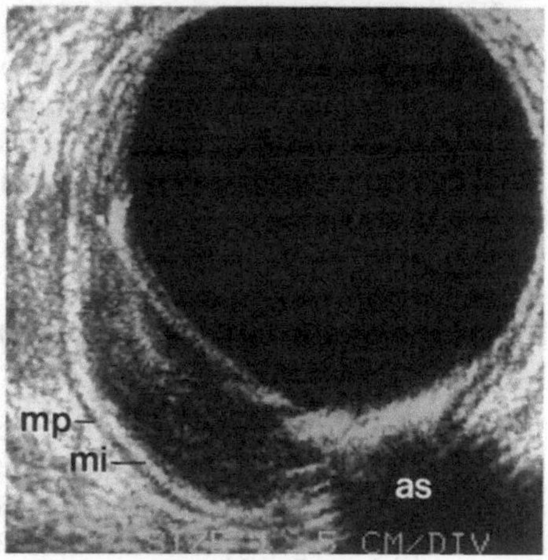

4.86

Fig. 4.83. The sonographic appearance of this adenoma is not uniform: it appears like a lobular or cystic tumour

Fig. 4.84. Sonogram of an apparently benign lesion. Histological examination revealed a villous adenoma with carcinoma in situ

Fig. 4.85. Sonogram of a mass confined to submucosa. Endoscopically the tumour resembled an adenoma. Histologic examination after removal instead revealed carcinoma in situ. Gas between water balloon and rectal wall produces an acoustic shadow (*as*). *mi*, middle interface; *mp*, muscularis propria

Fig. 4.86. Sonogram following transanal excision of an adenoma with transformation into carcinoma. The base of the excised specimen was not clear. The excision site appears hypoechoic. It is not possible to determine whether any tumour remains, because tumour and sutured muscularis propria cannot be differentiated from each other

4) Due to the heterogeneous echo patterns of benign adenomas, transformation into a malignant lesion cannot be assessed by ultrasound (Figs. 4.84, 4.85).
5) In scanning of pedunculated adenomas gas may remain between the water-filled balloon and the adenoma or the rectal wall. This causes artefacts (Fig. 4.84).

After excision of an apparently benign adenoma there is the problem of what to do if invasive carcinoma is found in the surgical specimen. Some authors advocate resection as treatment of choice in all cases, while others selectively advise resection in patients with poorly differentiated lesions or in young patients.

Does endosonography help when the pathologist thinks that some malignant tissue may have been left behind? Since the echo pattern even in benign adenomas is heterogeneous, a circumscribed area of malignancy will not be identified sonographically. If an excised adenoma is found on pathohistological examination to be malignant, it may be possible to visualize affected lymph nodes. This may help to establish the need for resection.

Following full-thickness excision biopsy of an adenoma the suture line appears sonographically thickened due to the double-layered muscularis. When an apparently benign adenoma is found to be invasive carcinoma, ultrasound cannot contribute to the evaluation of residual tumour (Fig. 4.86). Local recurrence may be detected only by repeated scanning over an extended period.

4.16 Malignant Tumours of the Anal Canal

The anal canal is bordered by the rectal mucosa above and the perianal skin below. It is divided into a proximal transitional zone encompassing the columns of Morgagni and a distal zone lined by squamous epithelium.

Three histologic types of tumours are identified in the anal canal: epidermoid carcinoma, cloacogenic carcinoma of the transitional zone and malignant melanoma. Because newer approaches combine local excision of anal canal cancers with chemo- and radiotherapy, it is necessary to assess the depth of invasion of the tumour. This can be achieved by endoanal ultrasound, which differentiates mucosa from the internal and external sphincters (Fig. 4.87).

4.16.1 Epidermoid Carcinoma

Epidermoid carcinoma of the anus is a rare tumour originating from the stratified squamous epithelium of the distal anal mucosa. Symptoms include rectal bleeding, tenesmus and change in bowel habit. The choice of therapy depends on the depth of tumour invasion. The latter is assessed more precisely by endoanal ultrasound than by digital examination (Fig. 4.88). Conventional surgical treatment is local excision for carcinoma invading the mucosa or internal sphincter and abdominoperineal excision for tumours invading the external sphincter.

4.87
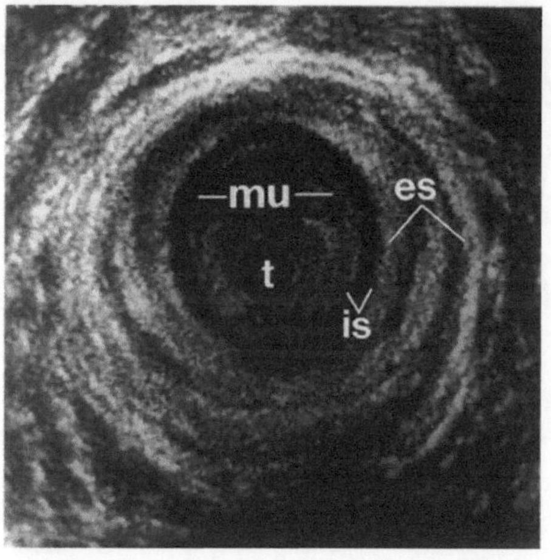

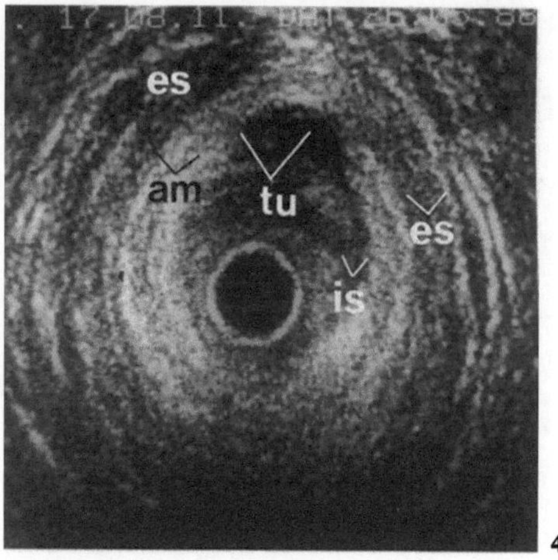

4.88

Fig. 4.87. Sonographic anatomy of the anal canal. *t*, transducer; *mu*, mucosa; *is*, internal sphincter; *es*, external sphincter with conjoined longitudinal muscle

Fig. 4.88. Sonogram of a histologically confirmed epidermoid carcinoma. The tumour (*tu*) invades the internal sphincter (*is*) and the adjoining longitudinal muscle (*am*). The external sphincter (*es*) is not infiltrated

In 1974 Nigro [27] reported treatment of epidermoid carcinoma of the anus by combined radio- and chemotherapy before operation. Following radio- and chemotherapy, patients mostly underwent only wide excision of the residual scar if there was no macroscopic evidence of tumour. In our opinion endoanal sonography adds to accurate assessment of the status of the tumour region after radio- and chemotherapy. With this advanced technique it will be possible to define the necessary extent of the excision or even to identify those residual tumours that are better treated by abdominoperineal excision.

4.16.2 Cloacogenic Carcinoma of Transitional Zone

Cloacogenic carcinomas of the transitional zone form a morphologically distinguished subgroup of anal canal carcinomas. They may be graded and staged in a similar way to epidermoid carcinomas. It seems sensible to apply the Nigro protocol also to these tumours. Non-invasive tumours (Fig. 4.89) are excised locally following radio- and chemotherapy. For invasive lesions abdominoperineal resection is more appropriate.

4.16.3 Malignant Melanoma

Malignant melanoma of the anal canal is an extremely rare condition with a poor prognosis [43]. The tumour is presumed to arise from melanocytes present in the squamous mucosa of the anal canal. Pigment is usually present, but about 30%

4.89 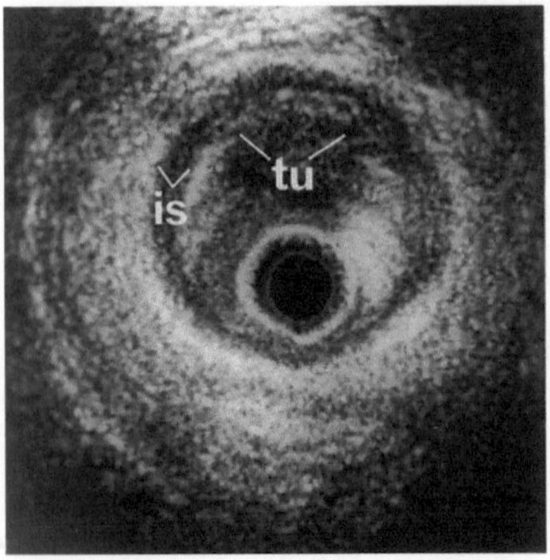

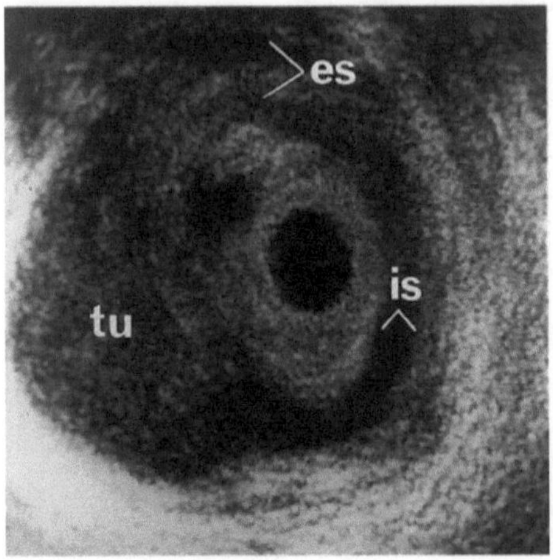 4.90

Fig. 4.89. Sonogram of histologically confirmed cloacogenic carcinoma of the transitional zone. The tumour (*tu*) invades the internal sphincter (*is*) but does not penetrate through it

Fig. 4.90. Sonogram of histologically confirmed malignant melanoma. The tumour (*tu*) has destroyed the internal sphincter (*is*) and is penetrating into the external sphincter (*es*)

of the lesions are histologically amelanotic. Rectal bleeding, change in bowl habit and the feeling of a mass are the clinical features. Abdominoperineal resection is the treatment of choice. In the case shown here (Fig. 4.90) we demonstrated sonographically that the tumour was invading the external sphincter. Because the prognosis is so poor, local excision is appropriate if not resulting in incontinence. Supplementary treatment of any other kind has been of no benefit. In our opinion, endoanal sonography can help to select patients whose lesions do not invade the external sphincter for local excision.

4.17 Impact of Endosonography on the Management of Rectal Cancer

The correct treatment for different stages of cancer of the rectum continues to be discussed. Any of a number of procedures available may be the optimal approach for an individual patient. In practice, the choice of treatment for rectal carcinoma is influenced by many factors. General considerations are age, general fitness, body habitus and metastatic or other systemic disease. Local factors affecting the choice of operation include the level, extent and histological grade of the tumour, the depth of penetration and lymph node involvement.

Sigmoidoscopy reveals the level of the tumour above the anal verge and the intraluminal appearance, but cannot assess the penetration depth or the presence of lymph node involvement.

The most promising method of obtaining this information has been for many years direct digital examination of the tumour and the perirectal area. Mason [23] introduced a clinical staging system with four stages as follows: stage 1: tumour freely moveable over underlying muscle wall of rectum; stage 2 tumour mobile but not movable separately from rectal wall; stage 3: tumour and rectum slightly fixed; stage 4 tumour and rectum firmly fixed. Nicholls et al. [25] modified the system in 1982 proposing four stages of local spread as follows: stage 1: tumour confined to rectum; stage 2: tumour confined to rectum or slight extrarectal spread; stage 3: moderate or extensive extrarectal spread; stage 4: involvement of other organs or unresectability. Lymph node status, negative or positive, was also proposed as a criterion. Stages 1 and 2 could be distinguished reliably from stages 3 and 4 in over 80% of patients. The concordance of clinical with pathological assessment of pararectal lymph nodes was 67%. Later Nicholls et al. [26] simplified the clinical staging system by differentiating only two groups: stage 1: tumour with no or slight spread; stage 2: moderate or extensive spread.

Computed tomography has been used to stage primary rectal cancer since 1981 [10, 38]. Experience with this modality suggests that it might be useful in assessing the resectability of tumours and in demonstrating unsuspected involvement of other organs. In less extensive tumours, however, CT fails to predict the degree of tumour penetration. Moreover, Dixon [10] considered it inadequate in the prediction of lymph node involvement. For these reasons, in our opinion CT has no place in the routine preoperative assessment of rectal cancer.

There are further deficiencies of CT compared with endosonography. As stated earlier, for good results it is essential that the tumour-bearing rectal wall is scanned at a 90° angle. This is not always achieved due to the fixed position of the scanner. Thus the tumour may be scanned tangentially, and invasion or organ penetration may be wrongly predicted. CT cannot differentiate individual layers of the rectal wall or detect slight invasion, and therefore cannot contribute to the choice of tumours for local treatment. Lymph nodes look the same on CT whether or not they are involved. A number of studies have revealed that there is no correlation between the diameter and the depth of penetration of the primary tumour and the status of regional lymph nodes. Hence neither palpation nor size as assessed by CT would be effective in selecting patients appropriate for sphincter-conserving operative procedures. It would be untrue to claim that endorectal sonography has entirely overcome these difficulties, but it has advantages over digital examination in that tumours out of reach of the palpating finger can be scanned. Objective evidence of a tumour's size and depth of invasion are very important when conservative surgery is being considered. Even the experienced surgeon who obtains a good correlation between digital and histological assessment of penetration depth has the disadvantage that his opinion is not pictorially documented.

The problem of lymph node assessment prior to therapy has not yet been solved. No method, digital palpation, CT or endosonography, can predict micrometastases. Even node size is not sufficient to differentiate involved from non-involved nodes. However, we have been able to demonstrate that lymph nodes may be differentiated on the basis of changing echo patterns. Hyperechoic lymph nodes visible sonographically are found to be non-specifically inflamed when revieved histologically. Normal non-involved nodes in individuals with no infection or tumour of the rectum are not visible. This is due mainly to their size, generally not more than 3 mm. The evaluation of hypoechoic nodes still remains a problem, since both metastatic infiltration and non-specific inflammation may have this appearance. Therefore, the likelihood of metastases being present is very low in patients with nodes that are hyperechoic or cannot be demonstrated, and very high in patients with hypoechoic nodes.

The preoperative assessment of tumour penetration depth and lymph node status by endorectal sonography provides a classification of rectal cancers into four therapy groups.

Group I: Tumour Stage uT1 N0. This group comprises tumours confined to submucosa with no suspicious lymph nodes seen on sonography. Other characteristics such as site, size, extent of circumferential involvement and degree of differentiation being favorable, patients in this group are ideally treated by local excision of the cancer. The incidence of lymph node metastasis in lesions confined to the submucosa ranges from 6% to 11%. Using ultrasound it seems possible to reduce the risk of undertreatment by the detection of some N1 tumours. With the objective sonographic assessment of tumour penetration depth and the exclusion of suspicious lymph nodes we have performed local excision of rectal cancer via the posterior approach in 22 patients. Two patients developed local recurrence within a 4-year follow-up period. One recurrence was obviously due to a surgical error at the time of primary treatment. None of the tumours in this group were understaged by ultrasound with respect to the T stage ascertained subsequently by histological examination.

Group II: Tumour Stage uT2 N0. Extension to the muscularis increases the risk of lymph node metastasis to 10%–20%. Using ultrasound this risk may be reduced, since some of the cases of node involvement will be detected sonographically. Nevertheless, there remains a more than 10% likelihood of metastasis. This has to be balanced, however, against the morbidity and mortality associated with the traditional therapy of rectal cancer – abdominoperineal resection and low anterior resection. In older patients especially, a colostomy, long hospitalization or complications can be anticipated and local excision in carefully selected patients would be a preferable alternative. When recurrence develops in patients treated by local excision it looks at first as if survival were worse, because the ideal radical treatment has not been employed. However, one must realize that local failure usually means that nodes are involved, and 5-year survival in many series of Duke's C patients is around 30%–40%, with many patients dying of disseminated disease rather than pure local progression. Hence local excision of a uT2 tumour and a risk of metastasis reduced by ultrasound but possibly still about 10% has to be balanced against significantly more morbidity and mortality by radical surgery with a still uncertain prognosis. The preferred therapy for stage uT2 N0 tumours is therefore local excision for older patients and radical surgery for younger patients. After local treatment careful follow-up is imperative to detect recurrence before it is beyond the reach of treatment. Endorectal sonography has proved to be effective in identifying early recurrence.

Group III: Tumour Stages uT2 N1 and uT3 N0. Extension through all layers of the rectal wall into the perirectal fat is associated with nodal metastasis in

33%–58% of cases. Tumour stage uT3 N0 will be identified endosonographically with a higher accuracy than with the conventional imaging techniques. The appropriate treatment for this group and for the occasional uT2 N1 tumours is anterior or abdominoperineal resection alone.

Group IV: Tumour Stage uT3 N1. In this group, which has the worst prognosis, survival rates have not improved in the last 30 years. Whilst surgery remains the definitive treatment, there must be further assessment of the role of adjuvant treatment in the hope of improving survival rates. The most complete series of adjuvant trials evaluated the role of preoperative radiotherapy in patients with operable rectal cancer [22]. In some studies there was a significant reduction in the number of patients with Dukes C cancers in the group given preoperative radiotherapy [34]. Others found no difference between the irradiated group and the control group [24]. A strong criticism of preoperative radiotherapy trials is that no one really knows how many patients with lymph node metastases enter the study. It is therefore important to pay particular attention to the selection criteria for adjuvant treatment. This does require that some simple pretreatment assessment be made before a program of combined management is decided upon. Endorectal sonography may potentially provide such a system by differentiating lymph nodes on the basis of varying echo patterns. The identification of the tumour stage uT3 N1 provides the criterion for selecting those patients who stand to profit from preoperative radiotherapy.

4.18 Endosonography and the Diagnosis of Recurrence

Perhaps one of the most important applications of endosonography will be in the diagnosis of local recurrence following surgery for rectal cancer. The currently available methods of routine follow-up have major shortcomings, and established local recurrence can be very difficult to manage.

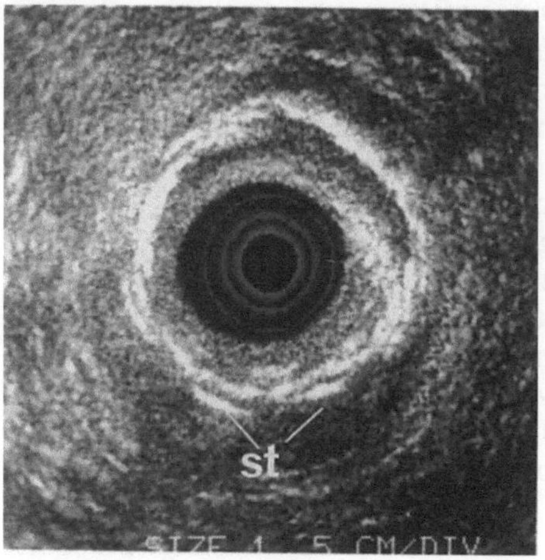

Fig. 4.91. Sonogram of stapled anastomosis. The staples (*st*) create bright echo without casting a shadow

4.92 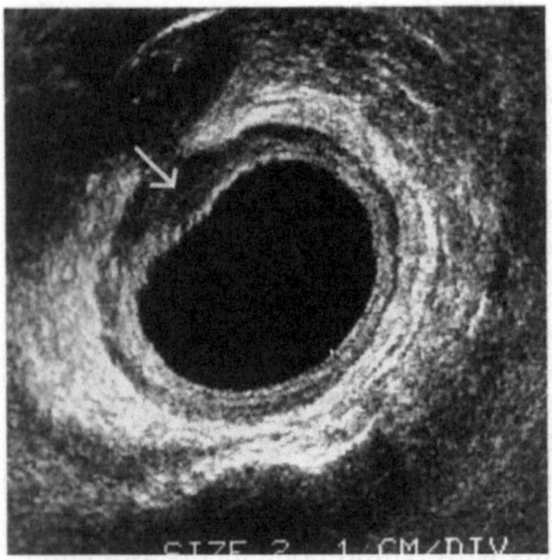

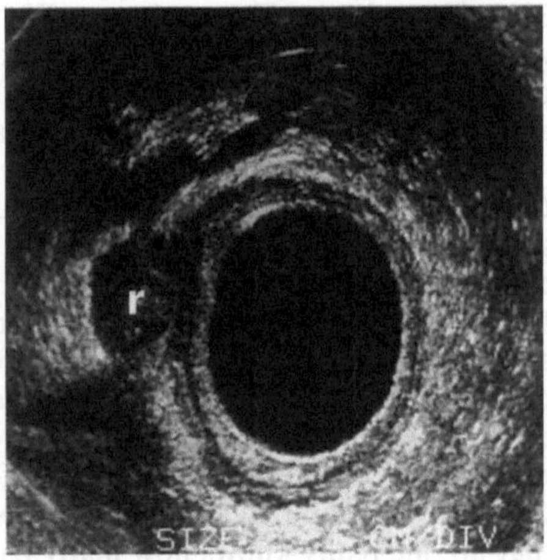

4.93

Fig. 4.92. Suture line recurrence (*arrow*). The area of the recurrence is hypoechoic

Fig. 4.93. Hypoechoic recurrence (*r*) of 2 cm diameter outside the anastomosis. The mucosa has not been invaded by the tumour

After an anterior restorative resection or a local excision procedure with an anastomosis at 15 cm or lower, the colon and rectal wall at the site of the anastomosis, together with the perianastomotic tissues, can be imaged. As endosonography is relatively cheap and the equipment is portable, it is easily incorporated into regular follow-up examinations by sigmoidoscopy or colonoscopy. Stapled anastomoses (Fig. 4.91) do not interfere with the interpretation of the sonographic image. The individual staples create a localized bright echo without casting a shadow to obscure the underlying perirectal tissues.

Local recurrence at a suture line disrupts the layers seen on a normal sonogram in a similar way to a primary tumour. If the mucosa is still intact or covered with granulation tissue, interpretation may be a little more difficult. The area of recurrence is hypoechoic (Fig. 4.92), and there may or may not be continuity with an area of extraluminal recurrence (Fig. 4.93). Recurrence outside the anastomosis also has an irregular hypoechoic or sometimes heterogeneous irregular appearance. This must be distinguished from a pelvic floor abscess, haematoma or fluid collection following surgery, which has a dark hypoechoic appearance similar to the water in the balloon around the transducer.

If there is any doubt about the diagnosis, such an area can be recorded, measured and rescanned after an interval or needle biopsied under ultrasound guidance. Since a lymphadenectomy is usually part of a radical excision, distinction between nodes and an area of recurrence presents no problem, although after local excision nodal enlargement may be the only sign of metastatic disease.

Following an abdominoperineal excision of the rectum in female patients the pelvis can be examined by passing the probe per vaginam.

4.18.1 Results

In Homburg 22 of the 123 patients followed endosonographically have developed local recurrence. Six of these had no symptoms, no clinical or endoscopic abnormality and a CEA level of less than 2.5 µg/l, and a further three had no symptoms and no clinical or endoscopic abnormality but CEA of up to 5 µg/l. The remaining 13 had either clinical or endoscopic signs or CEA elevated above 5 µg/l. In all 22 patients recurrence was detected or confirmed endosonographically, and in the six in the first group recurrence was diagnosed by endosonography alone. In Bristol and Oxford 90 patients have been scanned regularly and 13 local recurrences discovered. Two were detected by endosonography alone, and three suspicious lesions were confirmed endosonographically.

4.18.2 Discussion

Despite a seemingly successful operation with the complete removal of the primary rectal cancer, local recurrence is a depressingly frequent sequel to radical surgery, occurring in 5%–50% of patients [28]. True suture line recurrence – caused by implantation and readily seen at sigmoidoscopy – is rare, and the more usual, so-called anastomotic recurrence is actually an extrarectal local recurrence which ultimately presents at the anastomosis. This probably arises as a result of incomplete excision of the mesorectum.

Since local recurrence is so common, a number of methods have been employed with the aim of detecting recurrence at an early, treatable stage. In a scrupulous follow-up programme for colorectal cancer – including thorough history, sigmoidoscopy, barium enema and serial CEA estimations – Beart and O'Connell [3] found recurrence in 48 of 168 patients within 4 years of surgery. Although the patients had been examined at least every 15 weeks only one of the 48 recurrences was potentially resectable. Aggressive follow-up using CEA

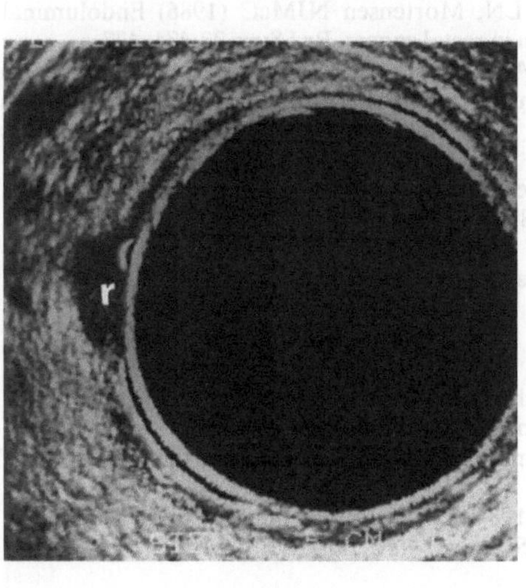

Fig. 4.94. Submucous hypoechoic recurrence (*r*) of 1 cm diameter at the left side of the sonogram

estimations and pelvic CT has been claimed by some [36] to reveal recurrences at a potentially resectable stage.

CT is certainly useful in the assessment of local recurrence, but the lesion has to be 2 cm or more in diameter for accurate diagnosis [47], and there may be difficulty in distinguishing between tumour and an inflammatory mass [48]. Tumour volumes can be calculated from CT and may assist treatment planning and help predict the outcome of treatment such as radiotherapy [19]. There are few reports of the routine use of regular pelvic CT scanning as a follow-up measure. Gualdi et al. [15] found four extraluminal recurrences, three of which were between 2 and 3 cm in diameter; radical excision was possible in all four cases. CT is expensive, however, and does not lend itself readily to the study of large numbers of patients.

Endosonography would seem to be the solution to the problem of accurate follow-up. It can be used either to image suspicious lesions found on routine clinical examination or as part of a regular follow-up programme with repeated examinations and the close scrutiny of suspicious areas. Recurrences smaller than 2 cm can be visualized (Fig. 4.94). Whether retreatment is effective with respect to long-term survival remains to be seen.

References

1. Aibe T, Ho T, Yoshida T, Noguchi T, Ohtani T, Fuji T, Takemoto T (1986) Endoscopic ultrasonography of lymph nodes surrounding the upper GI tract. Scand J Gastroenterol 21 (Suppl 12):164–169
2. Alzin HH, Kohlberger E, Schwaiger R, Alloussi S (1983) Valeur de l'échographie endorectale dans la chirurgie du rectum. Ann Radiol (Paris) 26:334–336
3. Beart RW, O'Connell MJ (1983) Post operative follow up of patients with carcinoma of the colon. Mayo Clin Proc 58:361–363
4. Beynon J, Foy DMA, Temple LN, Channer JL, Virjee J, Mortensen NJ McC (1986) The endosonic appearances of normal colon and rectum. Dis Colon Rectum 29:810–813
5. Beynon J, Foy DMA, Roe AM, Temple LN, Mortensen NJMcC (1986) Endoluminal ultrasound in the assessment of local invasion in rectal cancer. Br J Surg 73:474–477
6. Beynon J, Mortensen NJMcC, Foy DMA, Channer JL, Virjee J, Goddard P (1986) Endorectal sonography: laboratory and clinical experience in Bristol. Int J Colorectal Dis 1:201–226
7. Beynon J, Mortensen NJMcC, Foy DMA, Channer JL, Virjee J, Goddard P (1986) Preoperative assessment of local invasion in rectal cancer: digital examination, endoluminal sonography or computed tomography. Br J Surg 73:1015–1017
8. Boscaini M, Montori A (1986) Transrectal ultrasonography: interpretation of normal intestinal wall structure for the preoperative staging of rectal cancer. Scand J Gastroenterol 21 (Suppl 123):87–98
9. Boscaini M, Masoni L, Montori A (1986) Transrectal ultrasonography: three years' experience. Int J Colorectal Dis 1:208–211
10. Dixon AK, Kelsey Frey I, Morson BC, Nicholls RJ, Mason AY (1981) Preoperative computed tomography of carcinoma of the rectum. Br J Radiol 54:655–659
11. Dragsted J, Gammelgaard J (1983) Endoluminal ultrasonic scanning in the evaluation of rectal cancer. Gastrointest Radiol 8:367–369
12. Feifel G, Hildebrandt U, Koch B, Alzin H (1984) The ultrasonic imaging of the rectum. In: Givel JC, Saegesser F (eds) Coloproctology. Springer, New York Berlin Heidelberg

13. Feifel G, Hildebrandt U, Dhom G (1985) Die endorektale Sonographie beim Rektumkarzinom. Chirurg 56:398–402
14. Grabbe E, Lierse W, Winkler R (1983) The perirectal fascia: morphology and use in staging of rectal carcinoma. Radiology 149:241–246
15. Gualdi GF, Pappalardo G, Biase CD, Pitasi F (1982) The use of computerised tomography in the study of recurrent pelvic malignancy after surgical treatment of carcinoma of the rectum. Ital J Surg Sci 12:33
16. Hildebrandt U, Feifel G (1985) Pre-operative staging of rectal cancer by intrarectal ultrasound. Dis Colon Rectum 28:42–46
17. Hildebrandt U, Feifel G, Zimmermann FA, Goebbels R (1983) Significant improvement in clinical staging of rectal carcinoma with a new intrarectal ultrasound scanner. J Exp Clin Cancer Res (Suppl) 2:53
18. Hildebrandt U, Feifel G, Schwarz HP, Scherr O (1986) Endorectal ultrasound: instrumentation and clinical aspects. Int J Colorectal Dis 1:203–207
19. James RD, Johnson RJ, Eddleston B, Zheng GL, Jones JM (1983) Prognostic factors in locally recurrent rectal carcinoma treated by radiotherapy. Br J Surg 70:469–472
20. Koehler RP, Feldberg MAM, van Waes PFGM (1984) Preoperative staging of rectal cancer with computerized tomography. Cancer 54:512–516
21. Konishi F, Muto T, Takahashi H, Itoh K, Kanazawa K, Morioka Y (1985) Transrectal ultrasonography for the assessment of invasion of rectal carcinoma. Dis Colon Rectum 28:889–894
22. Lise M, Gerard A, Nitti D, Zane D, Buyse M, Duez N, Arnaud JP (1987) Adjuvant therapy for colorectal cancer: the EORTC experience and a review of the literature. Dis Colon Rectum 30:847–854
23. Mason AY (1976) Rectal cancer: the spectrum of selective surgery. Proc R Soc Med 69:237–244
24. MRC Working Party (1984) The evaluation of low dose preoperative x-ray therapy in the management of operable rectal cancer: results of a randomly controlled trial. Br J Surg 71:21–25
25. Nicholls RJ, Mason AY, Morson BC, Dixon AK, Fry IK (1982) The clinical staging of rectal cancer. Br J Surg 69:404–409
26. Nicholls RJ, Galloway DJ, Mason AY, Boyle P (1985) Clinical local staging of rectal cancer. Br J Surg 72 (Suppl):51
27. Nigro ND, Vaitkevicius VK, Buroker T, Bradley GT, Considine B (1981) Combined therapy for cancer of anal canal. Dis Colon Rectum 24:73–75
28. Philipps RKS, Hittinger R, Blesovsky FJS, Fielding LP (1984) Local recurrence following "curative" surgery for large bowel cancer. II. The rectum and rectosigmoid. Br J Surg 71:17–20
29. Rifkin M, Marks G (1985) Transrectal US as an adjunct in the diagnosis of rectal and extrarectal tumors. Radiology 157:499–502
30. Rifkin MD, Wechsler RJ (1986) A comparison of computed tomography and endorectal ultrasound in staging rectal cancer. Int J Colorect Dis 1:219–223
31. Rifkin MD, McGlynn ET, Marks G (1986) Endorectal sonographic prospective staging of rectal cancer. Scand J Gastroenterol 21 (Suppl 123) 99–103
32. Romano G, De Rosa P, Vallone G, Rotondo A, Grassi R, Santiangelo ML (1985) Intrarectal ultrasound and computed tomography in the pre- and post-operative assessment of patients with rectal carcinoma. Br J Surg (Suppl) 72:117–119
33. Ruf G, Hauenstein KH, Rudolf M, Schöffel U, Lausen U, Wimmer B (1986) Präoperatives Staging des Rektumkarzinoms mit der Computertomographie. Langenbecks Arch Chir 368:3–11
34. Ruff CC, Dockerty MB, Fricke RE, Wangh JM (1961) Preoperative radiation therapy for adenocarcinoma of rectum and rectosigmoid. Surg Gynecol Obstet 112:715–723
35. Saitoh N, Okui K, Sarashina H, Suzuki M, Arai T, Nunomura M (1986) Evaluation of echographic diagnosis of rectal cancer using interrectal ultrasonic examination. Dis Colon Rectum 29:234–242
36. Schiessel R, Wunderlich M, Herbst F (1986) Local recurrence of colorectal cancer: effect of early detection and aggressive surgery. Br J Surg 73:342–344

37. Spiessl B, Hermanek P, Scheibe O, Wagner G (eds) (1985) UICC TNM atlas, 2nd edn. Springer, Berlin Heidelberg New York
38. Thoeni RF, Moss AA, Schneyder P, Margulis AR (1981) Detection and staging of primary rectal and rectosigmoid cancer by computed tomography. Radiology 141:135–138
39. Thompson WM, Kalvorsen RA (1987) Computed tomographic staging of gastrointestinal malignancies. Part II. The small bowel, colon and rectum. J Invest Radiol 22(2): 96–105
40. Tio TL, Tytgat GNJ (1986) Endoscopic ultrasonography in analysing peri-intestinal lymph node abnormality. Scand J Gastroenterol 21 (Suppl 123):158–163
41. Tio TL, den Hartog Jager FCA, Tytgat GNJ (1986) Endoscopic ultrasonography of non-Hodgkin lymphoma of the stomach. Gastroenterology 91:401–408
42. van Waes PFGM, Koehler PR, Feldberg MAM (1983) Management of rectal carcinoma: impact of computed tomography. Am J Radiol 140:1137–1142
43. Ward MWN, Romano G, Nicholls RJ (1986) The surgical treatment of anorectal malignant melanoma. Br J Surg 73:68–69
44. Watanabe H, Ieari D, Ianahashi Y, Harada K, Saitoh M (1975) Transrectal ultrasonotomography of the prostate. J Urol (Paris) 114:734–739
45. Wild JJ, Reid JM (1956) Diagnostic use of ultrasound. Br J Phys Med 11:248–264
46. Yamashita Y, Machi I, Shirouzu K, Morotomi T, Isomoto H, Kakegawa T (1988) Evaluation of endorectal ultrasound for the assessment of wall invasion of rectal cancer. Dis Colon Rectum 31:617–623
47. Zaunbauer W, Haertel M, Fuchs WA (1981) Computed tomography in carcinoma of the rectum. Gastrointest Radiol 6:79–84
48. Zheng GL, Eddleston B, Schofield PF, Johnson RJM, James RD (1984) Computed tomographic scanning in rectal carcinoma. Proc R Soc Med 77:915–920

5 Endosonography of the Prostate and Associated Structures

W. H. Cooner

The development of an effective method for imaging the prostate has been a long-sought goal. Clinical assessment of the gland has relied historically upon digital rectal examination and cystoscopy. With the advent of transrectal endosonography, areas of the prostate and associated structures which previously were inaccessible to examination are now seen with unprecedented clarity.

5.1 History

Early efforts at visualization of the prostate with abdominal probes, utilizing the bladder as an acoustic window, were limited in their ability to discern internal prostatic architecture, principally because of the low frequency of the transducers which must be used for that application. In the 1950s, Wild and Reid [18] stimulated interest in the possibility of sonographic examination of the prostate with a transducer inserted into the rectum. While this early instrumentation did not provide images of the prostate which were suitable for clinical application, further refinements were to come.

In 1976 Watanabe et al. [17] reported the use of a chair-type scanner which permitted the prostate to be seen in transaxial views at 5-mm intervals. The prostate was displayed in bistable imaging until the application of gray-scale imaging to transrectal ultrasonography by Harada et al. in 1979 [1]. This development greatly improved the visualization of intraprostatic structures. The ensuing years have brought about technical refinements which permit detailed study of the prostate and its associated structures in virtually any plane.

5.2 Equipment

Transducer frequencies between about 5.5 MHz and 7.5 MHz provide good images of the prostate. Most instruments utilize frequencies in the upper part of that range, thus providing satisfactory penetration of the gland and better resolution of reflectors along the axis of the sound wave than would be possible with transducers of lower frequency.

Various transducer configurations permit the prostate to be seen transaxially, longitudinally, and, with some equipment, in an infinite number of planes between those two projections. The preferred configuration is largely a matter of user preference, although each has some advantages.

5.2.1 Orientation

The transaxial image is usually oriented with the right side of the prostate displayed on the viewer's left and the rectum at the bottom of the screen (Fig. 5.1). Longitudinal views are usually shown with the prostate base on the viewer's left and the rectum at the bottom of the screen (Fig. 5.2). While some equipment provides different orientation, this matters little unless one is using several different machines, in which case the correct orientation must be kept in mind in order to avoid confusion.

5.2.2 Transaxial Scanning

Examination of the gland in horizontal planes can be accomplished using either a rotary or a sector scanner.

Rotary scanners usually process 360° of the image. However, some instruments process only a portion of the image, with the result that the image looks much like a sector scan. In either instance, the image is sufficiently wide to permit simultaneous viewing of both sides of all except unusually large glands, a capability which is particularly helpful in comparing one side with the other when the examiner is faced with a subtle area of suspicion. In addition, the slow rotation of the radial transducer accommodates a high number of scan lines per degree of rotation, thereby providing enhanced spatial resolution. While temporal resolution is poor with a radial probe, this is of no consequence, since the prostate is a still organ. Blood flow cannot be seen because of the slow sweep speed, but any area in question can be evaluated subsequently with a longitudinal probe, which uses a more rapid sweep speed. A minor disadvantage of the rotary

5.1
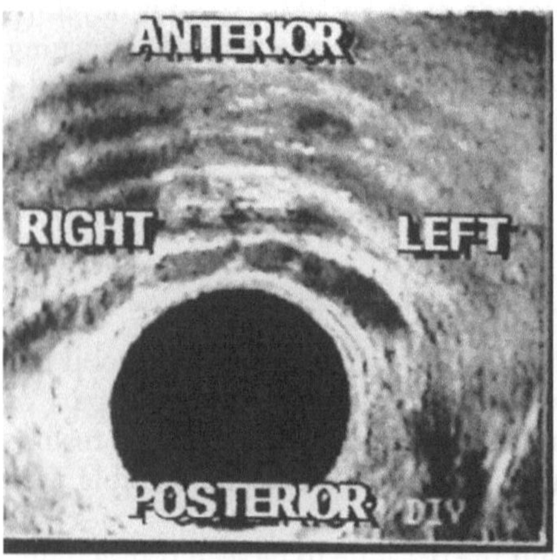

Fig. 5.1. Transaxial orientation

5.2
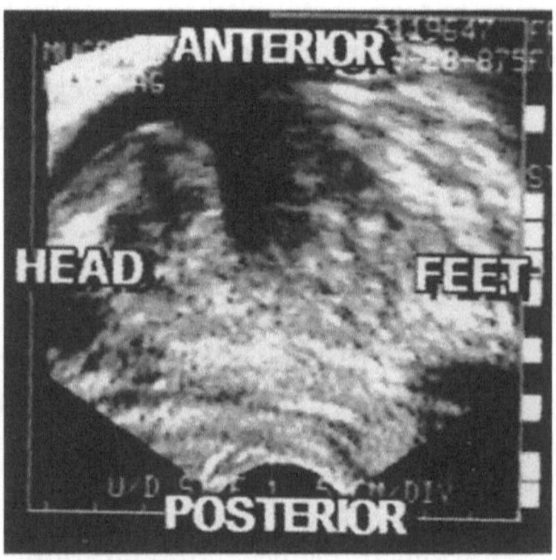

Fig. 5.2. Longitudinal orientation

scanner is the necessity that it be moved along the cephalocaudad extent of the prostate very slowly in order that portions of the gland not be skipped between the slow sweeps of the transducer.

Sector scanners produce a wedge-shaped image, either by the physical rotation or rocking of a single transducer through the sector (a mechanical scanner), or by the sequential electronic firing of individual transducers which are adjacent in a line or a curve (phased array). There appears to be little difference in image quality between the two. Mechanical scanners tend to be somewhat less expensive than phased array scanners, and, although they are proving to be quite durable, they may be less so than phased array scanners, which have no moving parts.

An advantage of the sector scanner is its ability to detect the flow of blood within vessels, a marginal help in evaluation of some questionable hypoechoic areas. The addition of Doppler scanning, available with some equipment, also assists in determining whether a suspicious area is vascular. An inherent disadvantage of sector scanners when used for transaxial viewing is that the sector angle may be so narrow as to preclude simultaneous viewing of both sides of the prostate. Often the gland can be elevated into a wider part of the sector, but care must be taken to assure that the gland remains within the focal range of the transducer. With some phased array sector scanners, the focal range is variable to a minor degree.

5.2.3 Longitudinal Scanning

The only true sagittal plane seen longitudinally is the midsagittal plane. As scanning proceeds laterally through the gland, the view becomes progressively more frontal if the probe is rotated on its axis within the rectum, or more nearly transaxial if the probe is levered using the anus as a fulcrum. Longitudinal scanning is performed either with a sector scanner or with a linear array scanner.

Sector scanners for longitudinal viewing share the same characteristics as those used for transaxial scanning. The inability to see seminal vesicles and prostate simultaneously with the apex of the gland is of no importance, since the two areas, being different in appearance, do not require simultaneous comparison. If the prostate is large, it may be necessary to scan in two segments, visualizing first the cephalad areas and then the caudad areas.

Linear array scanners provide a square or rectangular view of the prostate. An advantage of the linear array scanner is that the scanning lines are separated by equal distances in both the near and far fields. This affords slightly better resolution in the far part of the focal zone than is possible with a sector scanner, in which the lines at a distance from the transducer are farther apart than they are in the near field.

5.2.4 Probe Configuration

In some equipment used for endorectal sonography of the prostate, independent probes are used for viewing each plane, transaxial and longitudinal. In others, one probe bears two transducer configurations which permit both views to be seen without having to change probes. Still others use a transducer which can be rotated mechanically, thus affording views of the prostate in multiple planes from transaxial to longitudinal. In yet another instance, a sector scanner is used whose center of sweep is directly at the end of the probe, allowing transaxiofrontal and longitudinal views. The choice of transducer placement within the probe is largely a matter of personal preference, but the relative merits of transducer configuration must be kept in mind when making a choice of equipment.

Independent probes are designed to show the prostate in one view only, either transaxial or longitudinal. For thorough evaluation the gland must be examined in both planes, necessitating the sequential insertion of two probes. The minor inconvenience of using two probes is offset by the ease of manipulation and high image quality obtainable from an instrument designed for one specific purpose.

Biplane probes bear two sets of transducers (sector/sector, sector/linear array), which permit switching from a transaxial to a longitudinal plane without changing probes. This may be more a theoretical than a real advantage, since the transducers are not centered on a common line and require physical realignment of the probe each time a switch is made. Thus, it is not possible to see a suspicious area in bothplanes by rapidly switching back and forth.

A variant of the biplane probe is one which utilizes one mechanical transducer which is swept radially, but with limited sector processing, for the transaxial view, and then sweeps the same transducer at a right angle through a sector for the longitudinal view. In this configuration, the image can be centered along a line common to both viewing planes.

Some instruments utilizing biplane probes require employment of a separate probe for biopsy.

Multiplane probes which utilize mechanical rotation of a sector transducer in its horizontal plane allow visualization of an area through an infinite number of planes which rotate around a central axis. Instruments of this type do permit biopsy to be performed without the need for change to a separate probe.

In yet another form, multiplane viewing is possible by the axial rotation of a probe which bears an end-firing transducer at its tip. This probe does provide true longitudinal views of the prostate, but the transverse view varies from a nearly frontal one at the prostate base to a nearly transaxial view at the apex. The lack of ability to visualize the gland in a true transaxial view requires minor reorientation of the examiner's anatomical thinking.

5.3 Anatomy

Descriptions of intraprostatic anatomy have been varied and confusing. Much of the problem has arisen from the designation of lobes of the prostate based upon gross anatomical examination of glands in which there is benign hyperplasia. Clarification of the anatomy of normal and hyperplastic glands by McNeal [5, 6] has led to a better understanding of this subject, a particularly valuable contribution to the subject in view of the clarity with which we can now see the inner structure of the prostate sonographically.

McNeal utilizes as an anatomical reference point the urethra, which makes a 35° angle just cephalad to the verumontanum. He has described zonal anatomy as follows:

Nonglandular
Fibromuscular zone: fibrous tissue and smooth and skeletal muscle.

Glandular
Peripheral zone: ducts drain into prostatic urethra distal to verumontanum;
Central zone: ducts drain into verumontanum around urethral opening of ejaculatory ducts;
Transition zone: ducts drain into prostatic urethra proximal to verumontanum;
Periurethral glands: short ducts drain directly into urethra.

All of these zones can be seen sonographically.

5.4 Scanning Technique

The technique of scanning the prostate and adjacent structures may vary among examiners, but it is important that each examiner establish an examination sequence which seems best to him or her and to utilize it in a standardized manner. In our clinic, transaxial scanning begins superior to the seminal vesicles and progresses slowly toward the prostate apex. Longitudinal scanning begins at the midsagittal plane, with subsequent angling of the probe laterally first to the right lateral extremity of the gland, and then back through the midsagittal plane to the left extremity of the gland. Thorough attention is given to each zone of the prostate and to all associated structures which are within the focal range of the transducer.

Documentation is necessary, including appropriate marks to indicate location in the third, "invisible" plane of both transaxial and longitudinal views of the examination. Video-taping is strongly recommended, since static views do not allow the examiner to evaluate immediately adjacent planes. Additional documentation of still images is helpful, however, and this may be done with thermal prints, multiformat camera recording, or by the storage of digitized images on optical discs. The latter method is particularly useful and convenient, since the image is captured without degradation in quality and is subsequently transferrable to a thermal printer if desired.

5.5 Echogenicity of Prostate Zones

In order that there be a reference standard for the description of the amplitude of sound as reflected by the various zones of the prostate, isoechoic is the term which has been assigned arbitrarily to the appearance of the peripheral zone. Areas from which sound is reflected more intensely are hyperechoic, while those exhibiting less reflectivity than the peripheral zone are termed hypoechoic. Struc-

Table 5.1. Echogenicity of sonographically visible structures

Echogenicity	Structures
Isoechoic:	Peripheral zone
Hypoechoic:	Transition zone
	Fibromuscular zone
	Seminal vesicles
	Vasa deferentia
	Ejaculatory ducts
	Muscle
	Vascular structures
Hyperechoic:	Central zone
	Concretions
	Fat
Anechoic:	Cysts

tures from which there is no sound reflection are said to be anechoic. The reflectivity of areas visualized on transrectal ultrasonography is indicated in Table 5.1.

5.6 Prostate Cancer

In the early period of investigation of prostate ultrasonography, carcinoma was variously described as being hypoechoic, hyperechoic, isoechoic, or of mixed echogenicity [9, 14]. Uncertainty regarding the appearance of neoplasia led to considerable doubt as to whether this modality would ever be clinically useful. With improvement in equipment, especially the development of probes which permit visualization of the prostate in more than one plane and transducers whose frequencies are optimal for this application, there is now better awareness of the sonographic characteristics of prostate cancer.

Hypoechoicism as the hallmark of early prostate cancer has been established by Lee et al. [2], who have shown that in the overwhelming majority of instances prostate cancer is less echogenic than the surrounding tissue in which it develops (Fig. 5.3). Echogenicity has been reported to change in some instances as lesions age and involve adjacent areas of normal or hyperplastic prostatic tissue, with lesions becoming isoechoic, hyperechoic, or of mixed echogenicity [10, 12]. Advanced lesions are often difficult to detect by sonography, but the most reliable sign of advanced carcinoma is mixed echogenicity with loss of internal glandular architecture (Fig. 5.4). Secondary signs of cancer include asymmetry (Fig. 5.5 a) and loss of prostate boundary (Fig. 5.5 b).

The predilection for the development of carcinoma in the various zones of the prostate has been described by McNeal [6]. About 70% of neoplasias are believed to arise in the peripheral zone, and it is this zone which best lends itself to sonographic study. Less than 10% of cancers are thought to arise in the central zone, an area which also is well visualized sonographically. There is difficulty in

5.3

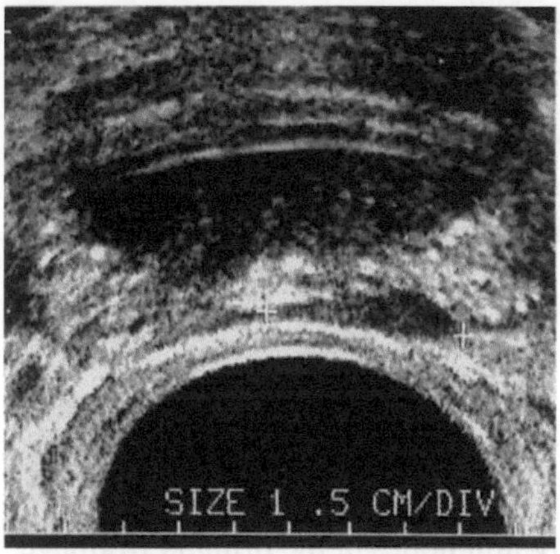

5.4

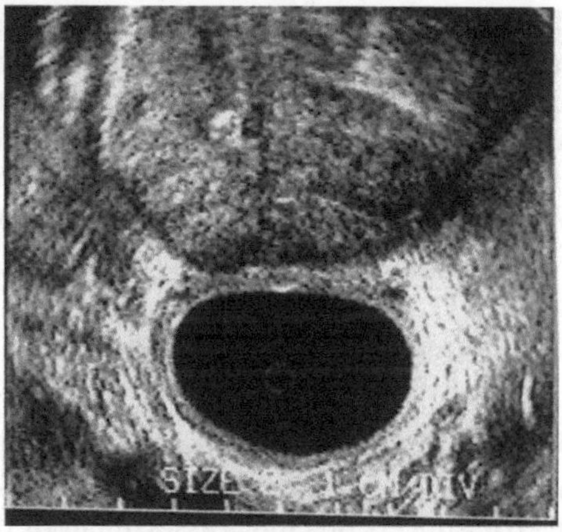

.5 a

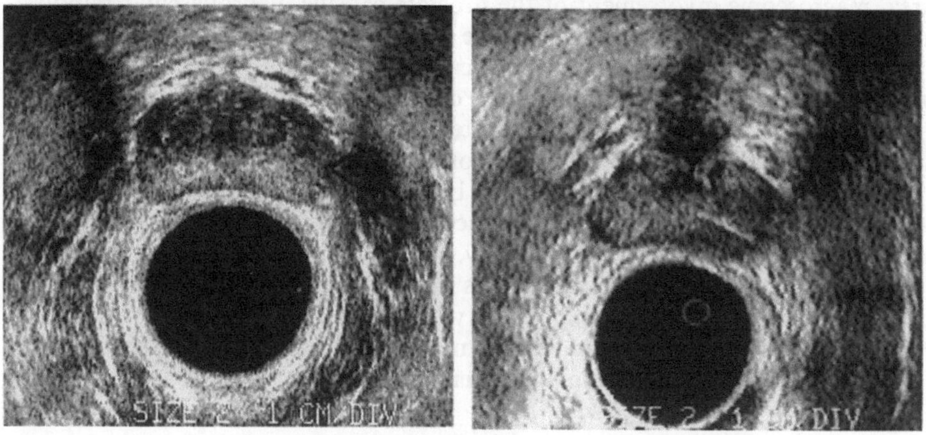

5.5 b

Fig. 5.3. Transaxial sonogram showing hypoechoic carcinoma (*between cursors*)

Fig. 5.4. Transaxial sonogram showing advanced carcinoma with loss of internal architecture

Fig. 5.5. a Transaxial sonogram showing asymmetry of the prostate due to carcinoma of mixed echogenicity in left posterior peripheral zone. **b** Transaxial sonogram showing loss of definition of left prostate boundary due to carcinoma which extends beyond the confines of the gland

sonographic visualization of early cancer in the transition zone, the apparent site of origin of malignancy in about 20% of instances. The reasons for this are several. Since the transition zone is sonographically slightly hypoechoic, early cancer may be masked by inability to visualize any disparity as compared to the surrounding hyperplastic tissue in the same zone. Additionally, if the cancer is in the anterior part of a very large hyperplastic transition zone, it may be more difficult to appreciate because it lies beyond the focal range of the transducer. Anterior lesions may be somewhat more difficult to see with sector scanners beause of the lower density of scanning lines as the examined area recedes from the transducer. Difficulty in the detection of cancer in the anterior part of the gland is somewhat disturbing in view of recent information indicating that about half of all prostate cancers develop in the anterior half of the gland [6]. While some tumors will be found sonographically in all areas of the gland which are subject to neoplastic change, the present stage of equipment development and image processing seem to afford the greatest chance of detecting early lesions which have developed in the central and peripheral zones.

5.7 Staging of Prostate Cancer

Prostate ultrasonography is often helpful in assessing the possible spread of prostate cancer beyond the confines of the gland. While the limited focal range of the transducers precludes assessment of the lymph nodes in the primary drainage area, macroscopic involvement of the prostate capsule, neurovascular bundles, and seminal vesicles is often visible. The absence of detectable microscopic involvement must not be construed as indicating that the disease is confined to the gland, however, since microscopic disease cannot be detected by this technique.

Seminal vesicle involvement is suggested by disparity in the appearance of the two vesicles in a given patient. It is far more important to compare the vesicles in the same patient than among patients, because of the marked interindividual variation in the structure and the difference in appearance between vesicles which are fluid-laden and those which are empty.

Involvement by tumor usually gives the seminal vesicle a more solid appearance than that of the normal vesicle, which has a more vacuolar appearance. Marked disparity in size of the vesicles may indicate macroscopic involvement (Fig. 5.6). Often an actual mass may be seen (Fig. 5.7).

5.6 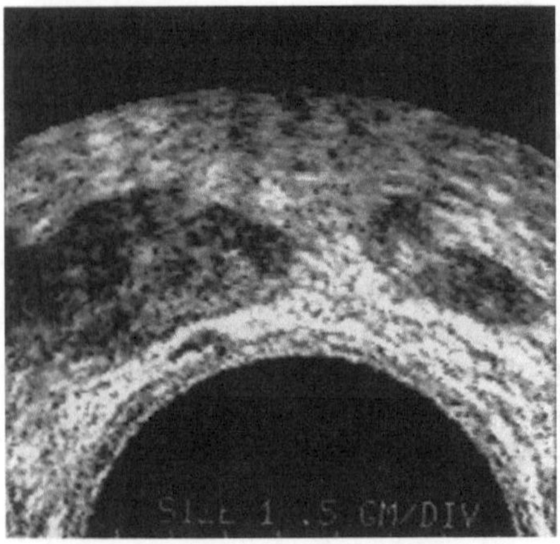

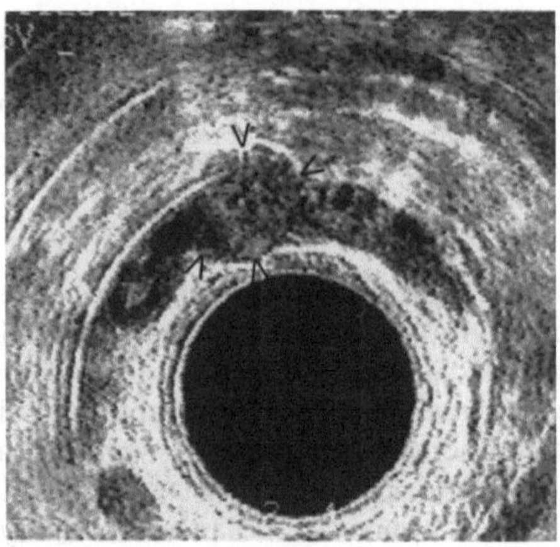 5.7

Fig. 5.6. Disparity in seminal vesicle size due to carcinoma in the right vesicle

Fig. 5.7. Mass effect due to carcinoma in right seminal vesicle (*between cursors*)

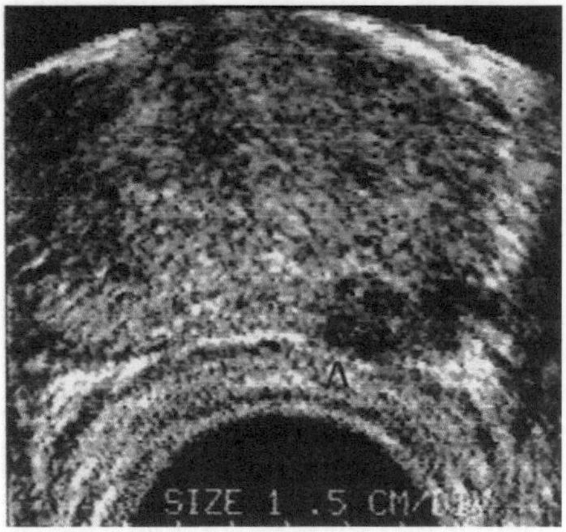

Fig. 5.8. Transaxial view showing disruption of prostate boundary posteriorly due to capsular penetration by carcinoma in left posterior peripheral zone (V)

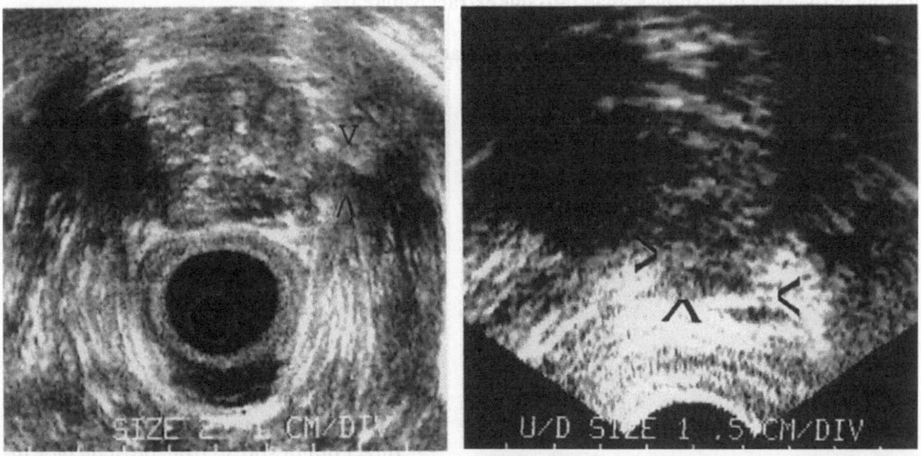

a b

Fig. 5.9.a Transaxial view showing tumor penetration into left neurovascular bundle (V). **b** Longitudinal view showing tumor penetration lateral to the prostate in the neurovascular bundle (V)

Tumor extension into the prostatic capsule is suggested by disruption or irregularity at the prostate boundary (Fig. 5.8). While the true capsule of the prostate is not often clearly discernible, the interface between the prostate and the surrounding fat can be seen clearly. Posteriorly, the boundary is easily identifiable as the fifth layer of the rectum, a hyperechoic band composed of sound reflection from the sonographic interface between the muscularis propria of the rectum and the adjacent fat, and the pararectal fat itself. Care must be taken not to ascribe disruption absolutely to tumor involvement because of the displacement of fat caught between a firm prostate tumor and the balloon inflated around the transducer in the rectum. Partial deflation of the balloon will often allow the fat to return to this area, thus avoiding a false determination of capsular involvement at that point.

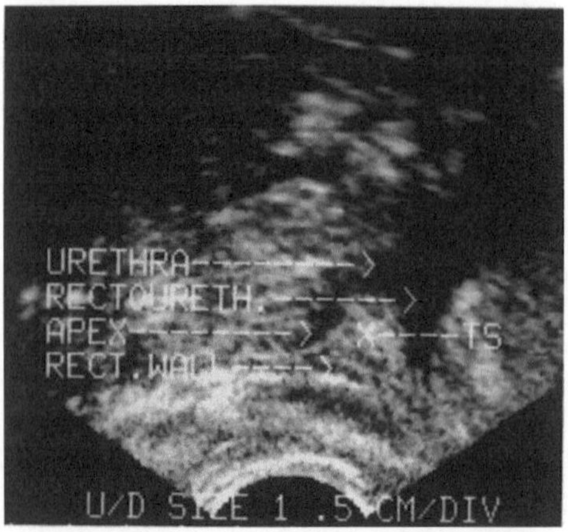

5.10

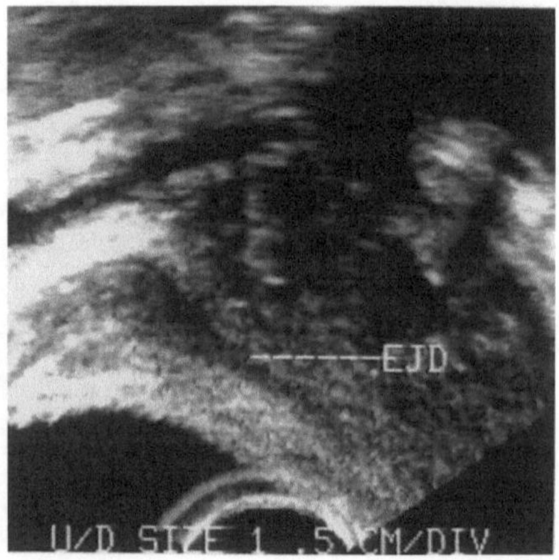

5.11

Fig. 5.10. Longitudinal view showing trapezoid space adjacent to prostatic apex. Carcinoma arising in the apex may show spread into this extracapsular area

Fig. 5.11. Longitudinal view showing course of ejaculatory duct through central zone of prostate

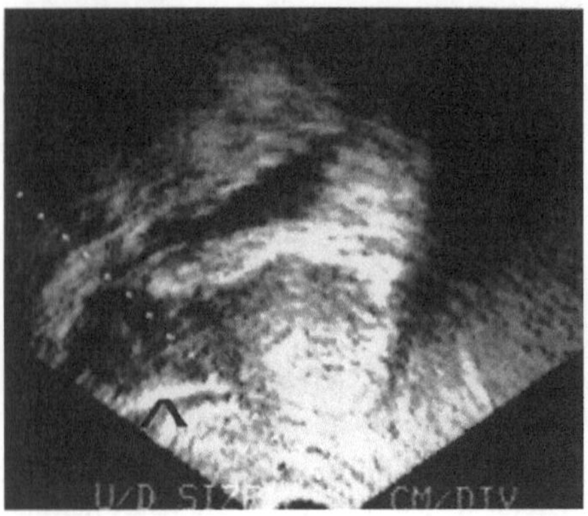

Fig. 5.12. Longitudinal view showing direct tumor spread from prostate base into seminal vesicle, with obliteration of fat between the two structures (V)

Tumor spread into the neurovascular bundles posteriolateral to the prostate is often visible. The appearance is that of direct continuity of tumor beyond the prostate boundary and can be appreciated on either the transaxial (Fig. 5.9 a) or longitudinal view (Fig. 5.9 b).

Tumor extension at the apex may be suspected sonographically. On midsagittal longitudinal views of the gland, a trapezoid space [4] is visible, the boundaries of which are the urethra anteriorly, the rectum posteriorly, the prostatic apex cephalad, and the rectourethral muscle caudad (Fig. 5.10). Biopsy of this space can be accomplished easily under sonographic guidance for confirmation of suspected involvement of this extraprostatic area by apical tumor.

Extraprostatic tumor spread may also occur in the area around the ejaculatory ducts as they course through the central zone from the seminal vesicles to the verumontanum. The ducts are surrounded by extraprostatic tissue which invaginates along the cephalad portion of the ducts for a variable distance into the prostate. This is termed by Lee [4] the invaginated extraprostatic space (IES). Obliteration of this space may occur if there is carcinoma in the ejaculatory duct region. This can be detected sonographically on longitudinal views as loss of the normal hypoechogenicity of the ejaculatory ducts as they course through the central zone of the prostate (Fig. 5.11).

Another route by which carcinoma may spread is directly from the base of the prostate into the seminal vesicles. In this circumstance, there is loss of the hyperechoic fat between the two structures. This is readily appreciated on comparison of the two sides on transaxial scanning, and may be seen as loss of the fat layer between the structures on the longitudinal view (Fig. 5.12). This phenomenon has been termed by Scardino the "adhesion sign" [13].

5.8 Volumetrics

There is increasing awareness of the relationship between the volume of prostate cancer and its grade and stage [7]. Estimation of cancer volume is possible by sonography, using one of several methods. The most accurate for relatively small lesions is measurement of its three dimensions. Width and height are obtained from the transaxial view (Fig. 5.13 a, b), and length is taken from the longitudinal view (Fig. 5.13 c). These measurements are used to calculate the volume mathematically, using any of several formulae. Two often employed are:

$$V = {}^{4}/_{3} \times \pi \times r^{3}$$

where V = volume and r = radius, and

$$V = 0.5(L \times W \times H)$$

where V = volume, L = length, W = width, and H = height. This second formula is actually a derivative of the first.

Since the specific gravity of prostate tissue is about 1.050, volume in cubic centimeters and weight in grams are approximately equivalent [16].

Volume determination also may be performed by planimetry using equipment which has accessories designed to provide this function (Fig. 5.14). Area measurements are made transaxially at predetermined intervals, and volume calculation is carried out automatically within the instrument. When dealing with small lesions, the closer the interval between area measurements the more accurate is the volume determination. However, measurements made with very small increments require an inordinate amount of time for performance. Sections made at greater intervals permit more rapid volume determinations to be done, but have the disadvantage of decreased accuracy.

A third method of volume calculation permitted by some equipment is elliptical voluming, a method which determines the volume of an ellipsoid by measurement of an area midway between its poles (Fig. 5.15). In this method, an assumption is made that the lesion to be measured is ellipsoidal in shape. Of course, this is rarely the case with prostate cancer.

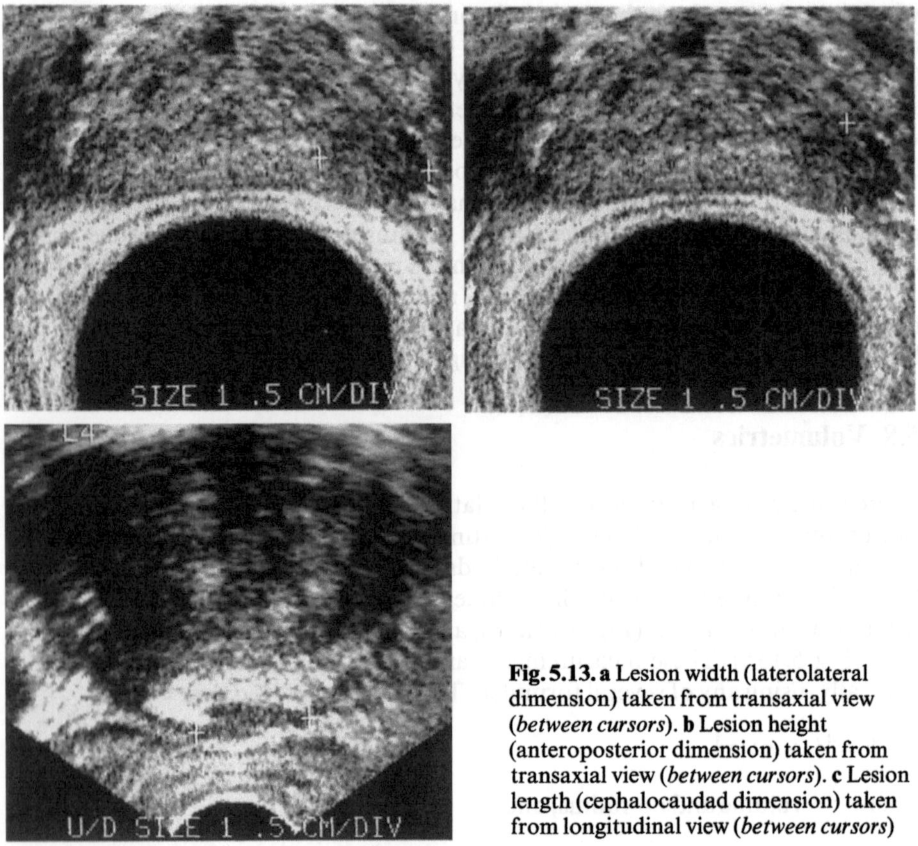

a b c

Fig. 5.13. a Lesion width (laterolateral dimension) taken from transaxial view (*between cursors*). **b** Lesion height (anteroposterior dimension) taken from transaxial view (*between cursors*). **c** Lesion length (cephalocaudad dimension) taken from longitudinal view (*between cursors*)

5.14
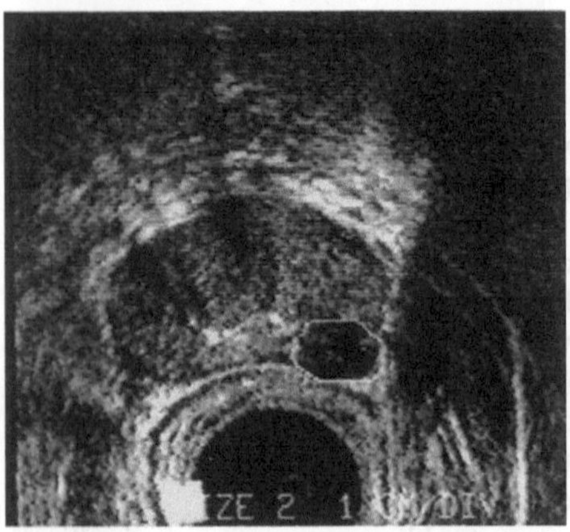

5.15
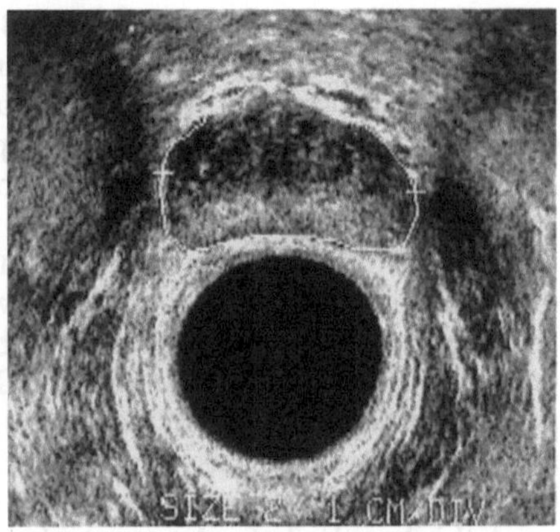

Fig. 5.14. Measurement of the volume of a lesion in the left posterior peripheral zone by planimetry. Areas of cross section are measured at predetermined cephalocaudad intervals

Fig. 5.15. Determination of the volume of the prostate elliptically on the basis of a cross section made about halfway between the base and apex of the gland

Lesions which are felt on digital rectal examination are almost always found on sonography to be larger than suspected. Pathologic examination always shows the lesions to be larger again than was suspected sonographically, since microscopic disease is not seen by sonography. It is important to realize that sonographically determined volume is always less than the true volume of the lesion.

5.9 Biopsy

Many prostate cancers are easily seen sonographically. However, others are quite subtle and may be suspected largely because the examiner has felt something suspicious in the same area. It is essential that the physician perform a digital rectal examination prior to sonography in order that he may compare the tactile examination with the sonogram and to ensure that there is no physical abnormality which would preclude the safe insertion of a probe.

The diagnosis of prostate cancer relies upon tissue identification, and an effective technique for biopsy is a necessity. Biopsy under ultrasonic guidance can be done easily, rapidly, reasonably innocuously, and with increased accuracy as compared with biopsy under tactile guidance. Most equipment permits biopsy to be done either transperineally or transrectally.

Transperineal biopsy requires the use of a needle guide which is attached to the probe in such a manner that the needle enters the perineum parallel to the long axis of the probe. When this is done with a transducer which produces a transaxial image, the needle is not seen until it penetrates the plane of the lesion. If the procedure is done with a longitudinal transducer, the progress of the needle can be monitored as it enters the prostate and approaches the area of suspicion. Generous infiltration of a local anesthetic agent is required into the skin, subcutaneous tissue, perineum, and prostatic capsule. In view of the depth of tissue which the needle must traverse transperineally, it may veer off the expected trajectory if a needle of small caliber is used. It is helpful to use a larger needle as a stabilizer. One technique is that of advancing a 14-gauge Tru-Cut needle into the lesion, withdrawing it slightly until it is no longer visible in the transaxial plane, removing the inner cutting element, and then passing the biopsy needle through the Tru-Cut sheath into the lesion.

Transrectal needle biopsy can be accomplished without sedation or anesthesia of any kind. This technique requires the use of a longitudinal transducer. Very accurate sampling of lesions within the prostate and seminal vesicles is possible via the transrectal route.

Administration of prophylactics antibiotics prior to biopsy, while not of proven efficacy, is prudent in view of the possible induction of septicemia by the needle puncture. This would seem to be particularly necessary if the biopsy is performed by the transrectal route.

A variety of needles for obtaining tissue are available. If aspiration of material for cytologic examination is desired, several satisfactory needles, such as the Lee-Ray and the Chiba, are available. For core biopsy, tissue may be obtained with a suction type needle, such as the Menghini. A particularly useful

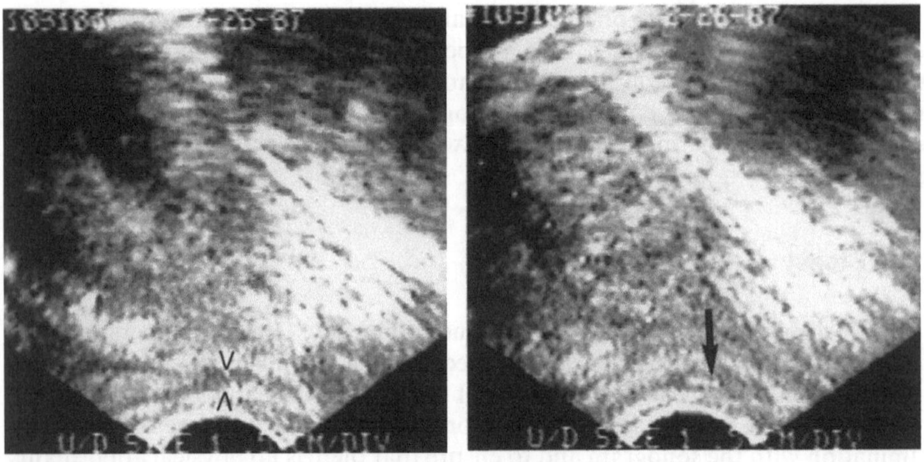

a b

Fig. 5.16. a Longitudinal view showing a carcinoma which measures only 3 mm anteroposteriorly (*between cursors*). **b** Longitudinal view showing needle tip within carcinoma (↓)

system is the Biopty needle, which permits the obtaining of cores nearly painlessly. The tissue obtained is of excellent quality, there being little crush artifact at the specimen edges due to the rapidity with which the tissue within the needle notch is severed by the rapidly advancing cutting sheath.

Biopsy of the seminal vesicles is easily accomplished, especially via the transrectal route. Since the seminal vesicles contain many lacunae, it is often helpful to obtain tissue from them with an aspiration type of core needle, since more tissue can be stacked within the needle than is possible with the Biopty system.

It has been suggested that sonographically guided biopsy offers no advantage over tactilely guided biopsy [8]. It is becoming clear, however, that especially with small lesions greater accuracy is possible with biopsy performed under sonographic guidance than from that performed under digital control (Fig. 5.16a, b) [3, 11, 15]. Of course, sonographic guidance is a necessity for biopsy of lesions which are visible sonographically, but which are not palpable.

The obtaining of negative tissue at biopsy of a palpable lesion has always presented a dilemma for the physician. It has been thought that this resulted from the bypassing of the suspicious area with the needle. A more likely explanation, however, is that the lesion is penetrated too deeply under tactile guidance. Many early lesions are quite thin and are located adjacent to the prostatic capsule. As the needle approaches the prostatic capsule, the capsule "tents up". When the needle finally penetrates the capsule, the latter springs back down and the tissue is taken from too deep a site, often from the transition zone.

5.10 Other Conditions

Although the diagnosis of prostatic carcinoma has become the focus of ultrasonography of the prostate and the seminal vesicles, other conditions lend themselves well to study by this method.

5.17
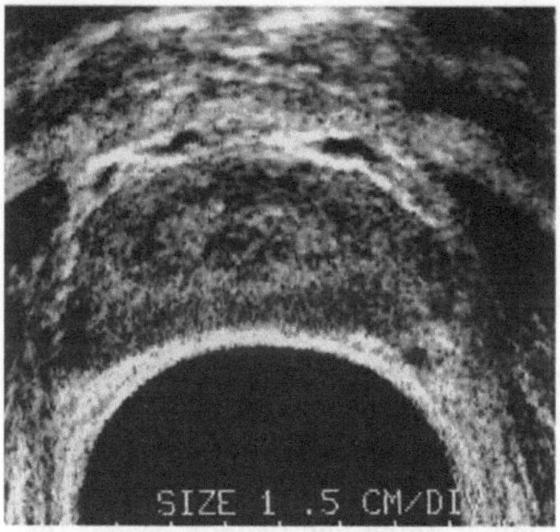

5.18
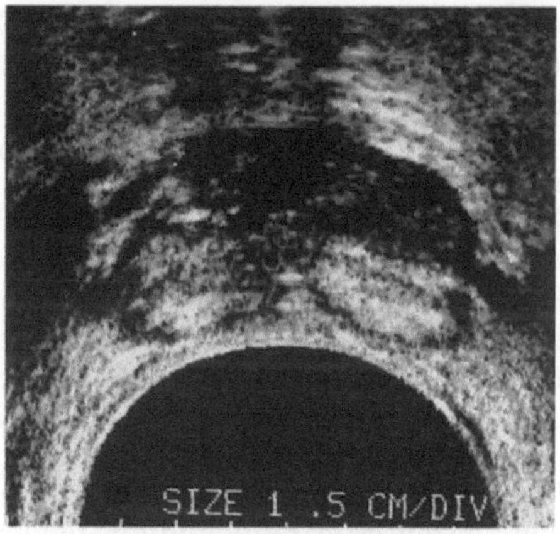

5.19
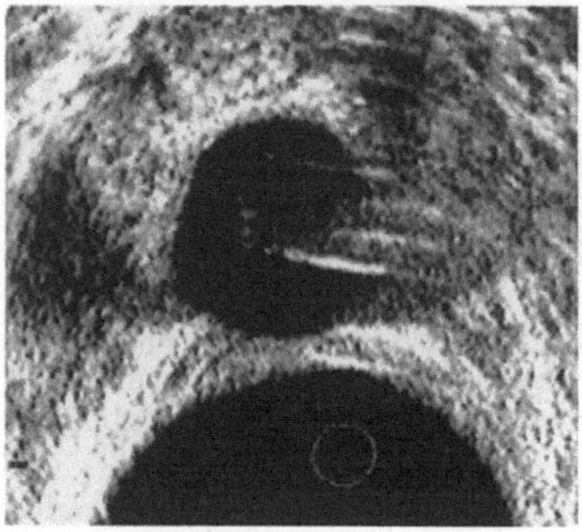

5.20
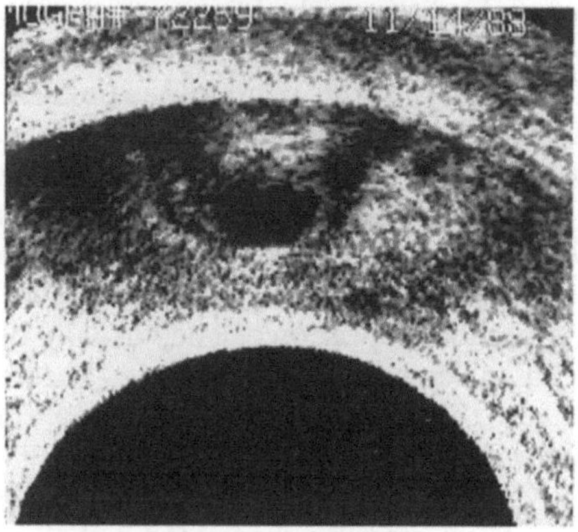

Fig. 5.17. Acute prostatitis showing diffuse mottling throughout peripheral zone

Fig. 5.18. Transaxial view showing areas of calcification throughout prostate, especially in peripheral zone

Fig. 5.19. Transaxial view showing large ejaculatory duct cyst near base of prostate

Fig. 5.20. Transaxial view of a Müllerian duct cyst in the midline at the verumontanum

5.10.1 Prostate

Acute prostatitis may appear in any portion of the gland, but it seems to have a tendency most often to involve the peripheral zone (Fig. 5.17). Characteristically the involved area is hypoechoic with indistinct margins, although diffuse mottling is often present. While acute prostatitis can look much like diffuse carcinoma, the latter is usually of somewhat mixed echogenicity by the time it reaches substantial size. Differentiation is also made easier by recognition of the clinical symptoms which accompany acute prostatitis.

Chronic prostatitis is markedly variable in appearance. It may resemble acute prostatitis, or, if long-standing, may show mixed echogenicity often interspersed with areas of microcalcification (Fig. 5.18). It has been our experience that hyperechoic areas confined strictly to the peripheral zone represent long-standing inflammatory areas rather than carcinoma.

Cysts of the prostate are commonly seen. Cystic disease displays the three signs of cystic changes seen anywhere in the body: (1) anechoic contents, (2) a sharply marginated distal wall, and (3) increased "through-transmission" of sound seen as a bright streak extending away from the distal margin of the cyst (Fig. 5.19). Cysts may occur anywhere in the prostate. Frequently they are seen in the ejaculatory duct and may be associated with concretions which lie adjacent to the ducts distal to the cyst. Müllerian duct cysts are occasionally encountered, and these lie just superior to or at the level of the verumontanum (Fig. 5.20). They are midline structures, a fact which helps to distinguish them from ejaculatory duct cysts. Although ejaculatory duct cysts may appear to be in the midline in many instances, careful study in the longitudinal plane will usually permit the two to be distinguished from one another. Cysts are also often seen near the apex of the gland, apparently representing dilation of ducts within this area (Fig. 5.21). The etiology of this condition is unknown. Often it appears in young men, beginning in about the third decade of life. Cysts located in this area frequently are palpable on rectal examination, particularly if they are fairly large.

Small cystic spaces within the transition zone are very common and likely represent dilated ducts within that portion of the prostate.

Prostatic abscesses are clearly visible by ultrasonography and exhibit a hypoechoic appearance. They usually display some internal echoes beause of the cellular elements within the fluid. The margins of abscess cavities are not as sharp as are those of a cyst. Increased "through-transmission" of sound is often present.

Concretions are often seen within the prostate. Para-ejaculatory duct calcifications may be associated with proximal ductal dilation if obstruction is present, but more often they are seen with no apparent effect on the ducts. The concretions may surround the duct (Fig. 5.22a), or they may be localized to only one margin of the duct, usually the posterior (Fig. 5.22b). Concretions within the ducts themselves are sometimes seen, most often within the course of the ducts through the verumontanum. Intraductal stones proximal to the verumontanum probably represent paraductal stones which have eroded into the ductal lumen (Fig. 5.23). If the duct containing the stone is dilated, migration of the stone can be demonstrated as the patient's position is changed.

Concretions are very often seen at the junction of the transition and peripheral zones. At other times, small concretions may be located within the periurethral glands, particularly those adjacent to the portion of the urethra proximal to the verumontanum. In this instance, they assume a linear appearance best seen in the longitudinal scan.

Although much has been written about sonographic visualization of corpora amylacea, these are recognized by the pathologist as microscopic structures which seemingly should not be well visualized by sonography. Stones characteristically produce shadowing, but not all concretions cast shadows. Therefore, use of the term "concretions" has been suggested by McNeal and would seem to encompass all such hyperechoic structures.

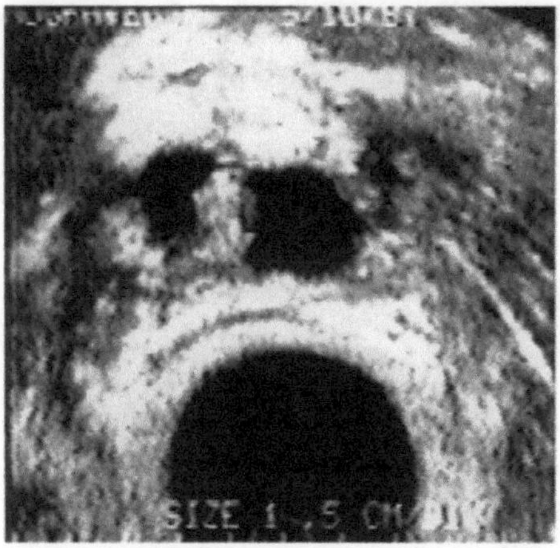

Fig. 5.21. Transaxial view showing multilocular cyst at prostate apex

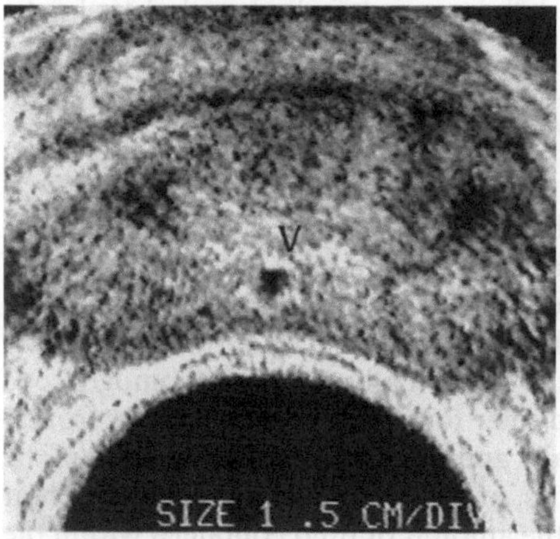

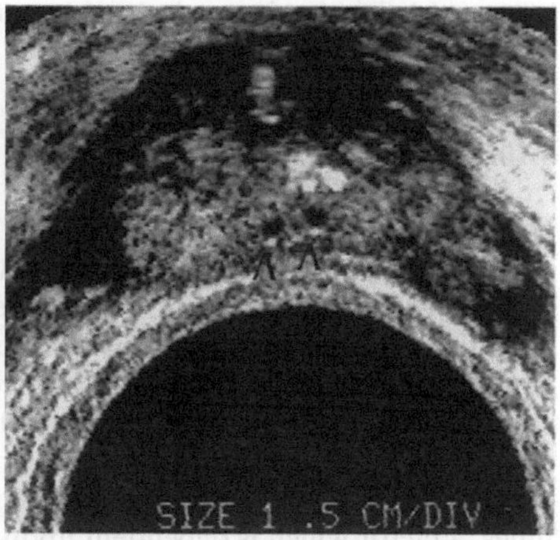

Fig. 5.22. a Transaxial view showing dilated right ejaculatory duct with circumferential concretions (V). **b** Transaxial view showing dilation of both ejaculatory ducts with small concretions just posteriorly (V)

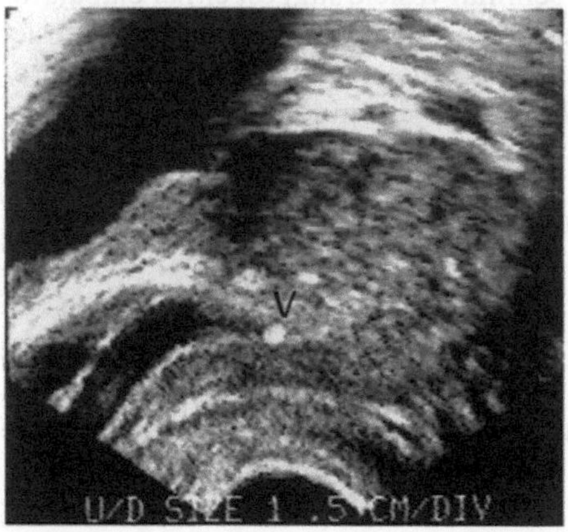

Fig. 5.23. Longitudinal view showing stone within ejaculatory duct (V)

a 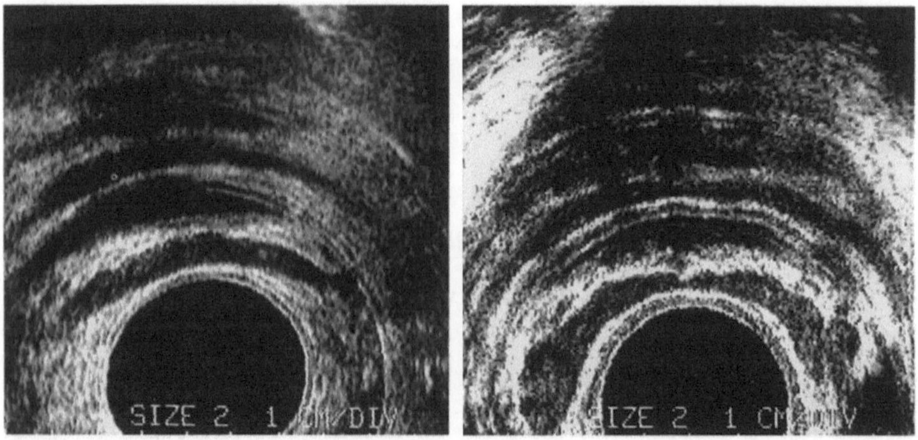 b

Fig. 5.24. a Transaxial view showing seminal vesicles which are situated in a nearly frontal plane. **b** Transaxial view showing seminal vesicles which lie more posteriorly along the lateral rectal wall

5.10.2 Seminal Vesicles

Until recently the seminal vesicles had been relatively inaccessible to examination, either physically or by means of various imaging modalities. A variety of imaging procedures now allows us to see these structures, and they are, indeed, exceptionally well seen by transrectal ultrasonography. The vesicles are highly variable in their anatomical appearance, but normally are fairly homogeneous and hypoechoic. Sometimes they lie with their long axes principally in a frontal plane (Fig. 5.24 a), or they may curl laterally and posteriorly along the sides of the rectum (Fig. 5.24 b). Vesicle size also varies, even in the same patient at different times, a factor which is dependent upon the amount of fluid contained within the structures. Because of these anatomical variations, it is much more important to compare vesicles for symmetry in the same patient than to compare vesicles among patients.

Dilated anechoic chambers within the seminal vesicle suggest either ejaculatory duct obstruction or vesicle abscess. These changes may involve the entire vesicle, or they may be focal. Aspiration of vesicle contents and injection of antimicrobial agents can be accomplished easily with sonographic guidance.

5.11 Clinical Indications for Performance of Transrectal Ultrasonography

As more experience is acquired with the use of transrectal ultrasonography, its use as a valuable adjunctive procedure in the management of a variety of clinical conditions is becoming apparent. In our hands, we have found it to provide unique information in a substantial number of instances and now utilize it in at least 18 situations:

1) Initially in patients aged 50 or above, along with rectal examination and determination of serum prostate specific antigen, for establishment of a baseline. Utilization of this tripartite approach has enabled us to identify a significant number of patients with cancer of the prostate at an early, potentially curable stage, when it was unsuspected by digital rectal examination alone.

2) In patients with an elevated prostate specific antigen.

3) In patients who have a palpable area of induration in the prostate.

4) In patients with a marginally suspicious area in the prostate which previously might have been followed up only by periodic rectal examination. Even following transurethral resection of the prostate (TURP), when slight irregularity in the feel of the gland might heretofore have been ascribed to "fibrosis," sonographic study will often show the irregularity actually to be due to cancer.

5) In patients who are to undergo TURP or prostatic enucleation for ostensibly benign disease. Previously, impalpable prostate cancer was found incidentally at the time of prostatectomy in about 20% of patients undergoing such procedures. Now we are often able to identify impalpable cancer prior to such surgery, permitting the correct procedure at the first surgical encounter and avoiding a needless interim operation.

6) Following the incidental discovery of prostate cancer at TURP or prostate enucleation. Postoperative blind biopsy or resectoscopic biopsy may fail to find residual cancer. Often it can be seen sonographically and confirmed by sonographically guided biopsy.

7) After obtaining negative tissue on tactilely guided biopsy. In the past, false-negative biopsies performed under tactile guidance have not been uncommon. By guiding the biopsy needle directly into a suspicious area under ultrasonic guidance, greater diagnostic accuracy is possible.

8) For the staging of prostate cancer preoperatively. Prostate cancer is often understaged clinically, leading unknowingly in some instances to inappropriate treatment. Prostate ultrasonography cannot show microscopic involvement of the prostatic capsule or seminal vesicles, nor does it always show even macroscopic disease. However, it often will indicate disease in these structures and facilitate confirmation by sonographically guided biopsy.

9) For monitoring the effectiveness of treatment (surgery, hormone therapy, irradiation). Prostate-specific antigen levels and prostate ultrasonography, along with rectal examination, provide more objective measures of the response to treatment than has previously been possible.

10) For monitoring the progression of cancer in patients whose disease is being followed without treatment. Again, more objective means are now available for determination of disease progression, allowing application of treatment appropriate to the patient's age and condition if advancement of disease is detected.

11) For evaluation of obscure symptomatology possibly related to prostate or seminal vesicles (cysts, abscesses, ejaculatory duct obstruction, prostatitis). Hitherto seminal vesicle disease has been difficult to diagnose. CT scanning has helped, but sonography shows these organs better, less expensively, and without irradiation.

12) In infertility. The seminal vesicles, distal vasa, and ejaculatory ducts are clearly seen. The ease with which they can be assessed sonographically often obviates the necessity for more invasive and expensive vasography.

13) In the cancerphobic patient. It must be emphasized to these men that, while sonography enhances our ability to diagnose prostate cancer, it does not exclude the possibility that cancer is present without being detectable.

14) As a help in the search for a possible prostate primary when metastatic adenocarcinoma is found at a distant site.

15) For greatly improved accuracy in placement of radioactive seeds for interstitial irradiation of prostate cancer in those patients for whom this form of treatment is indicated. Sonographic guidance permits this to be accomplished on an outpatient or short-stay basis.

16) For visualization of non-opaque distal ureteral calculi. Stones in the distalmost portion of the ureter are well seen by rectosonography. The fact that radiographically non-opaque stones cast shadows just as do opaque stones frequently circumvents the necessity for retrograde pyelography to confirm the presence of stones.

17) In men who have had an abdominoperineal resection. Evaluation of the prostate under this circumstance is a vexing problem for the physician. Application of the transducer to the perineum will accomplish visualization of the prostate reasonably well, although not nearly as clearly as by the transrectal route. Some degree of evaluation is also possible by utilization of transurethral transducers passed through a resectoscope sheath. Additionally, we now suggest to surgeons that, whenever feasible, transrectal ultrasonography of the prostate be performed prior to removal of the rectum in men over the age of 50 before the last opportunity to see the gland optimally is lost.

18) As a part of all teaching programs for urologists. Sonography provides better instruction in the internal anatomy of the prostate and in the natural history of early prostate cancer than any other available tool.

5.12 Early Detection of Prostate Cancer

The value of prostate ultrasonography as an independent screening procedure for the diagnosis of prostate cancer is questionable. No conclusive data are yet available which support its use in that role. However, when ultrasonography is combined with digital rectal examination and appropriate serum markers, the clinician may well find prostate cancer earlier than would be the case with rectal examination alone.

Should the sonogram present findings which are equivocal, biopsy is more likely to be performed if the clinician has felt a suspicious area in the same region or if the prostate specific antigen level is elevated.

References

1. Harada K, Tanahashi Y, Igari D, Numata I, Orikasa S (1980) Gray scale transrectal ultrasonography of the prostate. J Clin Ultrasound 7:45–49
2. Lee F, Gray JM, McLeary RD, Meadows TR, Kumasaka GH, Borlaza GS, Straub WH, Lee F Jr, Solomon MH, McHugh TA, Wolf RM (1985) Transrectal ultrasound in the diagnosis of prostate cancer: location, echogenicity, histopathology, and staging. Prostate 7:117–129
3. Lee F, Littrup PJ, McLeary RD, Kumasaka GH, Borlaza GS, McHugh TA, Soiderer MH, Roi LD (1987) Needle aspiration and core biopsy of prostate cancer: comparative evaluation with biplanar transrectal US guidance. Radiology 163:515–520
4. Lee F, Torp-Pedersen ST, Siders DB, Littrup PJ, Carroll JT, Mitchell AE (1988) Transrectal ultrasound examination and staging of prostate cancer with whole mount pathologic correlation. Presented at the 3rd international symposium on transrectal ultrasound, Chicago, Sept 23–24
5. McNeal JE (1968) Regional morphology and pathology of the prostate. Am J Clin Pathol 49:347–357
6. McNeal JE (1988) The prostate gland: morphology and pathobiology. Monogr Urol 9:36–54
7. McNeal JE, Kindrachuk RA, Freiha FS, Bostick DG, Redwine EA, Stamey TA (1986) Patterns of progression in prostate cancer. Lancet 1:60–63
8. Resnick MI (1988) Transrectal ultrasound guided versus digitally directed prostatic biopsy: a comparative study. J Urol 139:754–757
9. Rifkin MD (1985) Transrectal prostatic ultrasonography: comparison of linear array and radial scanners. J Ultrasound Med 4:1–5
10. Rifkin MD (1987) Endorectal prostate ultrasound: clinical implications. AJR 148:1137–1142
11. Rifkin MD, Kurtz AB, Goldberg BB (1983) Prostate biopsy utilizing transrectal ultrasound guidance: diagnosis of nonpalpable cancers. J Ultrasound Med 2:165–167
12. Salo JO, Rannikko S, Makinen J, Lehtonen T (1987) Echogenic structure of prostatic cancer imaged on radial prostatectomy specimens. Prostate 10:1–9
13. Scardino PT (1988) Transrectal ultrasonography of the prostate, diagnosis, localization and staging of prostate cancer. Presented at the state of the art summer conference, Bowman Gray School of Medicine, Winston-Salem, NC, Aug 27–28
14. Spirnak JP, Resnick MI (1984) Transrectal ultrasonography. Urology 23:461–467
15. Stamey TA (1987) Prostate cancer. Stanford Observer 22:8
16. Watanabe H (1974) Measurements of size and weight of prostate by means of transrectal ultrasonography. Tohoku J Exp Med 114:277–285
17. Watanabe H, Kaiho H, Tanaka M, Terasawa Y (1971) Diagnostic application of ultrasonotomography to the prostate. Invest Urol 8:548–559
18. Wild JJ, Reid JM (1957) Progress in techniques of soft tissue examination by 15 MC pulsed ultrasound. In: Kelly E (ed) Ultrasound in biology and medicine. American Institute of Biological Sciences, Washington, p 30

6 Endosonography in Gynecology – Hysterosonography, Rectosonography, Vaginosonography: Comparison with CT and MRI, Applications with Radiotherapy

H. HÖTZINGER

6.1 Introduction

Endosonography has gained considerable importance in gynecology. Depending on the structure to be investigated, different modalities are employed: hysterosonography (HS), rectosonography (RS) and vaginosonography (VS). These terms have been chosen to parallel those in endoscopy according to the placement of the probe – in the uterus, the rectum or the vagina. (Cystosonography has not assumed any importance in gynecology.) As each modality yields its specific information and has its own limitations, the indication for endosonography should be clearly defined. It must be decided first whether endosonography is likely to be helpful, and if so which procedure – HS, RS or VS – should be employed. Only in this way can optimal diagnostic results be obtained.

6.2 History of Endosonography in Gynecology

Since the introduction of sonography its noninvasive character has been emphasized. However, this very advantage brings with it a disadvantage, namely that the depth of penetration of ultrasound waves is dependent on the frequency used. Lower frequencies penetrate further, but display poor resolution. The logical consequence was to insert ultrasound probes into the natural body orifices, decreasing the distance from transducer to target structure and thus enabling the use of higher frequencies with their better resolution. Early trials were carried out by Kratochwil, who was the first to use the endosonographic principle in obstetrics – to document fetal heart action. As these first investigations were made using the A-mode system, the introduction of two-dimensional representation of the structures was a significant advance [23]. In the protocol employed by Kratochwil for VS and RS, a condom was placed over the probe for protection against infection. With smaller probes, first trials of cystosonography for the visualization of the ovaries were carried out [25].

Even at this early stage endosonography exhibited some distinct clinical advantages. Especially with RS, detection of local recurrences after radical hysterectomy was excellent, so much so that the findings could be used not only to establish the diagnosis but also to plan radiotherapy [26]. Another important step forward was the development of devices featuring automatic rotation of the transducer within a fixed tube, obviating the necessity for mechanical movement of the whole probe [48].

Further advances in the field of gynecology were made by the gynecologist Popp [36] and the radiologist/radiotherapist Hötzinger [20], who cooperated to establish the basic indications for HS. Popp took a particular interest in VS. He tested vaginal sector scanners with an antegrade field of view and an acoustic angle of 115°. With the help of these scanners he managed to perform transvaginal follicle puncture [35]. Hötzinger elaborated the basic applications of endosonography in individual radiotherapy planning [18].

6.3 Hysterosonography

6.3.1 Apparatus

Hysterosonography is performed with a sector scanner; the transducer (diameter 5 mm) is mounted on the tip of a steel rod (maximal diameter 7 mm). The frequency ranges from 5 to 10 MHz. In most cases 7 MHz seems to be optimal regarding depth of penetration and resolution. Because of the rotation of the probe and the possibility of damage to the uterus a sheath is necessary. This sheath also serves for introduction of isotonic salt solution to force the air out of the uterine cavity.

6.3.2 Method

Hysterosonography must be done under anesthesia because of the necessary dilatation of the cervical channel. In most cases we use general anesthesia, but spinal anesthesia may be employed. The combination of curettage and HS in one session has proved useful for primary diagnosis. In patients with known carcinoma of the uterine cervix or uterine corpus who undergo primary radiotherapy, HS may be performed directly before intracavitary radiotherapy.

The HS procedure is very short, the scanning itself taking only about 3 min. After dilatation of the cervical canal to Hegar 9 the whole probe is introduced gently into the uterine cavity. Via a bypass isotonic salt solution is filled into the uterine cavity to produce a water path. Transverse sectional images are generated by rotating the probe. The findings are documented every 0.5 cm, from the fundus to the cervix, and the distance from the external os should be displayed on the images. The exact position of the transducer can be read off a scale on the steel shaft of the probe in correlation to the external os. In general a quantity of 4–6 ml isotonic salt solution is sufficient to fill the uterine cavity to the desired level. The solution should be injected carefully, with little force, and injection should be stopped if liquid drips back through the cervical canal.

The best frequency for HS in general is 7 MHz, which combines sufficiently high resolution with adequate depth of penetration. The frequency of 10 mHz seems to be advantageous for imaging structures close to the transducer. Scanners with these two frequencies are already available.

Another important factor is the angle of emission of the ultrasound wave. For the visualization of the uterine cervix and corpus, 90° is optimal. For the uterine fundus, however, 45° in forward direction seems to be superior. This, too, has been incorporated into commercially available scanners.

Disinfection of the probe should be carried out according to the manufacturer's recommendations. For HS the probe has to be sterile.

6.3.3 Complications

The potential complications of HS are damage of the endometrium and myometrium, perforation and infection.

6.3.4 Contraindications

Contraindications to HS include gravidity, infections of the uterus, fallopian tubes or ovaries and inability to find the cervical canal.

6.3.5 Limitations

Visualization of the endometrium may be difficult or even impossible if there has been an injury of the endometrium resulting in bleeding from pieces of tissue floating freely within the uterine cavity. In this situation the rotation of the probe produces ill-defined echorich structures which prevent exact delineation of the endometrium (Fig. 6.1). One should wash out the uterine cavity with isotonic salt solution until clear liquid drips back.

6.3.5.1 Limited Depth of Penetration

Hysterosonography is performed using transducers of relatively high frequency (7–10 MHz), so that the depth of penetration of the ultrasound waves is limited.

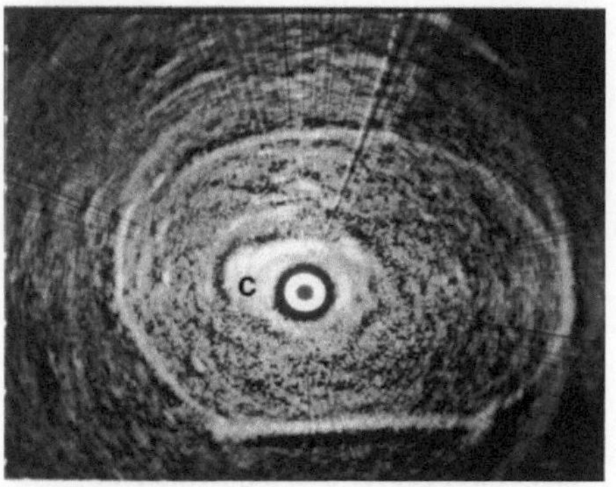

Fig. 6.1. HS: uterine cavity (*c*) filled by blood and tissue clots

6.2
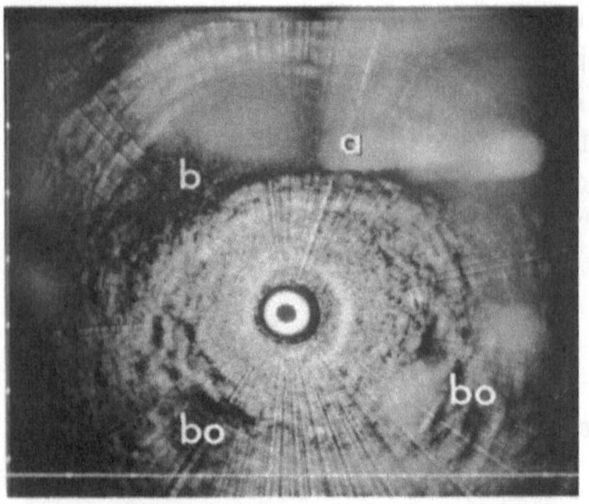

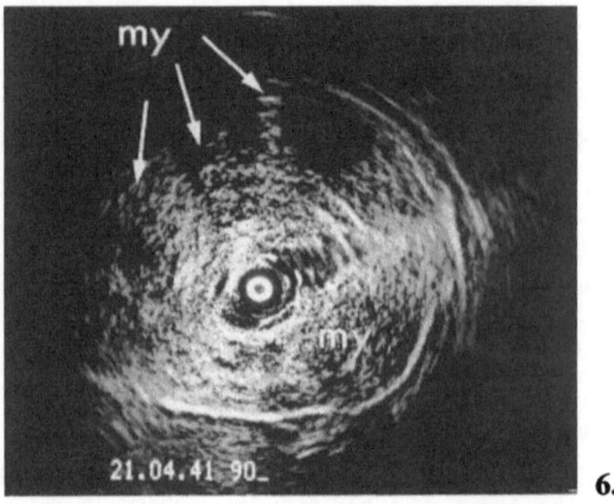

6.3

Fig. 6.2. HS: normal uterine corpus with partly visualized urinary bladder (*b*) and two loops of small bowel (*bo*). *a*, artifact

Fig. 6.3. HS: multiple large myomas (*my*), the lateral borders of which are not visualized clearly

This is the reason why adjacent structures like bladder or bowel cannot be visualized with sufficient clarity. In some cases parts of the urinary bladder or a piece of bowel can be differentiated, but normally HS is not the method of choice for their diagnostic workup (Fig. 6.2).

This limited depth of penetration makes it difficult to evaluate the lateral parts of a massively enlarged uterus as seen, for instance, in the case of large single or multiple myomas. HS fails to visualize pedunculated myomas in nearly all cases (Fig. 6.3).

6.3.6 Artifacts

In HS we have to deal with lots of artifacts, some of which may be avoided, some not. Considerably thickened endometrium may cast an acoustic shadow (Fig. 6.6). Image quality is badly disturbed by direct contact of the transducer with the endometrium, when an irregular acoustic pattern is seen (Fig. 6.4). The

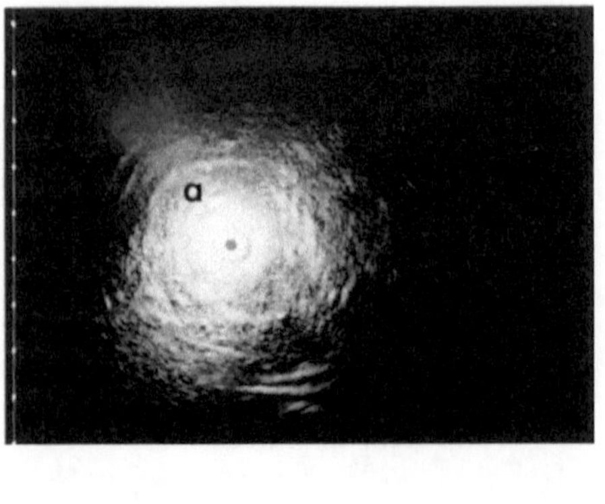

Fig. 6.4. HS: artifact (*a*) caused by direct contact of transducer with adjacent tissue

6.5 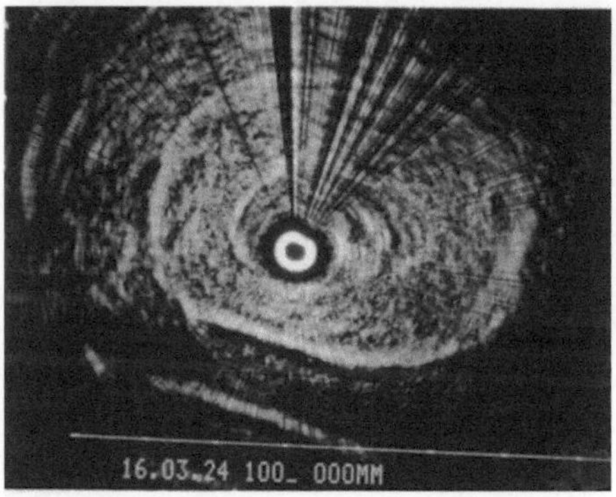

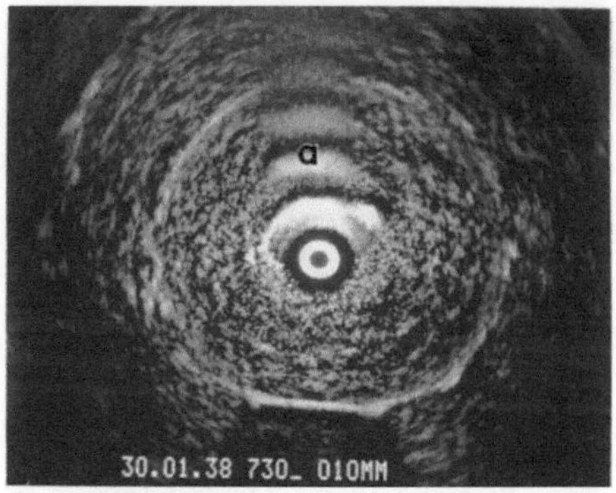 6.6

Fig. 6.5. HS: disturbance of image by sector artifacts caused by mechanical defects of wave transmission

Fig. 6.6. HS: artifact (*a*) caused by highly built-up endometrium

rotation of the probe should be stopped and the tip should be carefully moved away from the adjacent tissue so that isotonic salt solution comes between the probe and the endometrium. Image quality is also severely impaired by air within the uterine cavity. In this case isotonic salt solution should be given via the bypass until enough liquid drips back through the cervical canal. Mechanical disturbances of the scanner are characterized by typical sector artifacts (Fig. 6.5). Film artifacts are easily recognized (Fig. 6.2).

6.3.7 Findings

6.3.7.1 Normal Uterus

With HS one is able to define the macroscopic fine structure of the uterus, i.e., the uterine cavity, the endometrium, the myometrium and the serosa. On transverse sections of the uterus the probe can be seen inside the anechoic uterine cavity. The probe may be moved from side to side in the uterine cavity to help avoid compression of superficial endometrium layers.

The endometrium is hyperechoic (Fig. 6.7). HS does not allow differentiation between stratum basale and stratum functionale, nor does it show any correlation with microscopic changes in the endometrium. The myometrium, behind the endometrial layer, has medium echogenicity and appears homogeneous. The outermost layer of the uterine wall, the serosa, is hyperechoic. From the fundus to the cervix the uterine cavity gets smaller, and finally the cervical canal is totally filled by the HS probe. For this reason the upper 3 mm of the cervical epithelium cannot be adequately visualized using a 7-MHz transducer (Fig. 6.8). A 10-MHz transducer is able to achieve better visualization of this small area.

6.7 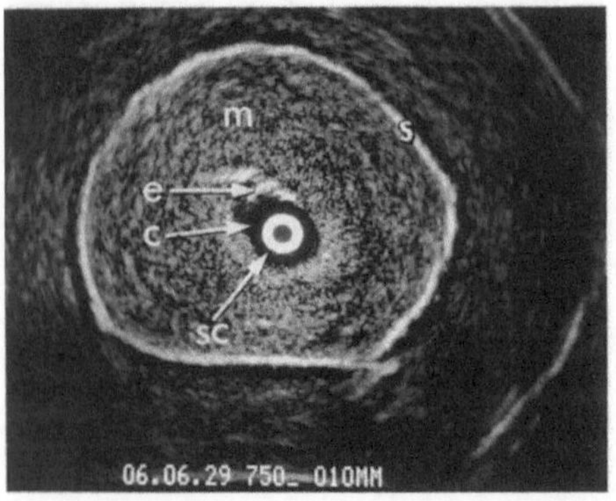

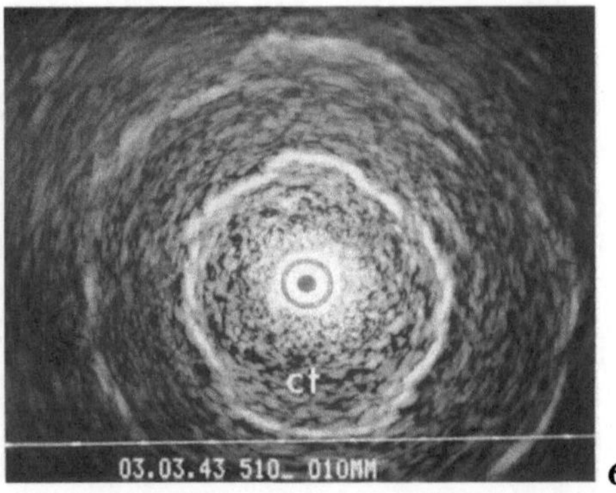 6.8

Fig. 6.7. HS: normal uterine corpus. The endometrium (*e*) of the anterior side of the uterine cavity (*c*) is higher than that on the posterior wall. *sc*, probe; *m*, myometrium; *s*, serosa

Fig. 6.8. HS: normal uterine cervix. The epithelium of the cervical canal in direct contact with the probe cannot be differentiated because of the near field of the transducer. *ct*, cervical tissue

6.3.7.2 Endometrium

The endometrium is visualized on HS as a hyperechoic layer clearly differentiated from the underlying myometrium (Fig. 6.9). The thickness of the endometrium varies depending on the menstrual cycle or secondary changes, and HS reflects this variation accurately, and reveals gross structure and surface configuration. However, HS is limited to these macroscopic features: it is unable to show only microscopic changes, and gives no pointers to the underlying histologic picture. Thickening of the endometrium may be caused by glandular-cystic hyperplasia (Fig. 6.10), adenomatous hyperplasia (Fig. 6.11) or adenocarcinoma. An atrophic endometrium shows up as a thin layer (Fig. 6.12).

Fig. 6.9. HS: endometrium in second half of menstrual cycle. The endometrium on the anterior wall of the uterine cavity shows up as a homogeneous, thick, hyperechoic layer. Discrete irregularities of the surface are normal. The endometrium on the posterior wall has already been removed by curettage

Fig. 6.10. HS: glandular-cystic hyperplasia. The anterior wall of the uterine cavity shows an irregular layer of highly built-up endometrium

Fig. 6.11. HS: adenomatous hyperplasia. The endometrium is irregular, especially on its surface, which shows a partly polypoid character. Anechoic areas corresponding to cystic degeneration are less evident than in Fig. 6.10

Fig. 6.12. HS: atrophic endometrium. The endometrium shows up as a thin layer surrounding the uterine cavity, the left anterior wall of which appears irregular. This is a typical finding after partial curettage. Blood clots (*bc*) and residual tissue within the uterine cavity

Fig. 6.13. HS: cyst of cervical epithelium. The cyst (*cy*) is visualized as a small hypoechoic area within the cervical tissue.

Fig. 6.14. HS: internal endometriosis (*ie*). Islands of endometrium within the myometrium have the typical appearance of highly echodense structures

6.3.7.3 Benign Cysts of the Cervical Epithelium

Cysts of the cervical epithelium are a common finding in adult women. Normally they have no clinical relevance. They appear on HS as areas of low echogenicity, in most cases nearly anechoic. They should, therefore, not be taken as signs of tumor invasion: infiltrating carcinoma is less echodense than normal myometrium but never shows a cystic appearance. Benign cysts usually have no visible direct connection to the cervical epithelium (Fig. 6.13).

6.9
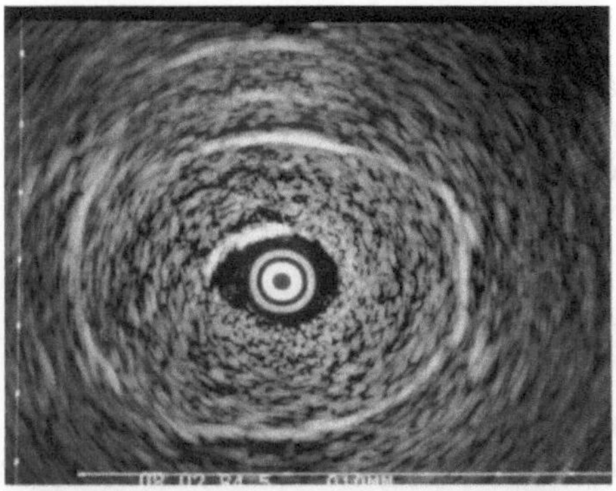

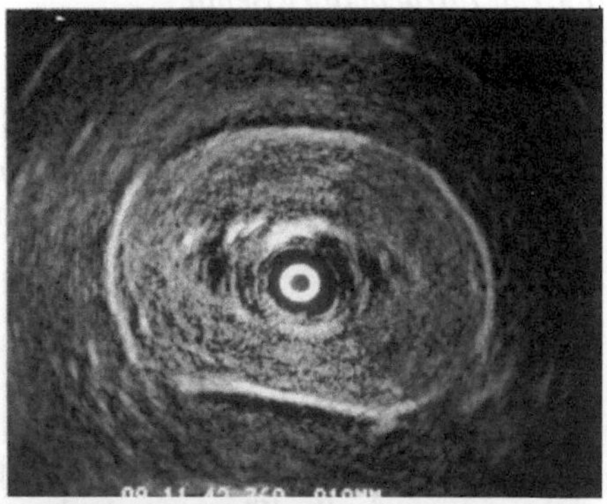
6.10

6.11
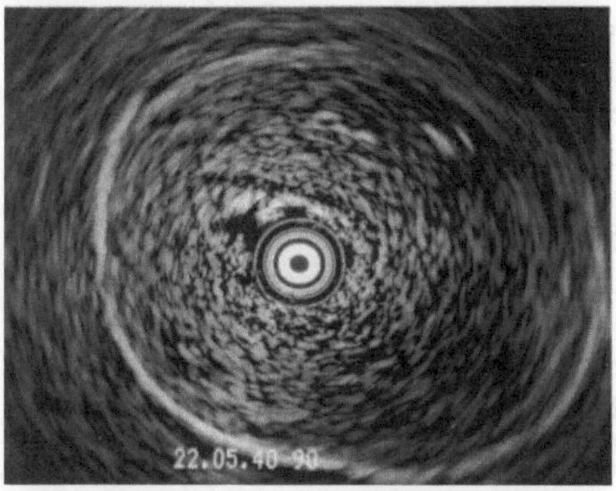

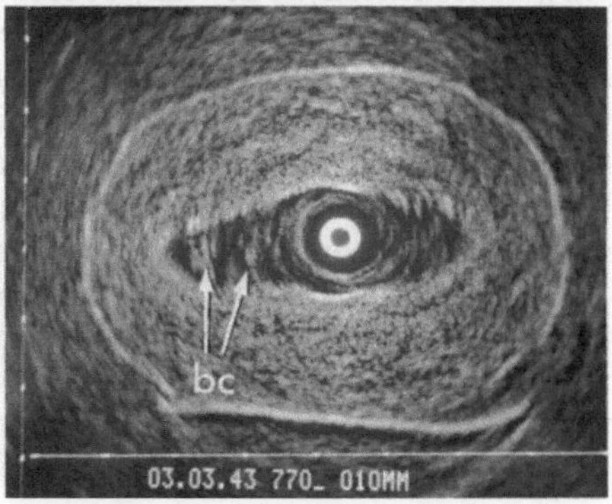

6.12

6.13
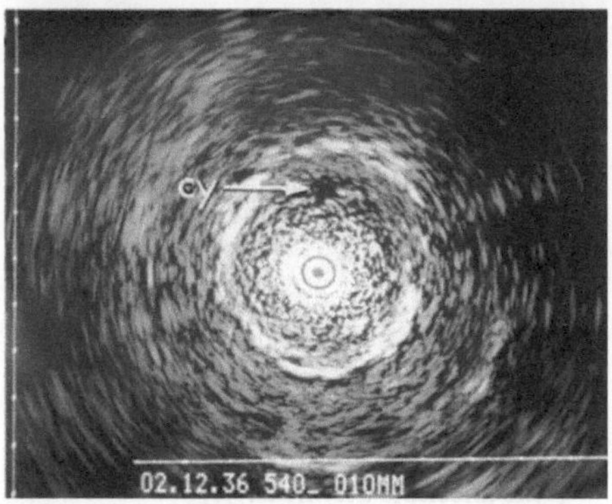

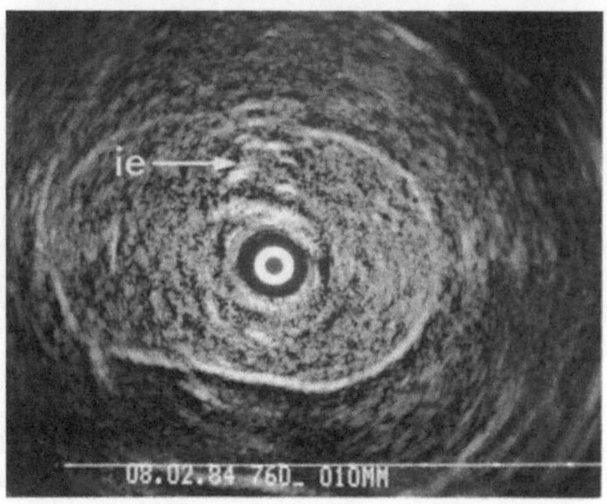

6.14

6.3.7.4 Endometriosis Interna

Endometriosis is the presence of endometrial tissue beyond its natural location. Endometriosis externa may involve the ovaries, fallopian tubes, bowel or bladder, while endometriosis interna affects the myometrium. HS is able to diagnose endometriosis interna by the typical hyperechoic appearance of endometrium (Fig. 6.14). With the course of the menstrual cycle the extension and diameter of areas of endometriosis interna may change.

6.3.7.5 Intracavitary Septa

Intracavitary septa may be congenital or acquired, in the latter case mostly after infections. These septa range from thin and fragile to broad and strong. Thin septa are missed with HS or destroyed during the examination, while thicker septa are visualized as bandlike structures within the uterine cavity (Fig. 6.15).

6.3.7.6 Myomas

Myomas appear less echodense than normal myometrium. The echo intensity may vary depending upon the proportion of connective tissue. Myomas tend to grow concentrically. They may be located submucously, intramurally, subserously or may be pedunculated. A complete or partial hyperechoic capsule may be seen (Figs. 6.16–6.19). Secondary degeneration may produce necrotic areas, which are anechoic (Fig. 6.20). Sometimes calcifications are seen with a typical hyperechoic rim and an acoustic shadow behind. It is difficult to visualize hysterosonographically the internal structure of the connective tissue within myomas. Some sort of septa are visible in most cases.

We performed HS in 42 patients with myomas of the uterus. The patients were then operated on and 129 myomas varying in diameter from 3 to 80 mm were found on histologic workup. Of these, 91 had been detected with HS. All were less echodense than normal myometrium. A capsule was clearly defined in 14.3% of lesions, partly present in 66.7% and absent in 19%. The myomas

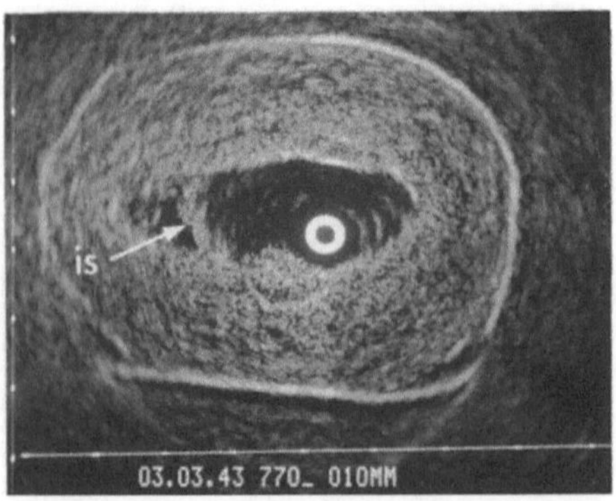

Fig. 6.15. HS: intrauterine septum. An intracavitary septum (*is*) characteristically shows up as a bandlike structure within the anechoic uterine cavity

6.16
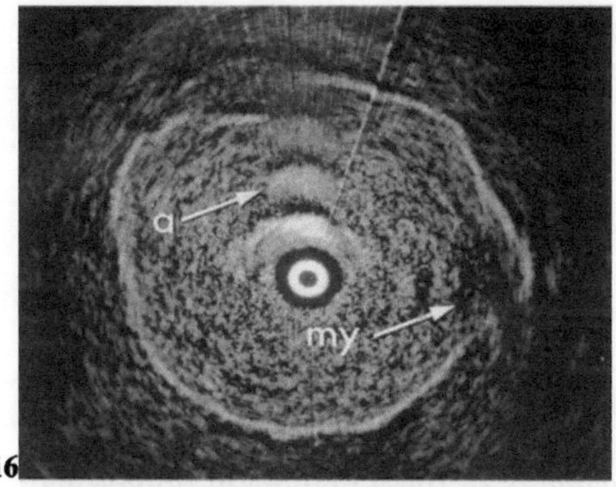

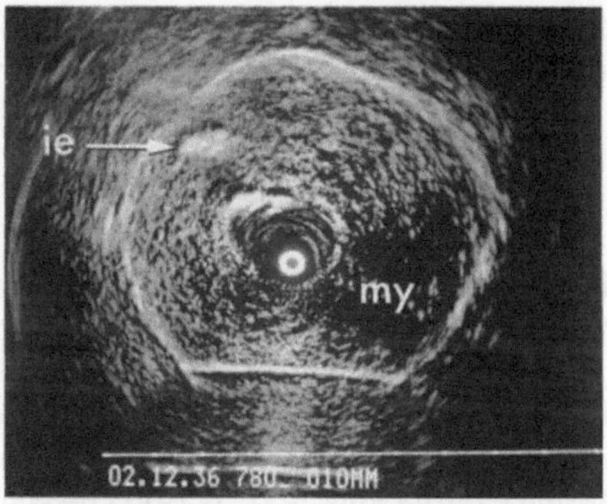

6.17

6.18
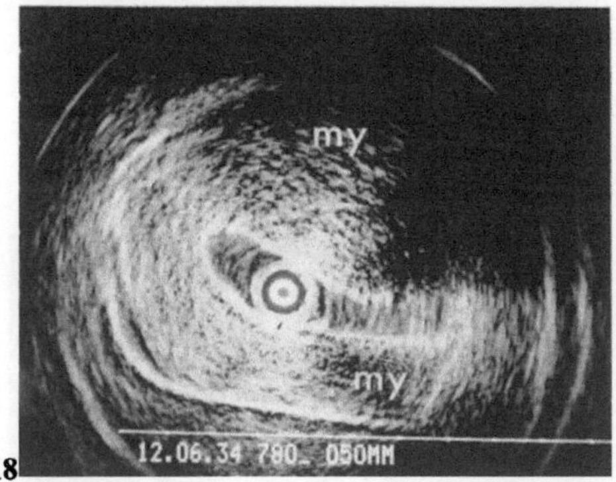

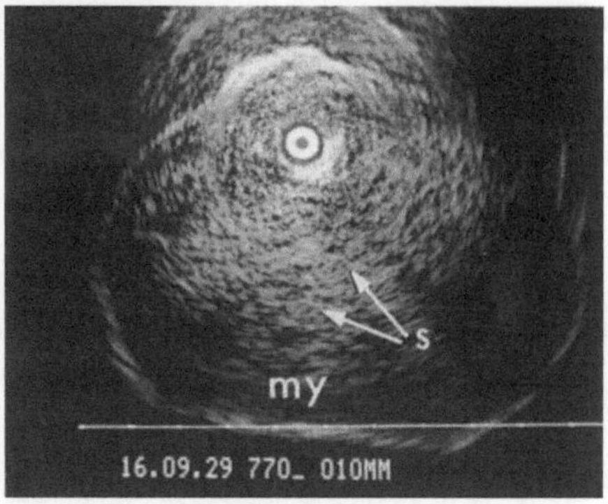

6.19

Fig. 6.16. HS: small myoma. On the left side of the uterus is a small subserous myoma (*my*). *a*, artifact

Fig. 6.17. HS: large left-sided myoma. The left dorsal portion of the myometrium is replaced by a myoma (*my*). The uterine cavity shows no deformation. On the right side ventrally is an island of internal endometriosis (*ie*)

Fig. 6.18. HS: myoma with deformation of uterine cavity. A large myoma (*my*) of the anterior wall of the uterus causes deformation of the anterior wall of the uterine cavity. A second, smaller myoma on the dorsal wall does not alter the shape of the uterine cavity

Fig. 6.19. HS: enormous myoma with replacement of normal myometrium of uterus. A huge myoma (*my*) of the dorsal side of the uterus has replaced the normal uterine architecture. Within the myoma septa (*s*) of connective tissue are visible

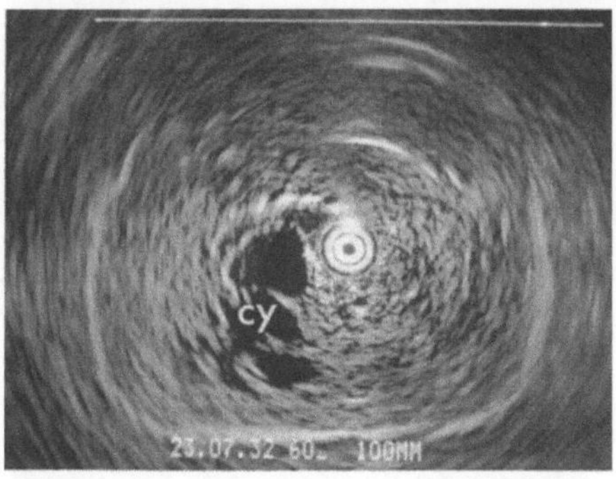

Fig. 6.20. HS: myoma with secondary cystic degeneration. Anechoic areas resulting from necrotic degeneration of myomas have replaced the normal appearance. *cy*, cyst

missed were either too small or were located between two of the transverse sections documented. Myomas under 0.5 cm in diameter are missed in most cases.

6.3.7.7 Carcinoma of the Endometrium

Hysterosonography shows thickening of the endometrium and thus reveals the macroscopic extent of carcinomas, but yields no information concerning histology. Carcinomas which are diagnosed only histologically, without macroscopic alteration, are missed with HS. Exophytically growing carcinomas of the endometrium present as polypoid hyperechoic structures protruding into the uterine cavity (Figs. 6.21, 6.22). The echogenicity of these malignant polyps may vary depending on their consistency. The basal parts of the tumors should be carefully evaluated for signs of myometrial infiltration (Fig. 6.23). The size of the tumors in the sagittal axis can be measured easily using the external os as a reference point, and the axial extent can be determined from the transverse HS

6.21
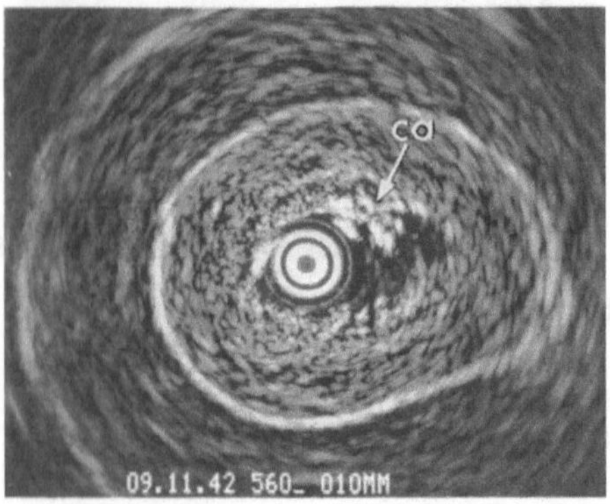

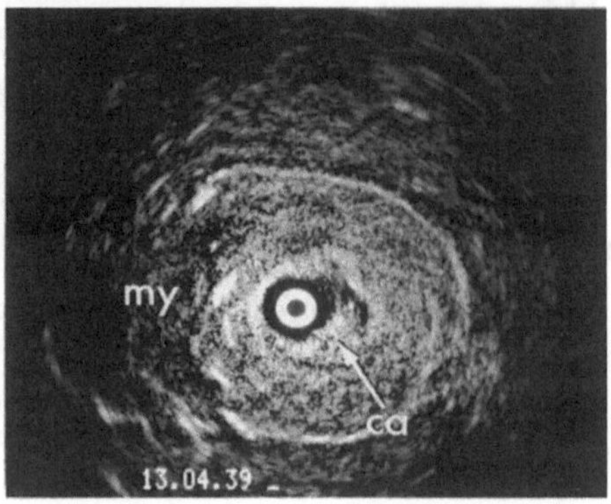

6.22

Fig. 6.21. HS: small exophytically growing carcinoma of endometrium (*ca*). The ventral portion of the endometrium shows a polypoid lesion with irregular surface

Fig. 6.22. HS: exophytic carcinoma of endometrium (*ca*). The dorsal wall of the endometrium shows a polyp with a broad base. The surface is partly compressed by the scanner. *my*, myoma

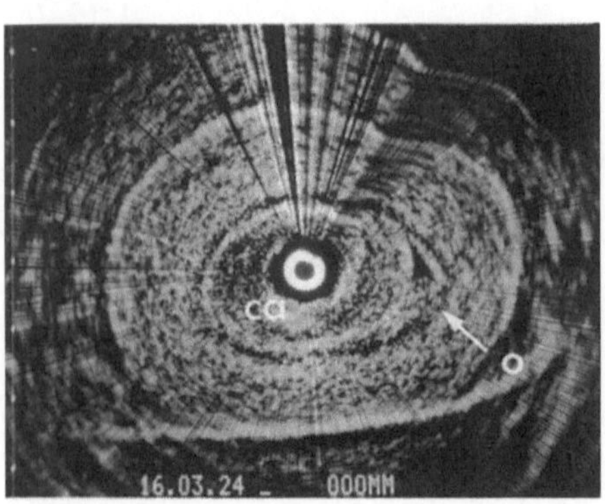

Fig. 6.23. HS: large exophytic carcinoma filling whole uterine cavity. The malignant tumor (*ca*) has filled the entire uterine cavity so that the probe is enclosed by the tumor. The endometrium is preserved except for a small area at the left dorsal site which seems to be the origin of the carcinoma (*o*)

6.24 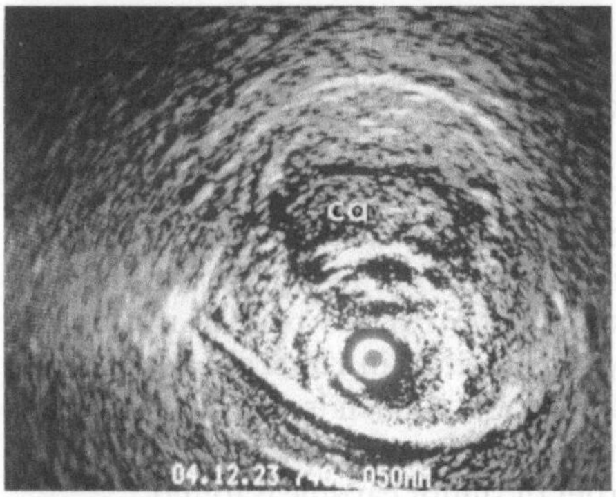

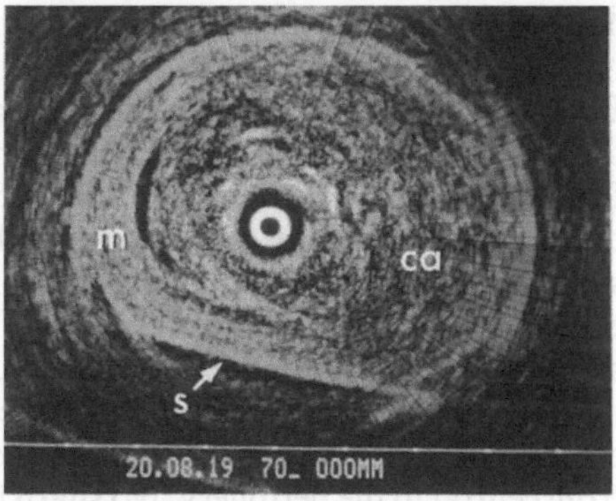 6.25

Fig. 6.24. HS: infiltrative carcinoma of endometrium. Infiltrative growth into the myometrium is visualized as an area of tissue less echogenic than normal myometrium. In this case the tumor (*ca*) has invaded the ventral wall. The outer border of the myometrium is preserved, however

Fig. 6.25. HS: carcinoma of endometrium with infiltration to serosa. The exophytically growing part of the tumor has filled the whole uterine cavity so that the probe is surrounded by the carcinoma (*ca*). In addition there is broad tumor invasion into the myometrium (*my*) as far as the serosa (*s*) on the left side. The myometrium on the right side shows no sign of infiltration

images. Polypoid lesions may reach a considerable size, and the tumor surface may be partly compressed by the rotating probe. Sometimes the whole uterine cavity is filled with carcinomatous tissue so that the probe is enclosed by the tumor.

Carcinomas of the endometrium with infiltration into the myometrium are characteristically less echodense than normal myometrium. In contrast to the concentric growth tendency of myomas, infiltrating carcinomas of the endometrium extend from the central endometrium into the periphery. The depth of infiltration can be directly measured from the HS images (Figs. 6.24, 6.25).

We performed HS in 60 cases of carcinoma of the endometrium. All patients then underwent hysterectomy. In 36 there was only exophytic tumor growth (thickness of endometrium more than 4 mm). Eleven patients exhibited tumor invasion into the myometrium, while in 13 tumor extension was only microscopic. A statistical comparison between the macroscopic findings and the appearance on HS was carried out (Table 6.1).

Table 6.1. Tumor invasion: correlation between macroscopic specimen and findings of HS

		Regression line	Residual mean square error
Depth of infiltration	0.99	x=1.0 y−0.2	0.3
Sagittal extension	0.99	x=1.0 y−0.7	0.1
Exophytic growth, axial	0.84	x=1.2 y−0.6	8.5
Exophytic growth, sagittal	0.98	x=1.0 y−0.8	0.1

6.3.7.8 *Carcinoma of the Cervix*

Because of the narrowness of the cervical canal the probe is in close contact with the cervical epithelium. Since, depending on the frequency used, no reliable information can be obtained within 2–5 mm lateral from the transducer, only tumors infiltrating the cervix to a depth of at least 5 mm can be identified with sufficient confidence. Tumor infiltration is characterized by an appearance less echodense than that of normal cervical tissue (Fig. 6.26). HS permits no conclusions concerning the underlying histology. Infiltration in cervical cancer looks just like that seen in carcinoma of the endometrium (which is usually adenocarcinoma). Also like carcinomas of the endometrium, cervical cancers tend to grow from central to the periphery. No sharp border or tumor capsule is found.

We operated on 29 patients with FIGO stage Ib carcinoma of the cervix and compared the macroscopic findings to the appearance on HS. The results are shown in Table 6.2.

Tumor growth beyond the natural organ borders can be diagnosed by HS (Fig. 6.27). Because of the limited depth of penetration of the sound waves, the

Table 6.2. Infiltrating carcinoma of the cervix: correlation between macroscopic specimen and findings of transverse HS

		Regression line	Residual mean square error
Depth of infiltration	0.9	x = 1.0 y − 1.7	1.3
Sagittal extension of infiltration	0.9	x = 1.0 y − 0	1.3

6.26
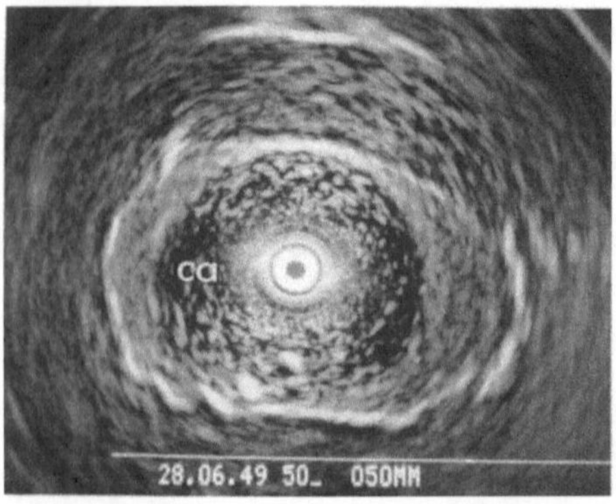

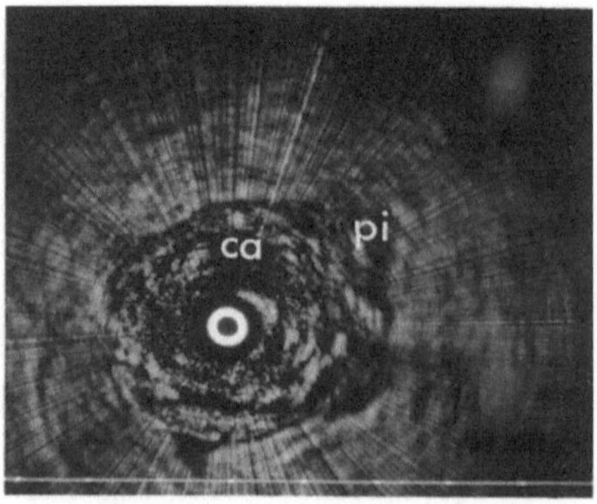

6.27

Fig. 6.26. HS: carcinoma of cervix stage Ib. There is concentric tumor invasion into the cervical tissue with a clearly defined rim of normal cervical tissue around the tumor. The tumor itself (*ca*) has an irregular appearance

Fig. 6.27. HS: carcinoma of cervix stage IIb. On the left side there is tumor invasion beyond the natural borders of the uterine cervix into the paracervical tissue. The whole cervical tissue is replaced by the carcinoma (*ca*). *pi*, paracervical infiltration

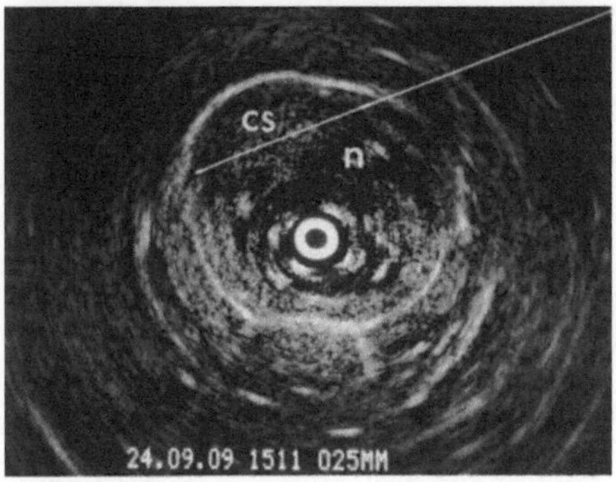

Fig. 6.28. HS: carcinosarcoma of uterus. The tumor (*CS*) has invaded the ventral wall of the uterus to the serosa. On the left side of the tumor is a large area of necrosis (*n*)

lateral portions of far advanced tumors infiltrating as far as the pelvic wall (stage III b) cannot be visualized.

6.3.7.9 Carcinosarcoma

Carcinosarcomas of the uterus are rare. The hysterosonographic criteria for exophytic or infiltrative tumor growth are identical to those described already. We have examined two cases in both of which there were zones of necrosis within the tumor mass (Fig. 6.28).

6.4 Rectosonography

6.4.1 Apparatus

Rectosonography may be performed either with sector scanners or with linear scanners. The latter have only a small field of view, and for this reason their routine clinical application in gynecology has not been successful. Sector scanners, on the other hand, are widely used. A frequency of 5–7 MHz has proved to provide the best combination of resolution and depth of penetration. The sector scanners used for RS are constructed like those for HS (see Sect. 6.3.1), but the diameter of the probe is greater (about 1 cm).

6.4.2 Method

No special preparation is necessary for RS of the female internal genitalia, but an enema should be administered before the examination. RS is started at the level of the pelvic floor and transverse sectional images are produced. The scanner is then moved deeper into the rectum, with documentation of the findings usually every 0.5 cm from the anal sphincter. The scanning plane may be shifted to the left or to the right according to the clinical situation. Rectosonograms are oriented like CT scans, so that direct comparison is possible.

6.4.3 Complications

No severe complications of RS have yet been described. The probe must be inserted carefully to avoid unnecessary pain. The danger of perforating the rectum should be kept in mind.

6.4.4 Contraindications

No contraindications to a carefully performed RS examination are known. RS may be impossible in cases of anal or rectal strictures or in patients with a stenosing tumor of the rectum.

6.4.5 Capabilities and Limitations

Rectosonography is able to visualize the vagina, the uterus (cervix, corpus and fundus) and the paracervical area. The ovaries may be seen if they are enlarged. The resolution of RS is limited, so that in contrast to HS the macroscopic fine structure of the uterus cannot be discerned. The probe cannot be inserted more than 16–18 cm into the rectum, so no information can be gained above this level. RS is the diagnostic method of choice for pathologic processes with which the probe may be brought into close approximation. These include especially car-

6.29

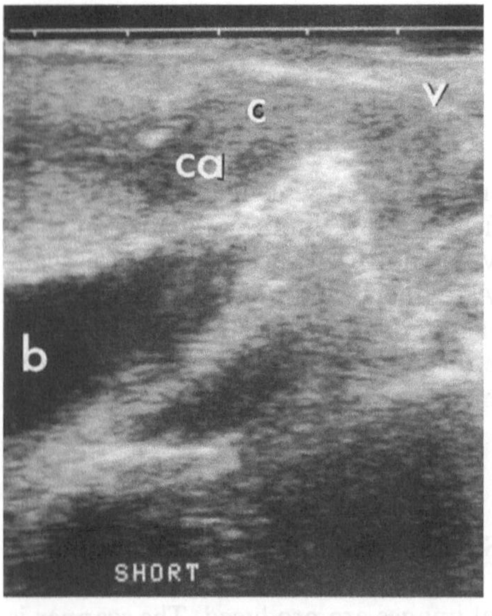

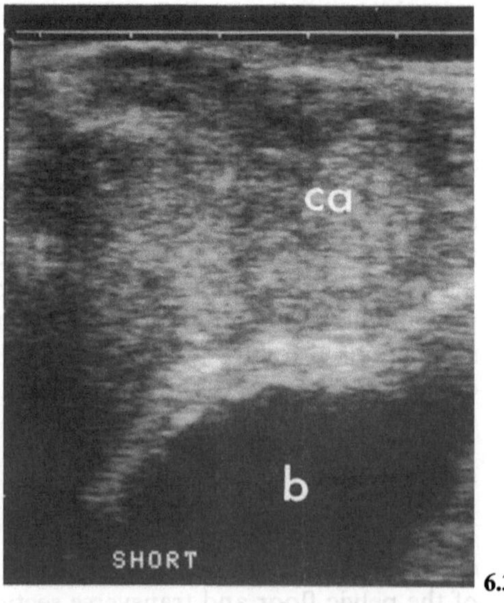

6.30

Fig. 6.29. RS with linear scanner: carcinoma of cervix stage Ib. The small cervical carcinoma (*ca*) is hypoechoic. *v*, vagina; *c*, cervix; *b*, bladder

Fig. 6.30. RS with linear scanner: carcinoma of cervix stage IIb. Irregular tumor mass (*ca*) with extension to the bladder (*b*)

cinomas of the cervix with extension into the parametrium or, generally, the region of the upper vagina, the cervix and the parametrium. RS is not an adequate diagnostic tool for areas with which the probe cannot be brought into close approximation, i.e., the ovaries, or even the uterine corpus or fundus in the case of enlargement or marked anteflexion.

6.4.5.1 RS with a Linear Scanner

As already mentioned, linear scanners are not widely used for RS. The main reason is the limited field of view, so that orientation is difficult and only a small portion of the region of interest may be visualized at any one time (Figs. 6.29, 6.30).

6.4.6 Findings

6.4.6.1 Normal Female Internal Genitalia

The *vagina* is visualized as a sickle-shaped area in front of the probe. It appears less echodense than the paravaginal tissue. Centrally within the vagina is the bright reflection of the vaginal epithelium. Located in front of the vagina is the hyperechoic vesicovaginal septum. The paravaginal tissue has an equal echodensity. Sometimes bowel loops may be seen deep in the small pelvis (Fig. 6.31). The *cervix* appears with its typical round appearance. The cervical epithelium has the same bright aspect as the vaginal epithelium (Fig. 6.32). As the probe is advanced, the *uterine corpus and fundus* appear with an increasing diameter. Lateral position of the uterus may be diagnosed, but it should be considered that the probe may displace the uterus (Fig. 6.33).

6.31
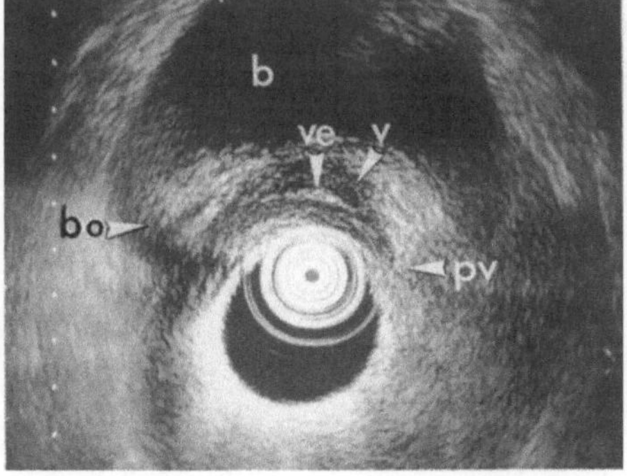

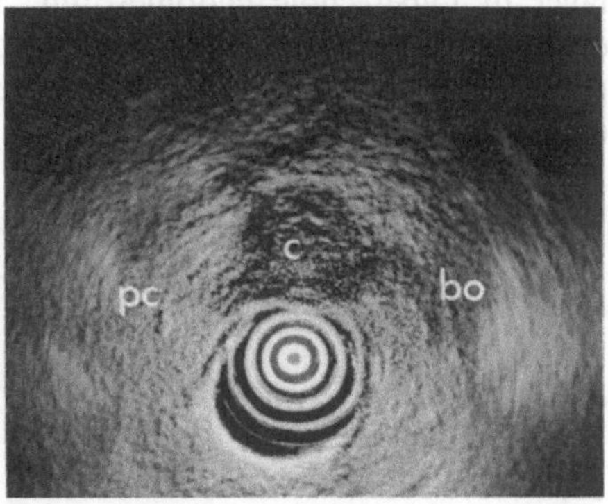

6.32

Fig. 6.31. RS: normal vagina. *v*, vagina; *ve*, vaginal epithelium; *b*, bladder; *bo*, bowel; *pv*, paravaginal space

Fig. 6.32. RS: normal uterine cervix. *c*, cervix; *pc*, paracervical tissue; *bo*, bowel

6.33 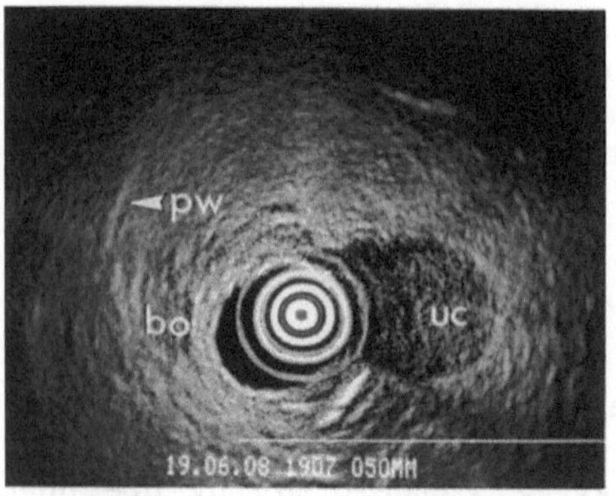

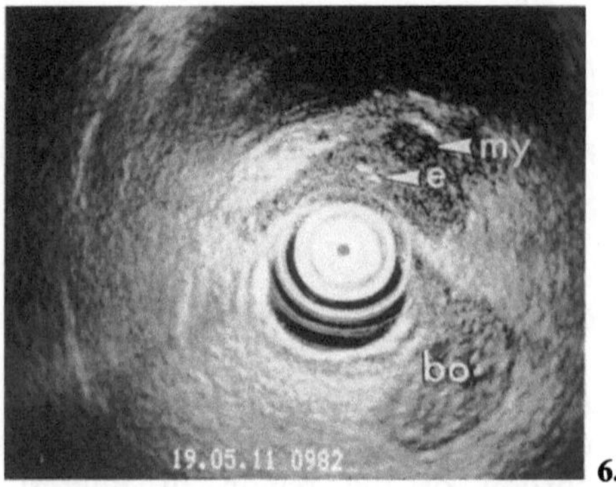 6.34

Fig. 6.33. RS: normal uterine corpus. Left-sided position of uterus. *uc*, corpus; *bo*, bowel; *pw*, pelvic wall

Fig. 6.34. RS: subserous myoma. *my*, myoma; *bo*, bowel; *e*, endometrium

6.4.6.2 Myomas

RS should not be used for the routine diagnosis of myomas. As the depth of penetration of the ultrasound waves is limited, rectosonographic information about structures which cannot be brought into close approximation with the probe is suboptimal. The rectosonographic picture of a myoma resembles the hysterosonographic appearance (Sect. 6.3.7.6). Myomas appear less echodense than normal myometrium. Depending on the site, mild to marked deformation of the outer contour of the uterus is seen (Fig. 6.34).

6.4.6.3 Retention Within the Uterine Cavity

Fluid retentions within the uterine cavity have a typical ultrasonic appearance: a hypoechoic area located centrally within the myometrium is surrounded by a layer of hyperechoic endometrium. The endometrium should be thoroughly evaluated if a fluid retention is diagnosed, because carcinomas of the endometrium or of the cervix often cause secondary obstruction of the cervical canal (Fig. 6.35).

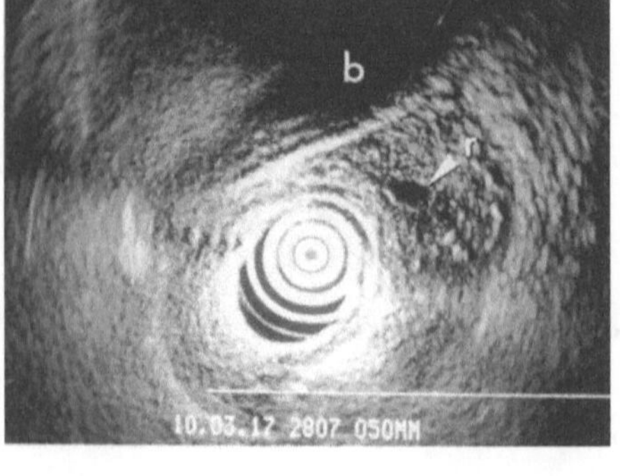

Fig. 6.35. RS: fluid retention (*r*) within uterine cavity. *b*, urinary bladder

6.4.6.4 *Carcinoma of the Cervix*

Tumor growth limited to the uterus is classified according to FIGO as stage Ia (preinvasive) or Ib (invasive). Stage Ia is always missed with RS and in most cases also stage Ib cannot be diagnosed. More advanced cervical cancer is manifested on RS by deformation of the outer organ contour, different echogenicity from the normal cervical tissue and secondary necrotic zones around the cervical canal. As the natural organ borders are respected in stage Ib, if RS reveals the lesion at all the diagnosis is based on the detection of necrotic areas around the cervical canal or an altered appearance of the carcinomatous tissue. In most cases the carcinoma is less echodense than normal cervical tissue.

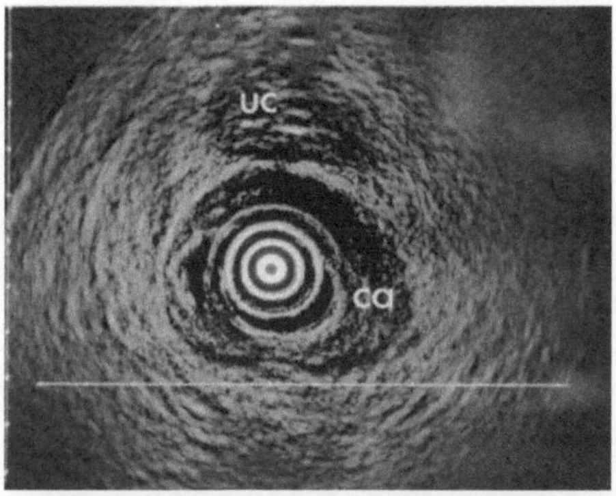

6.36

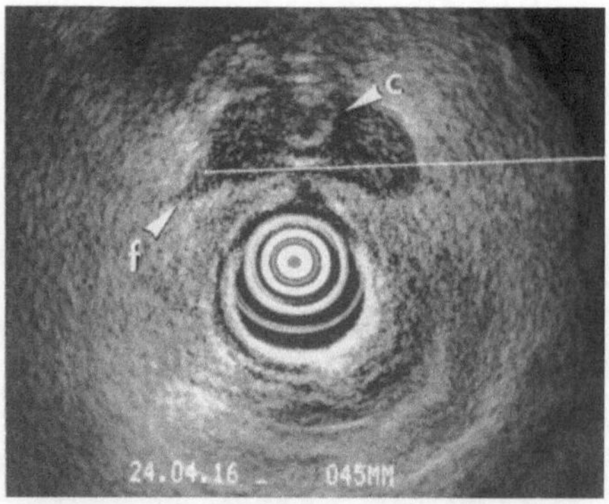

6.37

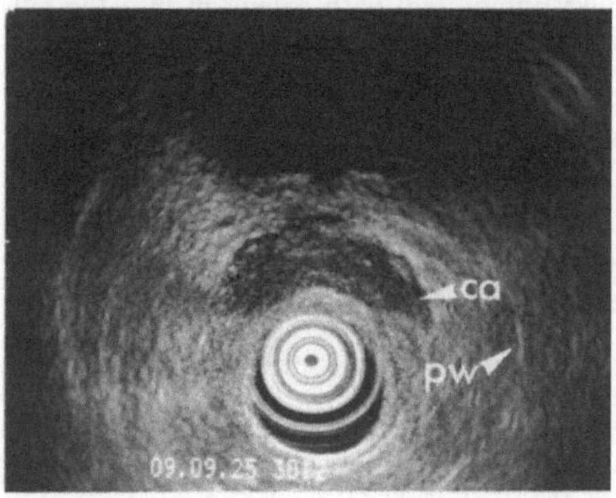

6.38

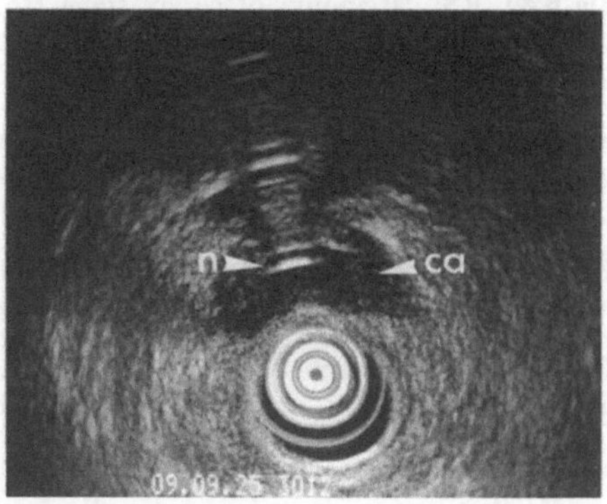

6.39

Fig. 6.36. RS: carcinoma of cervix stage IIa. The examination was performed with the probe in the vagina, not the rectum. The vaginal wall is thickened by concentric tumor growth. *ca*, carcinoma; *uc*, uterine corpus (partially visualized)

Fig. 6.37. RS: carcinoma of cervix stage Ib. Irregular appearance of the cervix (*c*), with hyperechoic and hypoechoic areas. Nearly symmetrical fornices (*f*) lateral to the cervix

Fig. 6.38. RS: carcinoma of cervix stage IIb. Asymmetrical appearance of the fornices with tumor extension into the left parametrium. No further differentiation or tissue characterization is possible. *ca*, carcinoma; *pw*, pelvic wall

Fig. 6.39. RS: carcinoma of cervix stage IIb. Necrotic destruction of the cervical canal (*n*) with early tumor involvement of the left parametrium. *ca*, carcinoma

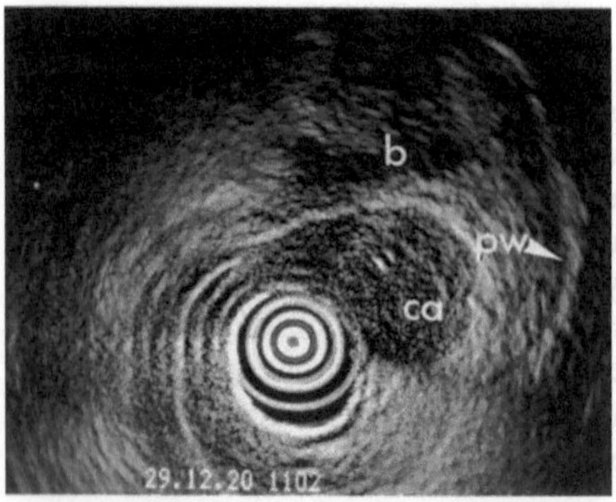

6.40

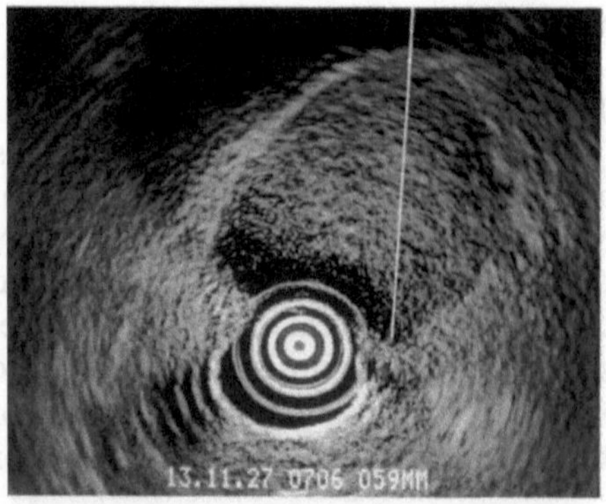

6.41

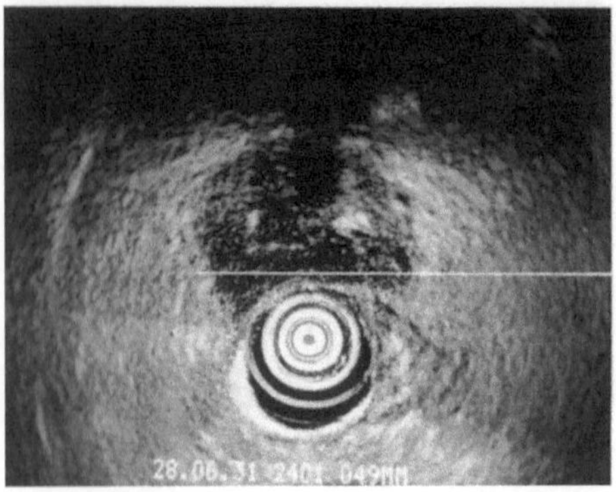
6.42

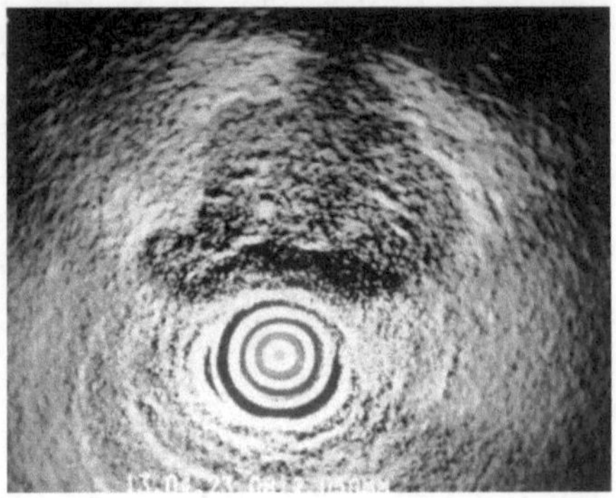
6.43

Fig. 6.40. RS: carcinoma of cervix stage IIb. Bulky tumor (*ca*) with extension into the left parametrium. Asymmetrical position of the cervical canal. Healthy parametrial tissue between the tumor and the pelvic wall (*pw*). *b*, bladder

Fig. 6.41. RS: carcinoma of cervix stage IIb with anterior extension. The tumor mass appears homogeneous. The left lateral border shows irregular tumor invasion into the residual parametrium. The pelvic wall is not reached

Fig. 6.42. RS: carcinoma of cervix IIb with necrotic degeneration of tumor. The carcinoma has an irregular appearance. Delineation of the bladder wall may be difficult in cases such as this

Fig. 6.43. RS: carcinoma of cervix stage IIb. Growth of the carcinoma to the right and anteriorly. The central parts of the tumor are inhomogeneous

With tumor extension laterally beyond the natural organ borders, first the parametrium is invaded (stage IIb). RS is very sensitive in the diagnosis of parametrial carcinomatous growth. As normal parametrium has a high echogenicity, carcinomatous invasion is easily detectable by the typical hypoechoic appearance. The pelvic wall is reached in stage IIIb. Infiltration of the vagina (stage IIa and IIIa) is diagnosed by clinical examination. RS is able to determine the depth of tumor invasion of the vaginal wall (Figs. 6.36–6.44).

Stage IVa is characterized by infiltration of the urinary bladder or the rectum. RS shows direct tumor invasion into the bladder wall or the rectum. It may be difficult, however, to decide whether there is only reactive swelling of the bladder wall (Figs. 6.45, 6.46).

6.44

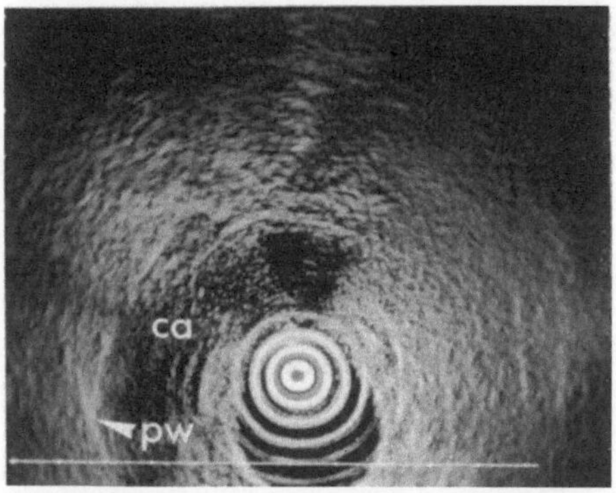

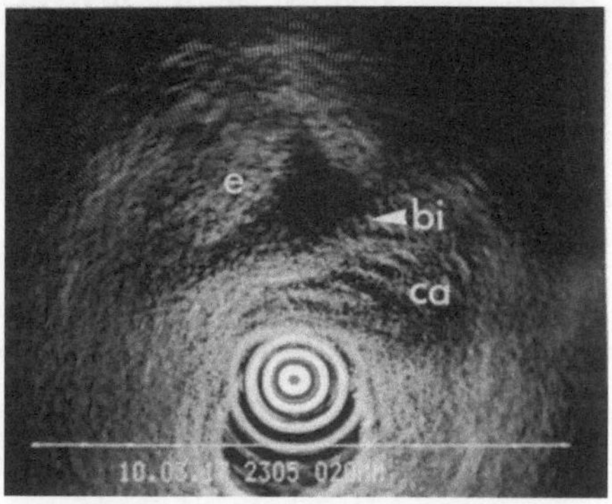

6.45

6.46

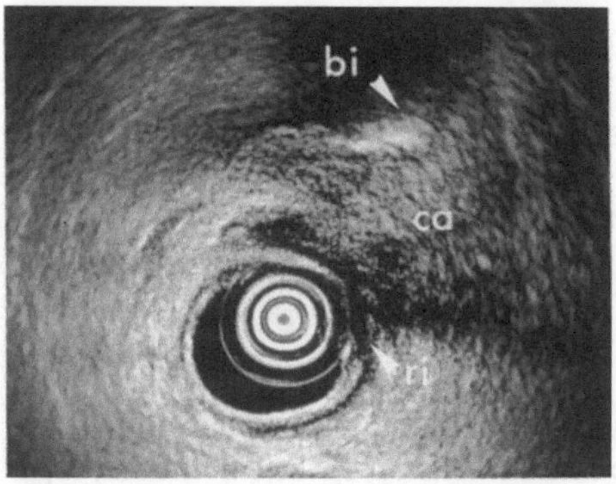

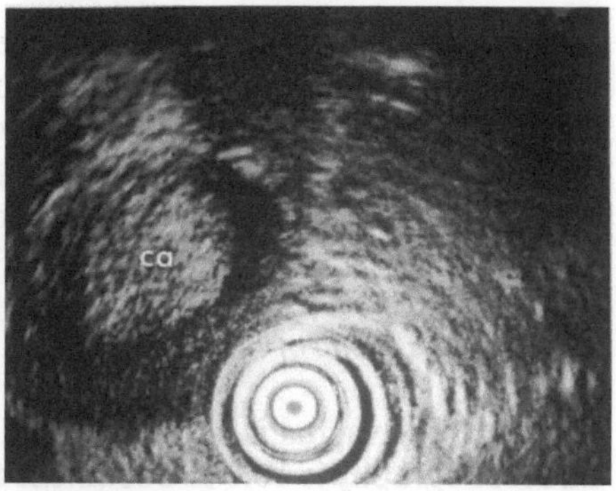

6.47

Fig. 6.44. RS: carcinoma of cervix stage IIIb. Tumor involvement of the right parametrium and the right uterosacral ligament till the pelvic wall (*pw*). *ca*, carcinoma

Fig. 6.45. RS: carcinoma of cervix stage IVa. Tumor invasion of the posterior wall of the urinary bladder (*bi*). Extensive edema of the right and left anterior bladder wall (*e*). *ca*, carcinoma

Fig. 6.46. RS: carcinoma of cervix stage IVa. Tumor invasion of the urinary bladder (*bi*) and the rectum (*ri*). Ill-defined tumor mass (*ca*) with extension to the pelvic wall. No delineation from the dorsal bladder wall and the left anterior wall of the rectum. Irregular appearance of the carcinoma with hyperechoic structures near the bladder wall.

Fig. 6.47. RS: carcinoma of uterine corpus. Enlargement of the whole organ with dextroposition. Highly built-up endometrium with irregular appearance. *ca*, carcinoma of endometrium with exophytic growth

A statistical evaluation of 150 patients with histologically verified carcinoma of the uterine cervix showed that RS estimated the stage according to FIGO with an accuracy of 84% relative to the clinical examination. These findings are confirmed in the literature [1, 2].

6.4.6.5 *Carcinoma of the Endometrium*

RS should not be applied for the routine diagnostic workup of patients with a carcinoma of the uterine corpus. In about 30%–40% of cases the whole corpus

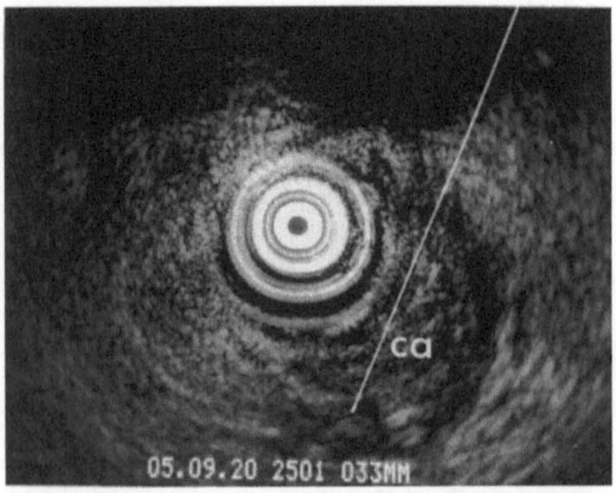

Fig. 6.48. RS: cancer of vagina. Deep tumor invasion into the left paravaginal tissue (*ca*). For this examination the rectal probe was positioned in the vagina

may not be visualized, especially when the uterus is enlarged, so that reliable diagnostic information about the whole uterus cannot be obtained. Within the diagnostic range, rectosonographic signs of carcinoma of the endometrium are thickening, irregular appearance, cystic degeneration, irregularity of the basal border and, in advanced cases, enlargement of the uterine corpus (Fig. 6.47).

6.4.6.6 Carcinoma of the Vagina

Cancer of the vagina is best diagnosed by inspection and bimanual examination. Endosonography is able to document the exact extension of the carcinoma, especially the tumor spread beyond the vaginal wall. This may be done with conventional RS, but in this specific situation more accurate results are obtained by positioning the rectal probe in the vagina. Infiltrating cancer of the vagina is characterized by hypoechoic tissue with extension into the paravaginal space (Fig. 6.48).

6.4.6.7 Ovarian Tumors

While normal ovaries cannot be detected with RS, ovarian tumors may be visualized when they have reached a size of more than 4 cm. Ovarian tumors often become very large, however, and it is then impossible to visualize the whole tumor mass. This is the main reason why RS is not used for basic diagnosis of ovarian tumors. There are no absolutely reliable criteria for the differentiation of benign and malignant tumors, but benign tumors appear homogeneous (Fig. 6.49), whereas malignant tumors often show heterogeneous tissue with irregular solid parts (Fig. 6.50–6.52).

6.4.6.8 Follow-up After Hysterectomy

The rectosonographic appearance after hysterectomy depends upon how much time has elapsed since operation. In the early postoperative phase edematous

6.49
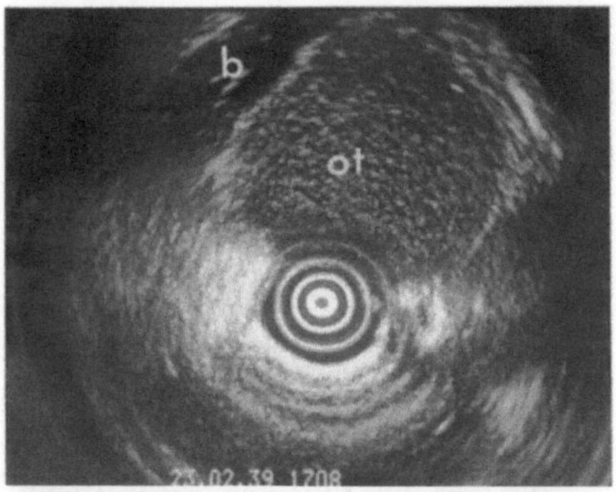

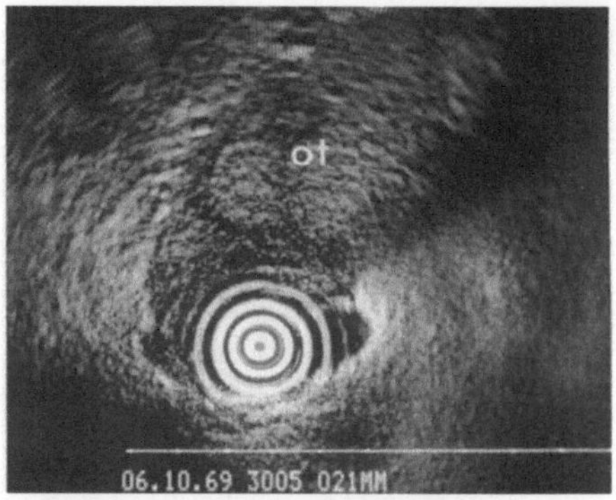

6.50

6.51
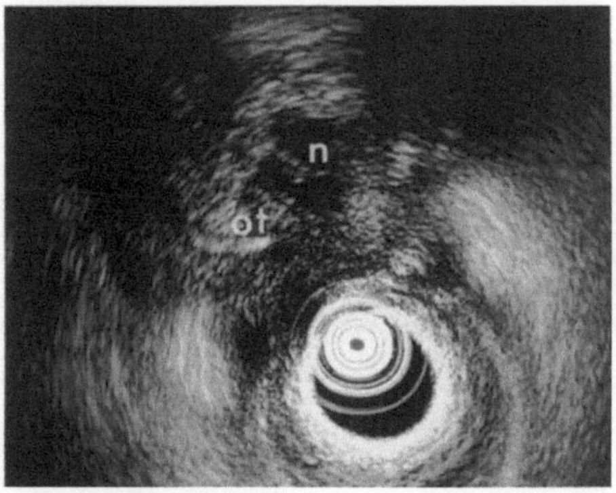

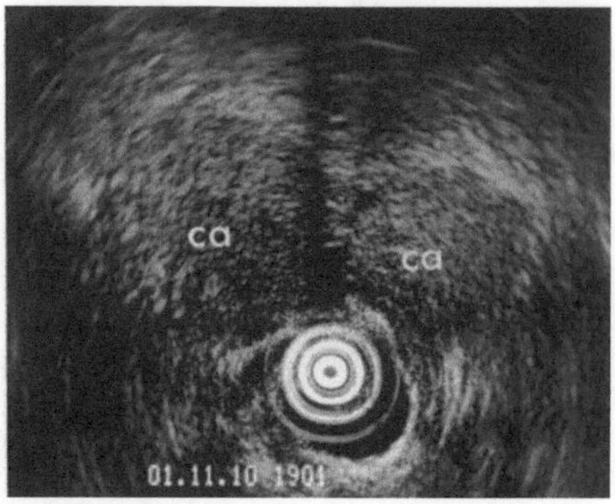

6.52

Fig. 6.49. RS: benign cystadenoma. Homogeneous appearance of the ovarian tumor mass (*ot*) behind the bladder (*b*)

Fig. 6.50. RS: malignant teratoma. Large ovarian tumor (*ot*) with irregular appearance. The uterine corpus cannot be differentiated from the teratoma

Fig. 6.51. RS: ovarian carcinoma. Ill-defined tumor mass (*ot*) with hypoechoic areas because of tumor necrosis (*n*)

Fig. 6.52. RS: carcinoma of both fallopian tubes. Relatively homogeneous appearance of the tumor (*ca*). On the left side the border of the tumor is clearly delineated, whereas on the right side the lateral border is ill-defined

swelling of the tissue at the end of the vagina presents as an ill-defined area of relatively low echogenicity (Fig. 6.53). Within the 1st to the 2nd week the edema vanishes and the hypoechoic tissue components become smaller (Fig. 6.54). The final postoperative status is characterized by no definite rectosonographic structures. Not uncommonly, hematomas complicate the postoperative phase (Fig. 6.55). Those located at the blind cranial end of the vagina are easily detected by RS. Hematomas appear as hypoechoic areas which become anechoic if the hematoma becomes liquid. If the hematoma becomes organized it will appear more and more echodense (Fig. 6.56). Definite diagnosis is possible only with follow-up examinations.

6.53
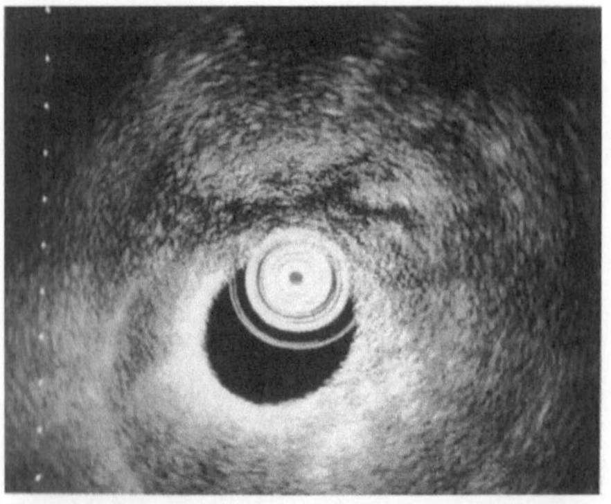

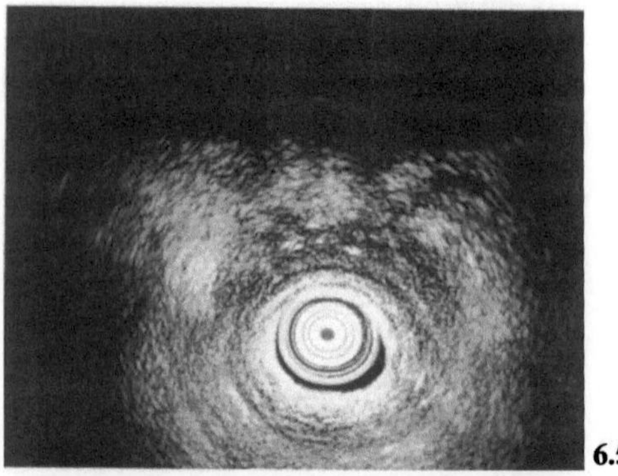
6.54

6.55
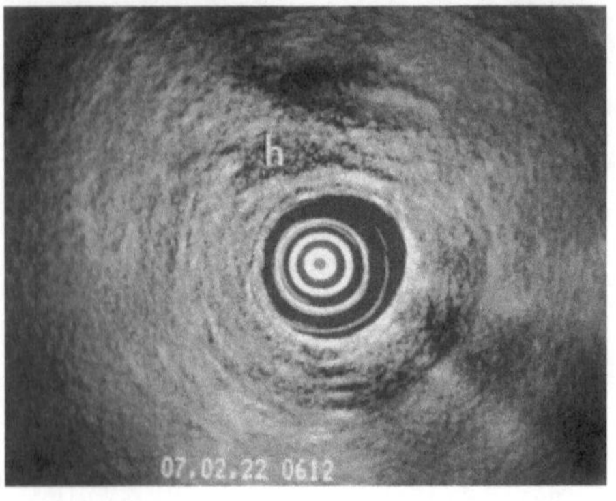

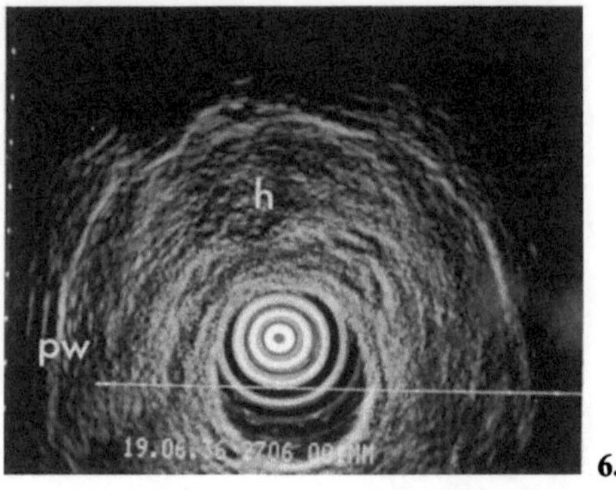

6.56

Fig. 6.53. RS: early postoperative status after hysterectomy. There is marked edema at the end of the vagina

Fig. 6.54. RS: status 2 weeks after hysterectomy (same patient as Fig. 6.53). The edema at the end of the vagina has diminished. Scar formation is not yet complete

Fig. 6.55. RS: small hematoma (*h*) at end of vagina after hysterectomy

Fig. 6.56. RS: old large hematoma at end of vagina after hysterectomy. The hematoma (*h*) already shows a relatively echodense structure, a sign of increasing organization. *pw*, pelvic wall

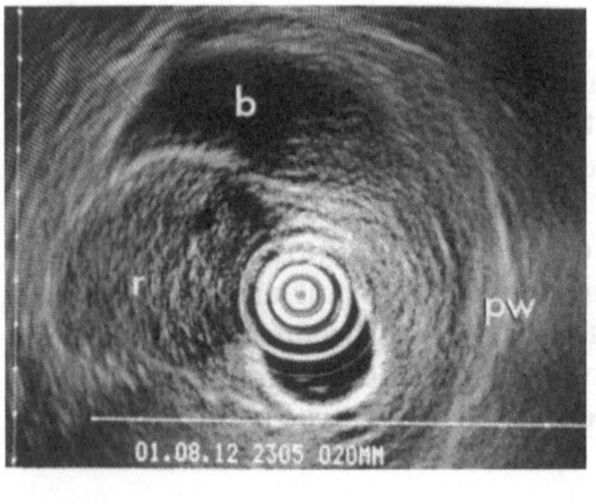

Fig. 6.57. RS: local recurrence at cranial end of vagina with lateral extension to right side. The urinary bladder (*b*) is indented but no sign of infiltration is visible. *r*, recurrence; *pw*, pelvic wall

6.4.6.9 Local Recurrence After Hysterectomy

Local recurrences after hysterectomy for carcinoma of the uterine corpus, the cervix or the ovaries present a major therapeutic problem. They should be diagnosed as early as possible. RS is able to diagnose recurrences at the cranial end of the vagina by their typical appearance (Fig. 6.57). They present as a hypoechoic mass in direct contact with the blind-ending vagina. The borders of the recurrence are clearly defined in most cases. RS is able to show the extent of the recurrence and its relation to the bladder and to the pelvic wall. Secondary signs of necrosis can be easily recognized by their typical anechoic appearance.

For a recurrence to be detected with RS it must have a minimal diameter of about 2 cm. Space-occupying lesions at the cranial end of the vagina after hysterectomy are not always local recurrences, as unspecific granulation tissue after hematoma or after local infection has the same sonographic appearance. RS can detect a lesion and describe its size and location, but the final diagnosis is made by cytology or histology.

Pathologically enlarged lymph nodes may be detected from a diameter of 1.0 cm on. Like local recurrences, they appear hypoechoic. No specific diagnosis is possible with RS, as pathologic and merely reactive lymph node enlargement cannot be differentiated (Fig. 6.58).

6.4.6.10 Local Recurrence After Radiotherapy

Local recurrences after radiotherapy are characterized by a hypoechoic appearance on RS. They are more difficult to detect than local recurrences after hysterectomy because of the necessity of differentiating them from uterine tissue after irradiation. In general, the presence of a local recurrence after irradiation is strongly suggested by an irregular contour of the uterus, irregularity of the echo pattern and a tendency to grow. Regular RS is of great importance for the diag-

6.58
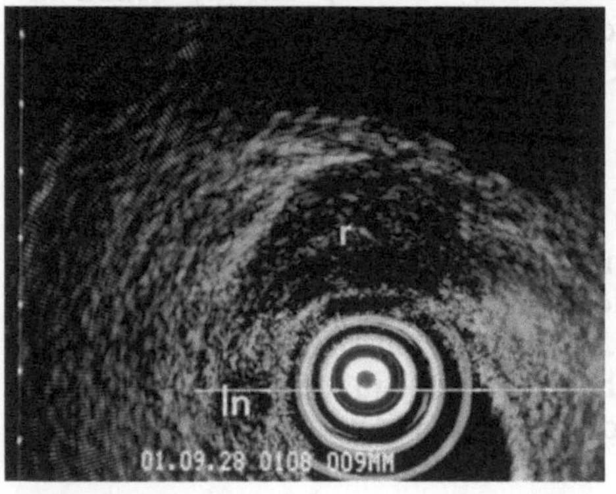

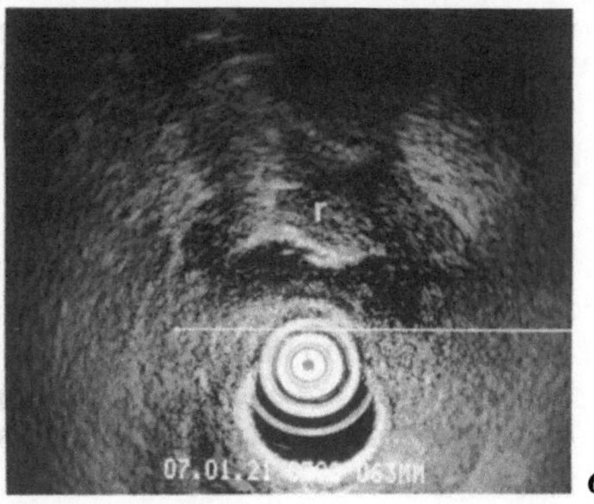

6.59

Fig. 6.58. RS: local recurrence (*r*) of carcinoma of carvix stage IIb treated with irradiation. *ln*, lymphnode

Fig. 6.59. RS: large local recurrence 1 year after irradiation of carcinoma of cervix stage IIb. Irregular appearance of tumor (*r*) with ventral extension

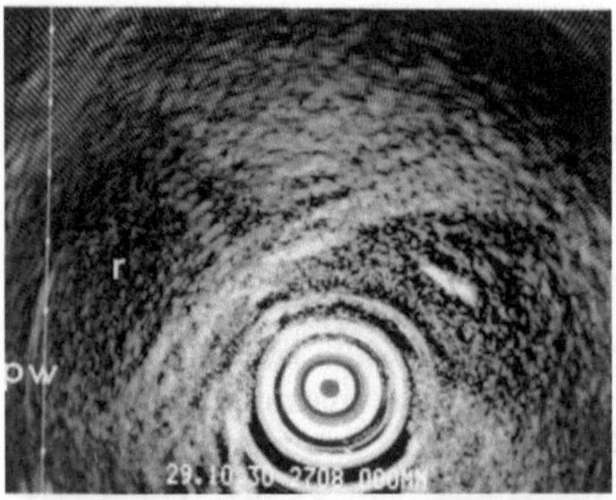

Fig. 6.60. RS: recurrence (*r*) on the pelvic wall (*pw*) of carcinoma of cervix stage IIb treated with irradiation

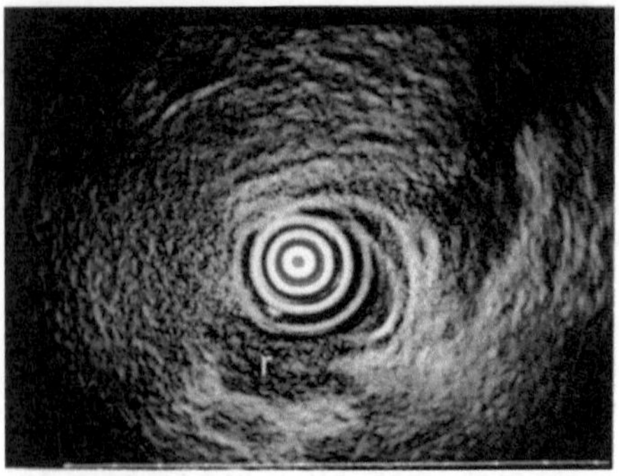

Fig. 6.61. RS: recurrence after irradiation. A tumor mass (*r*) is seen dorsal on the right side with finger-like extension into the paravaginal tissue. For this examination the rectal probe was placed in the vagina

nosis of local recurrences after radiation therapy. Recurrences detected rectosonographically are more than 2 cm in diameter in most cases. Identification of recurrences very early (within 6 months) after irradiation may be impossible because early edematous reaction cannot be differentiated from recurrent carcinoma. Local recurrences after irradiation may develop directly within the uterus or at the pelvic wall; in both cases they may be visualized only partially because of the limited field of view with RS (Fig. 6.58–6.60).

6.4.6.11 *Recurrence in the Vagina*

Vaginal recurrences of gynecologic tumors are not infrequent. They are diagnosed by inspection and palpation. Endosonography is able to define the depth of infiltration into the paravaginal tissue. As with primary carcinomas at this site, the best results are obtained by placing the rectal probe in the vagina. In this way direct assessment of tumor extension is possible (Fig. 6.61).

6.4.6.12 *Response of Carcinoma of the Cervix to Therapy*

Rectosonography is a cheap, reliable modality for checking the efficacy of therapy for carcinoma of the cervix. During radiotherapy the size of the tumor

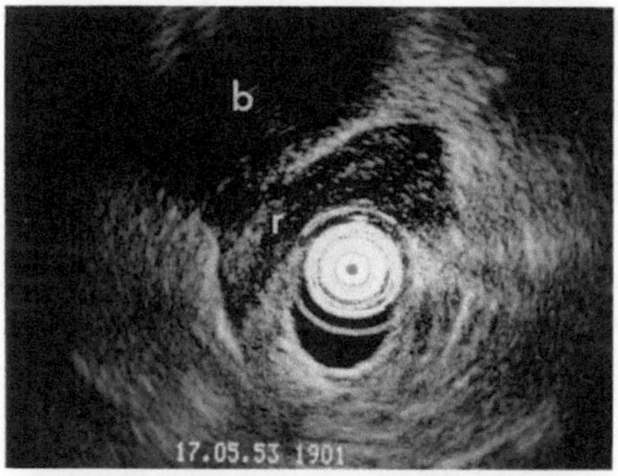

6.62

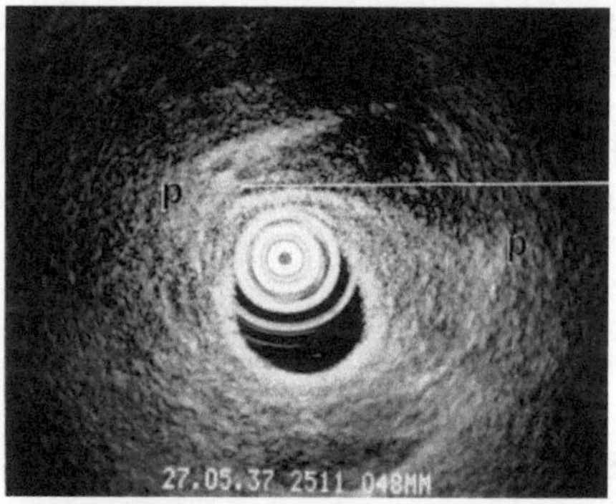

6.63

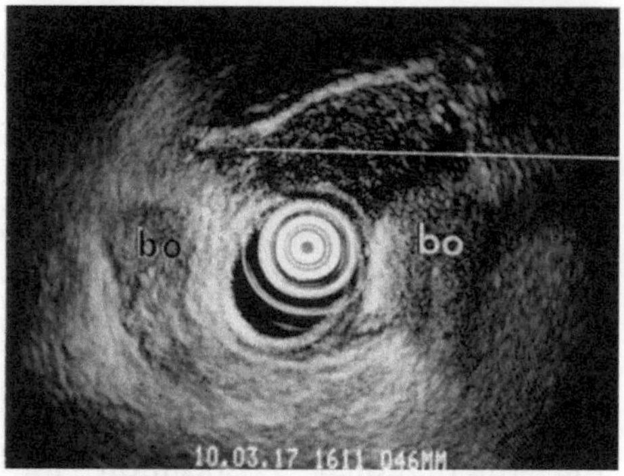

6.64

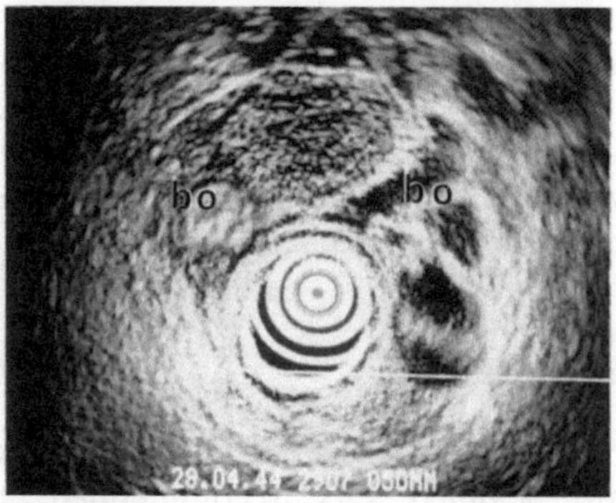

6.65

Fig. 6.62. RS: status of primary carcinoma of cervix stage IIIb after four courses of chemotherapy. The relatively hyperechoic residual tumor is already shrunken with residual extension to the right uterosacral ligament and to the dorsal bladder wall. *r*, recurrence; *b*, bladder

Fig. 6.63. RS: status 5 years after radiotherapy of carcinoma of cervix stage IIIb with massive parametrial scarring. RS of the parametrium (*p*) shows no abnormalities except a left-sided uterus

Fig. 6.64. RS: status after radiotherapy of carcinoma of cervix. Clinically massive parametrial scarring. RS shows adherent loops of small bowel (*bo*)

Fig. 6.65. RS: status after radiotherapy of carcinoma of uterine corpus. Numerous loops of small bowel (*bo*) adherent to the uterine body

remains constant in most cases during the first two thirds of the course of treatment. There are considerable reactions within the tumor, however, reflected by increasing areas of necrosis. Only slowly does the tumor mass diminish. The same development can be observed on RS during chemotherapy (Fig. 6.62).

6.4.6.13 Control After Irradiation

The status after irradiation of carcinomas of the cervix or, to a lesser degree, carcinomas of the corpus, is often characterized clinically by considerable parametrical scar formation. Thus it may be difficult to exclude or confirm a local recurrence. RS is extremely helpful in this situation because scars have a typical rectosonographic appearance unlike that of local recurrences. As already mentioned, local recurrences are hypoechoic, while scars resemble normal parametrium (Fig. 6.63). Loops of small bowel directly adherent to the parametrium after irradiation may alter the appearance of parametrial scarring (Figs. 6.64, 6.65).

6.5 Vaginosonography

(Sects. 6.5.1–6.5.7 in collaboration with L. W. Popp)

6.5.1 Apparatus

Vaginosonography (VS) is performed with sector scanners with a field of view varying from about 100° to 270° depending on the model used. The frequency used for VS is usually 5–7 MHz.

6.5.2 Method

No specific preparation of the patient is necessary for VS. First, sagittal planes are scanned. As recommended by the International Association for Endosonography (IAE), for reasons of standardization the bladder should be depicted on the left side of the image. Scans in the second, coronal plane should be oriented in such a way that the right side of the patient is shown on the right of the vaginosonogram.

6.5.3 Complications

No complications of VS have been reported to date.

6.5.4 Contraindications

An intact hymen normally prevents VS, as do vaginal strictures such as are seen after radiotherapy. A narrow vaginal lumen in older patients cannot be penetrated by the probe. In these circumstances, VS may be tried from the lower third of the vagina which is often wider, or from the introitus. The diagnostic results are often poor, however.

6.5.5 Capabilities and Limitations

VS is able to visualize the whole uterus from the cervix to the fundus. In contrast to RS, the fallopian tubes and the ovaries can also be seen. As a result of the necessary compromise between resolution and depth of ultrasound penetration, the macroscopic fine structures of the uterus are not demonstrated as clearly as with HS. On the other hand, VS is much less intrusive than HS, causing little discomfort to the women examined. For this reason, VS is the basic examination for the uterus and especially for the ovaries, which cannot be visualized sufficiently either with HS or with RS. Because of the close approximation between the transducer in the lateral vaginal vault and the ovaries, VS not only provides diagnostic information but also allows the performing of invasive diagnostic and therapeutic procedures such as punctures.

The main limitation of VS is that inherent in all imaging systems: no conclusions can be drawn regarding histology. However, with experience certain VS features may turn out to be associated with particular types of tumors.

6.5.6 Findings

6.5.6.1 Normal Uterus

The VS examination starts with a *sagittal* section of the small pelvis. The whole uterus is visualized in its typical anteflexed position. Centrally within the uterus is the hyperechoic layer of the endometrium. Sometimes even a small uterine cavity may be depicted. Near the fundus parts of the iliac vessels can be differentiated easily from adjacent tissue by their typical pulsation in rhythm with the heartbeat. In front of the sacrum and behind the uterus the middle third of the rectum is visualized (Fig. 6.66). The *coronal* section provides a good overview of the fundus, fallopian tubes and ovaries (Fig. 6.67). Sometimes it is difficult to obtain coronal scans more caudally in the region of the cervix, a section which is of great interest in cases of carcinoma of the cervix for detection or exclusion of parametrial infiltration.

6.66

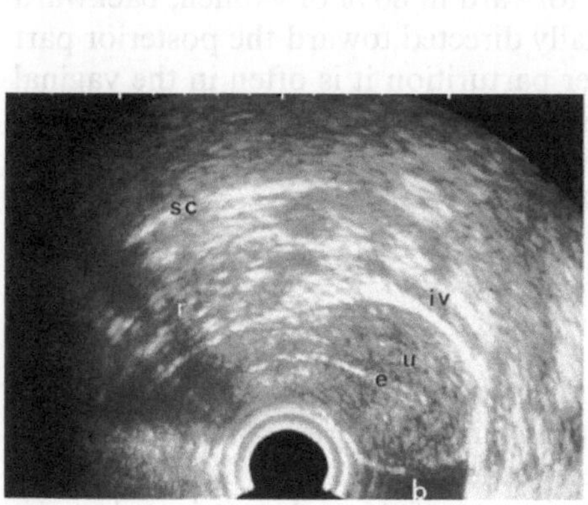

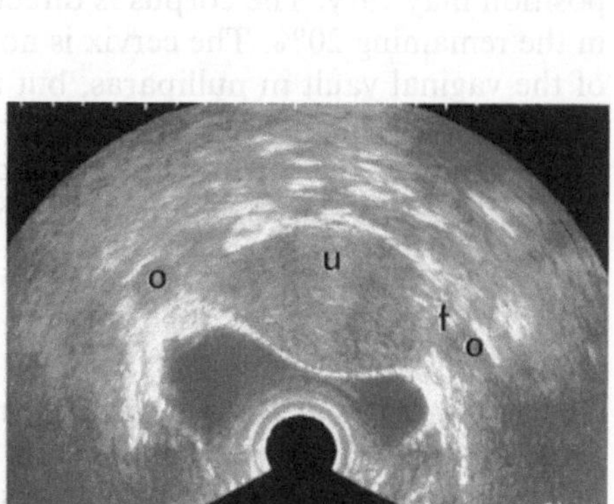

6.67

Fig. 6.66. VS: normal uterus (sagittal section). *u*, uterus; *e*, endometrium; *b*, bladder; *iv*, iliac vessels; *r*, rectum; *sc*, sacrum

Fig. 6.67. VS: normal uterus (coronal section). *u*, uterus; *t*, fallopian tubes (partly visualized); *o*, ovaries

6.68
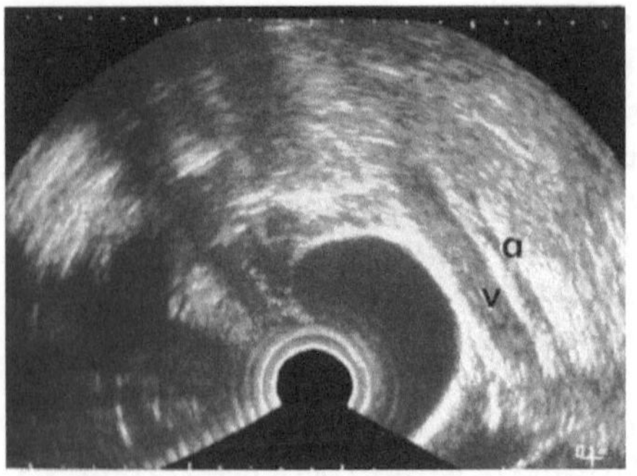

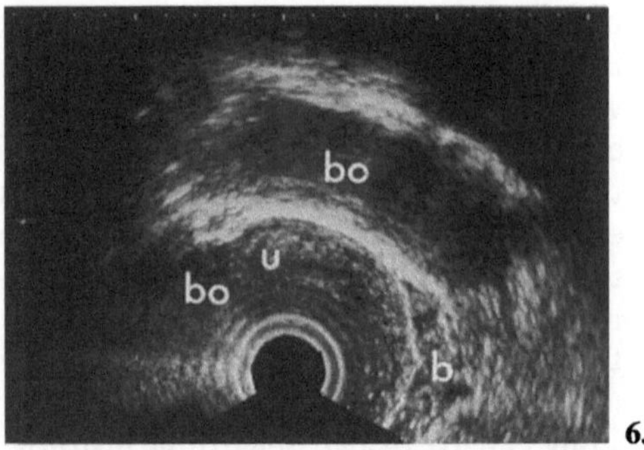

6.69

Fig. 6.68. VS: iliac vessels. Visualized are parts of the iliac artery (*a*) and vein (*v*) behind the bladder

Fig. 6.69. VS: retroflexion of uterus. *u*, uterus; *bo*, bowel; *b*, bladder

6.5.6.2 Iliac Vessels

On sagittal sections VS is able to visualize parts of the iliac vessels (Fig. 6.68). Usually the artery has a smaller diameter than the vein; this finding is pronounced in the case of venous dilatation. The vessels are easily identified by virtue of their typical pulsation.

6.5.6.3 Malposition of the Uterus

Displacement of the uterus may be lateral, anterior or posterior. Slight lateral displacement cannot be diagnosed with VS, while massive lateral displacement requires modification of the direction of the probe. As the uterus is not fixed, its position may vary. The corpus is directed forward in 80% of women, backward in the remaining 20%. The cervix is normally directed toward the posterior part of the vaginal vault in nulliparas, but after parturition it is often in the vaginal axis. If there is angulation between corpus and cervix, this is called retroflexion. The position of the corpus is revealed by VS, but no information about the position of the cervix can be obtained (Fig. 6.69).

6.5.6.4 Endometrium

The endometrium is characterized by rapid, cyclic variation of its structure and function during reproductive life. For optimal diagnostic results morphological and physiological features must be considered together.

VS is able to visualize the *macroscopic* aspects of the endometrium, but microscopic changes are not detected. No differentiation between stratum basale and stratum functionale is possible (Fig. 6.70). The normal endometrium is seen as a *hyperechoic layer* lying centrally within the myometrium. The basal border between endometrium and myometrium is clearly defined in most cases. A *hypo-*

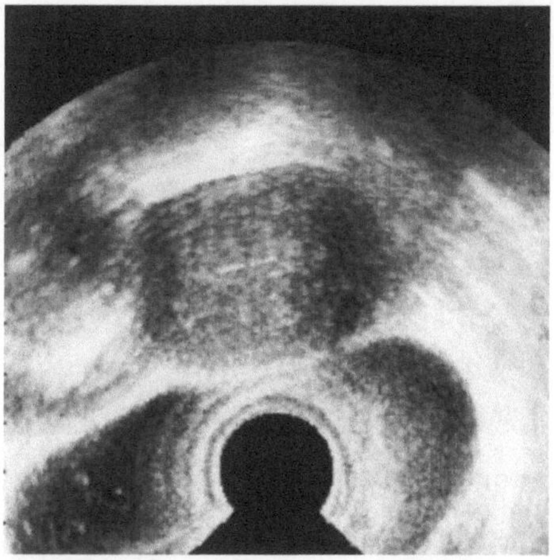

Fig. 6.70. VS: endometrium, 5th day of menstrual cycle. Early proliferation phase with a thin layer of hyperechoic endometrium

6.71

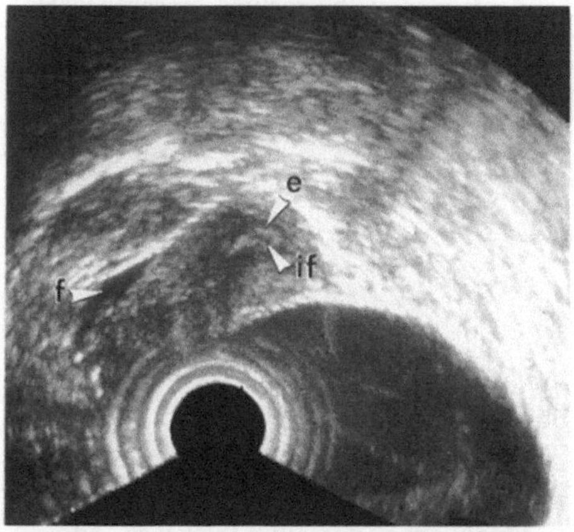

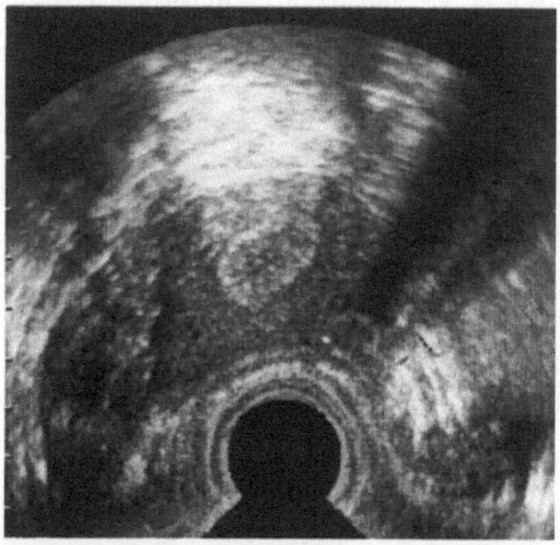

6.72

Fig. 6.71. VS: endometrium, 14th day of menstrual cycle. Moderately built-up endometrium (*e*) with a small amount of fluid within the uterine cavity (*if*), which is often found at the time of ovulation. As a sign of ovulation we see a little free fluid in the cul-de-sac (*f*)

Fig. 6.72. VS: endometrium, 25th day of menstrual cycle. Late secretory phase with a highly built-up endometrium. Not unusual is the partly ill-defined border of the endometrium on the anterior wall

echoic rim reminiscent of the junction zone known from MRI (see Sect. 6.8.2.1) is sometimes seen below the endometrium.

The *variability* of the endometrium is characterized physiologically by differences in thickness, histologically by differences in gland activity. In the secretion (premenstrual) phase the endometrium may be as much as 10 mm thick, compared with 1–2 mm at its thinnest in the reparative (postmenstrual) phase. The border between the stratum basale and the myometrium may appear irregular even histologically. The surface of the endometrium may appear irregular physiologically due to local differences in fluid or glands (Figs. 6.71–6.75).

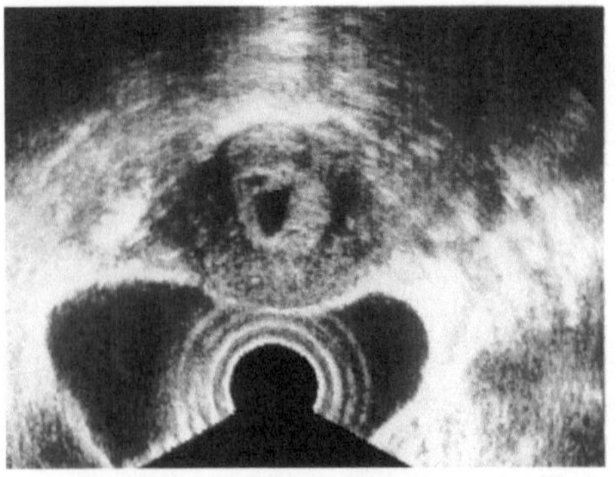

6.73

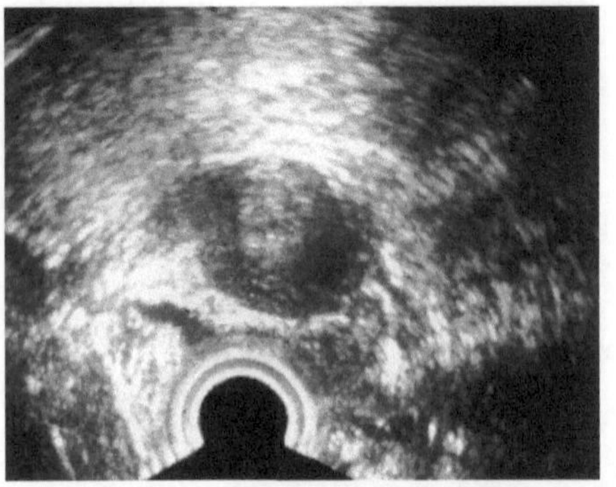

6.74

Fig. 6.73. VS: glandular-cystic hyperplasia of endometrium. The endometrium is highly built-up. Its surface appears slightly inhomogeneous. The basal border of the anterior wall is ill defined. There are several cystic areas within the endometrium and free fluid within the uterine cavity

Fig. 6.74. VS: adenomatous hyperplasia. Ill-defined endometrium with irregular appearance. No cystic structures of any great size

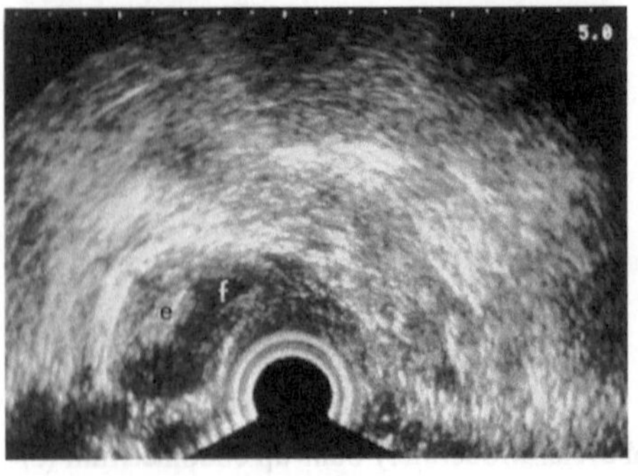

Fig. 6.75. VS: localized glandular-cystic hyperplasia. The sagittal section of the fundus shows dorsally a thickened endometrium (e). *f*, fluid within uterine cavity

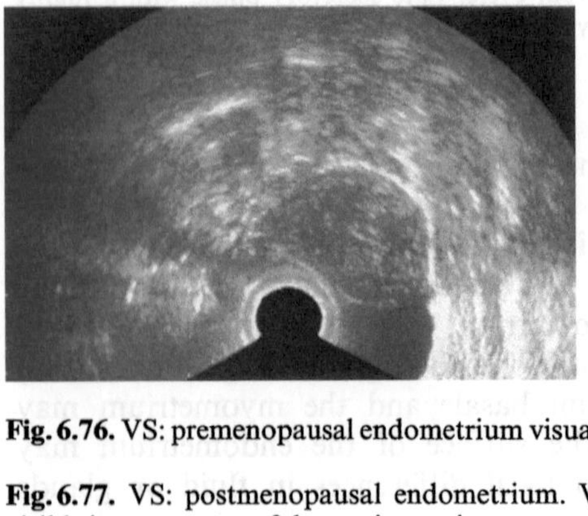

6.76

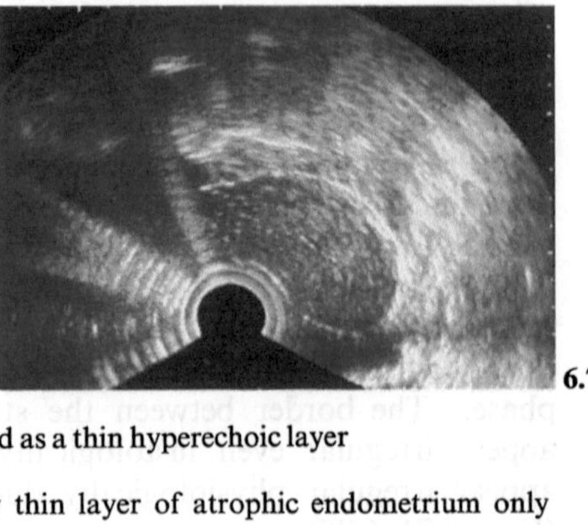

6.77

Fig. 6.76. VS: premenopausal endometrium visualized as a thin hyperechoic layer

Fig. 6.77. VS: postmenopausal endometrium. Very thin layer of atrophic endometrium only visible in some parts of the uterine cavity

6.78

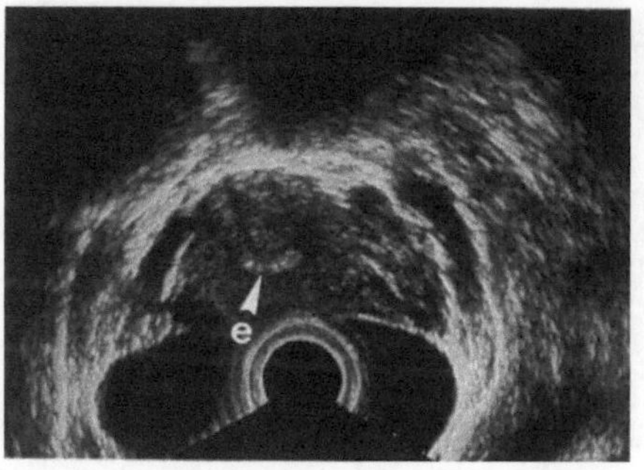

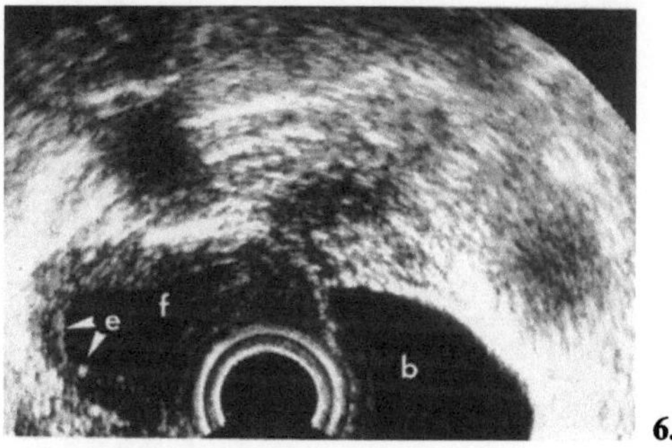

6.79

Fig. 6.78. VS: superficial endometrial carcinoma. Early exophytic tumor growth in the uterine fundus. No infiltration into the myometrium. VS is unspecific, but a highly developed endometrium (*e*) after the menopause is suspicious

Fig. 6.79. VS: endometrial carcinoma. Retroflexion of the uterus. Enlarged uterine corpus with central fluid retention (*f*). Only a small rim of hyperechoic endometrium (*e*) which shows no specific signs of endometrial carcinoma. *b*, bladder

Pre- and Postmenopausal State: Premenopausal endometrium shows local differences in thickness. After the menopause, in the absence of ovarian hormones, the now functionless endometrium becomes thin and eventually atrophic.

With VS one can determine the thickness of the endometrium as an indicator of the hormonal status (Figs. 6.76, 6.77). VS yields information on the *surface of the endometrium* (smooth/irregular), its *structure* (homogeneous/inhomogeneous) and the *basal border* (clearly defined/poorly defined). The relevance of a poorly defined basal boundary is not yet clear.

6.5.6.5 Carcinoma of the Endometrium

The primary criteria of carcinoma of the endometrium on VS are a highly developed endometrium, irregularity of the endometrial surface, a poorly defined basal border and extension of hyperechoic endometrium into the myometrium. A secondary sign is fluid retention within the uterine cavity. All these features are nonspecific, as they may also be seen in benign hyperplasia of the endometrium. In patients with known endometrial carcinoma, only very rough estimation of tumor extension is possible with VS. In contrast to HS, the exact depth of tumor infiltration cannot be determined reproducibly. Tumor growth beyond the natural organ borders may be identified, however (Figs. 6.78–6.83).

6.5.6.6 Carcinoma of the Cervix

The VS criteria for carcinoma of the cervix are an irregular echo pattern of the cervical epithelium, enlargement of the cervix and deformation of the natural organ borders. With VS it is not always possible to differentiate between normal

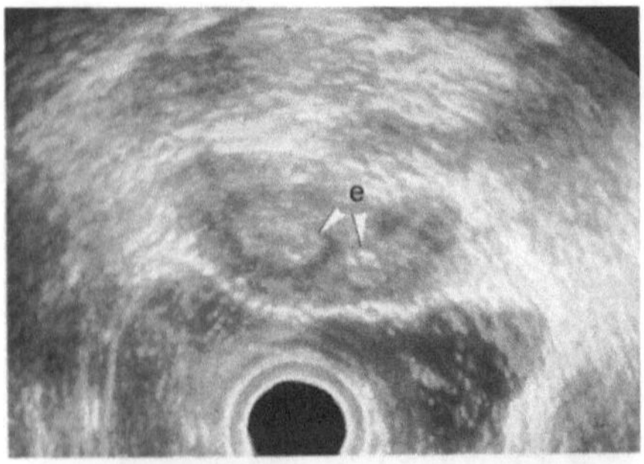

6.80

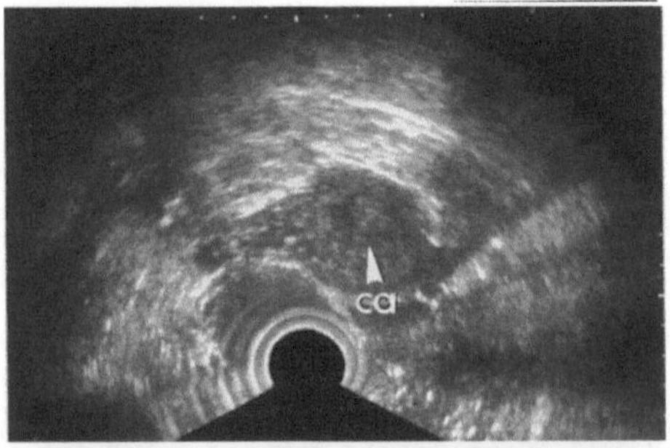

6.81

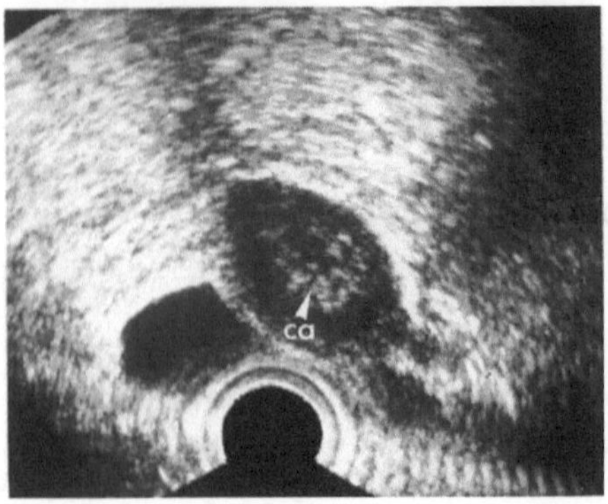

6.82

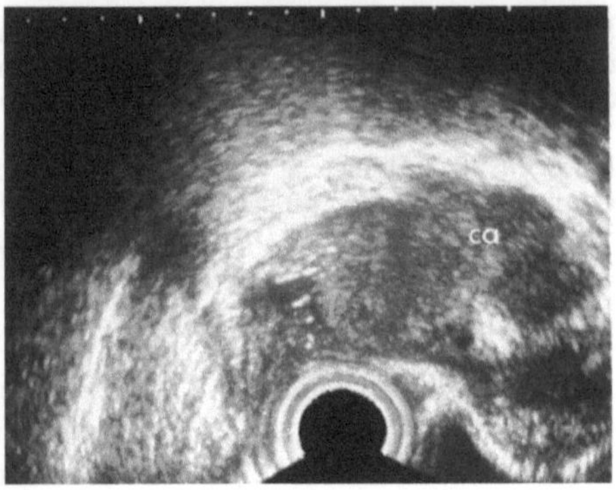

6.83

Fig. 6.80. VS: endometrial carcinoma with exophytic growth in uterine fundus. On the right side the surface is irregular. Small fluid retention. No signs of myometrial infiltration. *e*, endo metrium

Fig. 6.81. VS: endometrial carcinoma with predominantly exophytic growth but early myometrial infiltration. The hyperechoic part of the exophytically growing carcinoma (*ca*) has an ill-defined basal border, sign of early infiltrative growth

Fig. 6.82. VS: endometrial carcinoma with infiltrative growth. The hyperechoic endometrium shows an irregular basal border. Ventrally, a ring of myometrium is preserved. Dorsally, hyperechoic structures nearly reach the serosa, suggesting deep infiltration. *ca*, carcinoma

Fig. 6.83. VS: endometrial carcinoma, FIGO stage III. The coronal section shows tumor masses (*ca*) beyond the organ borders with extension towards the left side of the pelvis

Fig. 6.84. VS: cervical carcinoma stage Ib. The cervix is not enlarged but an irregular, hyperechoic cervical epithelium is demonstrated. *ca*, carcinoma

Fig. 6.85. VS: cervical carcinoma stage Ib with enlarged cervix. No infiltration of the parametrium is seen. *ca*, carcinoma; *pw*, pelvic wall

Fig. 6.86. VS: cervical carcinoma stage IIb. Large tumor mass (*ca*) with irregularities and a central necrosis. The pelvic wall is free. *bo*, bowel

Fig. 6.87. VS: cervical carcinoma stage IIIb (sagittal section). Besides an enlarged cervix the uterine corpus is infiltrated too, with irregular tumor mass (*ca*) within it. Marked swelling of the bladder wall (*bw*)

Fig. 6.88. VS: cervical carcinoma stage IIIb, same patient as in Fig. 6.87 (coronal section). The tumor extension has reached the pelvic wall

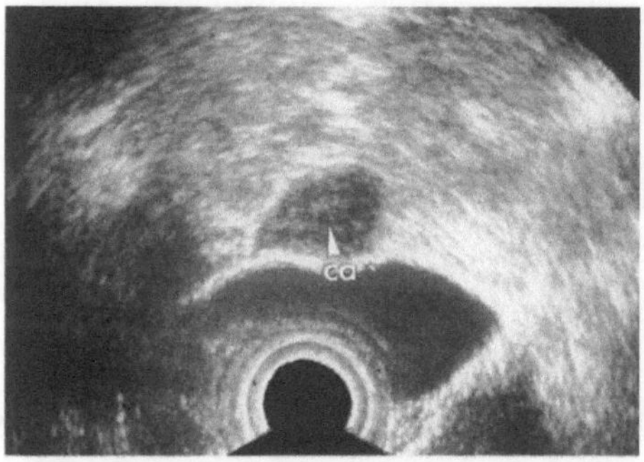

6.84

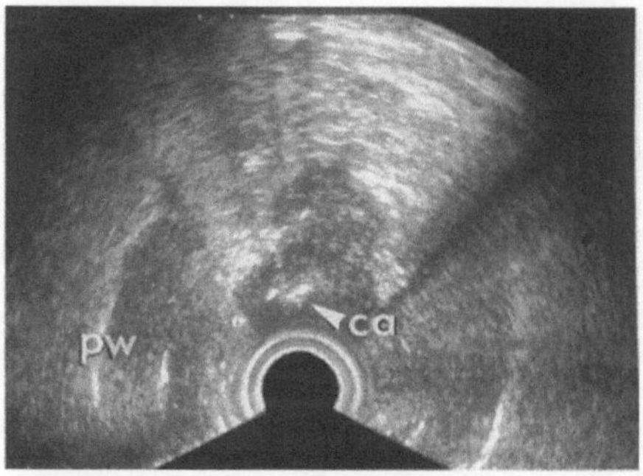

6.85

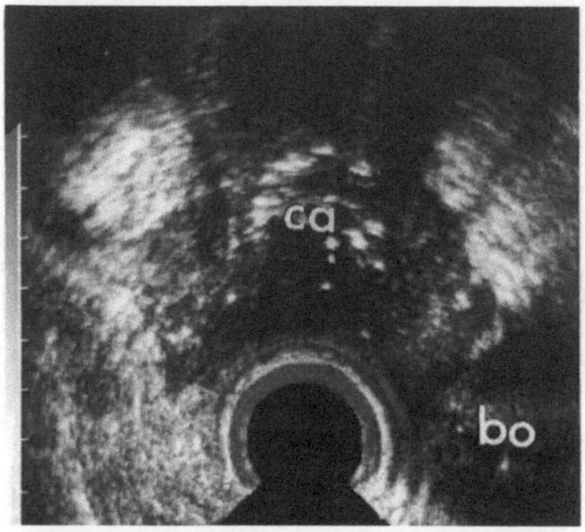

6.86

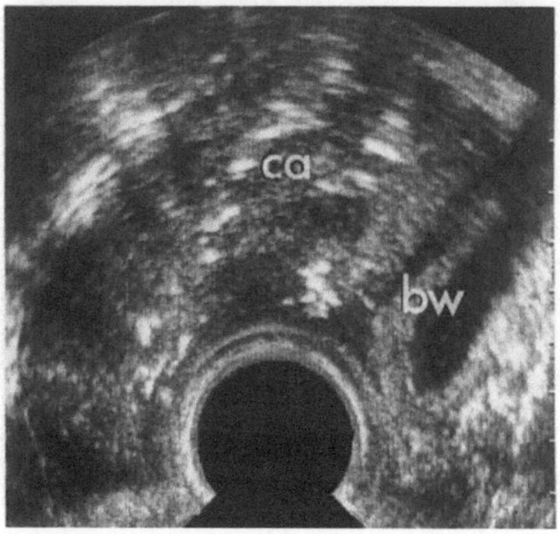

6.87

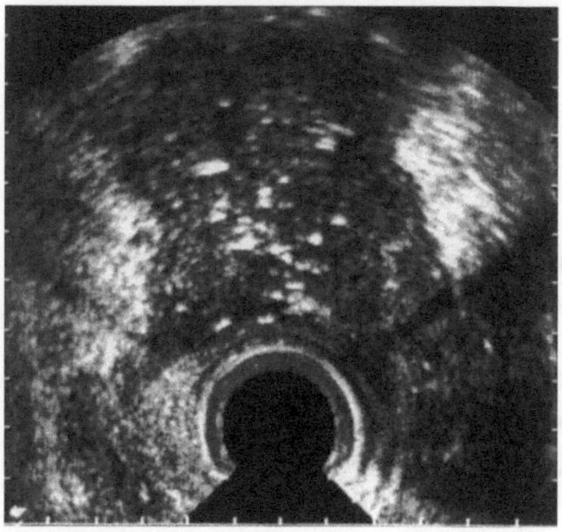
6.88

cervical tissue and carcinoma, so that it may be impossible to diagnose a carcinoma stage Ib. In addition to the information afforded by RS, VS can yield sagittal scans which are useful for demonstrating the relation of the cervix to the bladder and to the rectum. The accuracy of staging of carcinomas of the cervix by VS seems to be slightly inferior to that by RS or CT, but no comparative study has yet been published (Figs. 6.84–6.88).

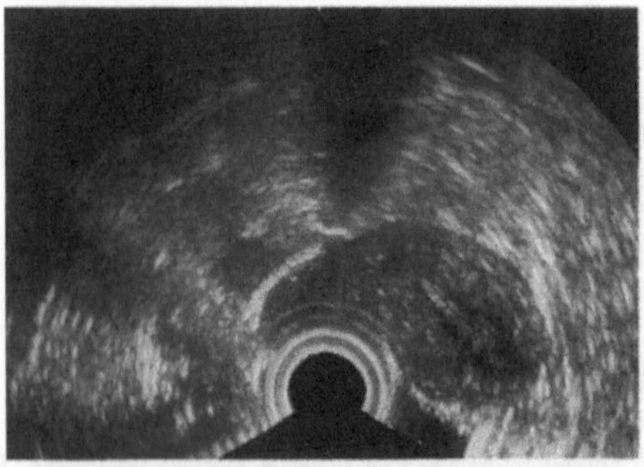
6.89

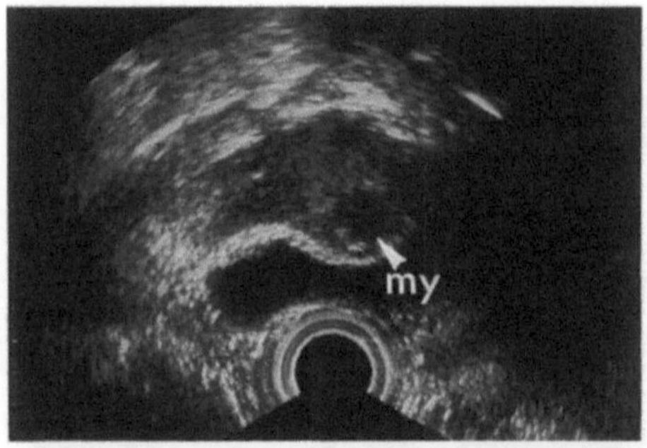

6.90

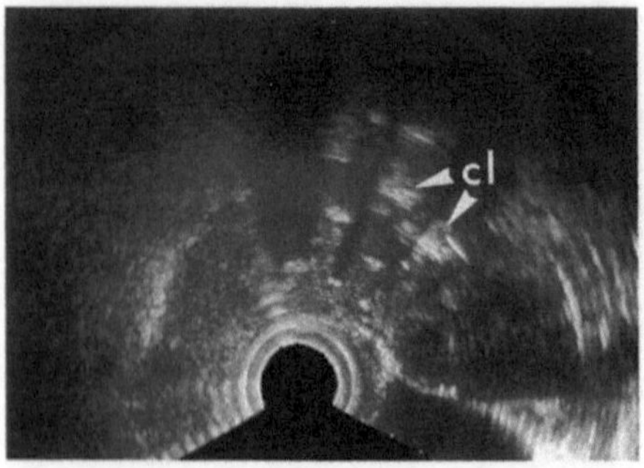

6.91

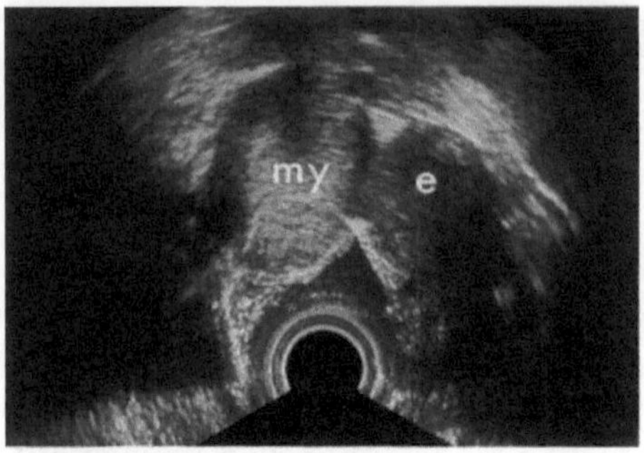

6.92

Fig. 6.89. VS: diffuse myohyperplasia. Slight irregularities within the myometrium

Fig. 6.90. VS: single myoma (*myoma*)

Fig. 6.91. VS: large myoma with calcifications (*cl*)

Fig. 6.92. VS: pedunculated myoma. On the right side of the uterus is a big pedunculated myoma (*my*). *e*, endometrium

6.5.6.7 Myomas

Diffuse hyperplasia within the myometrium is characterized by an altered echo pattern (Fig. 6.89). The appearance of myomas on VS does not differ from that known from percutaneous ultrasound. Because of the higher frequency (5–7 MHz) used for VS, myomas may be detected down to a diameter of 1 cm if their echo pattern differs from that of normal myometrium (Figs. 6.90–6.92). Anechoic areas are typical of secondary liquefication, whereas hyperechoic structures with dorsal acoustic shadow are typical of calcifications.

6.5.6.8 Ovaries

The ovaries can be visualized in about 95% of premenopausal women and about 75% of postmenopausal women. They are ovoid, flattened, solid organs whose size varies but is generally about 1.5 × 3 × 3.5 cm. Enlargement of the ovaries may be caused by solid or cystic processes. While cystic changes of the ovaries may be diagnosed from a diameter of 0.3 cm, solid changes are much more difficult to

6.93
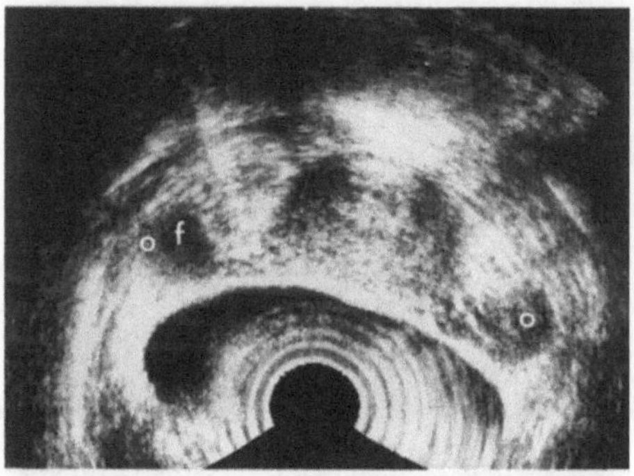

6.94
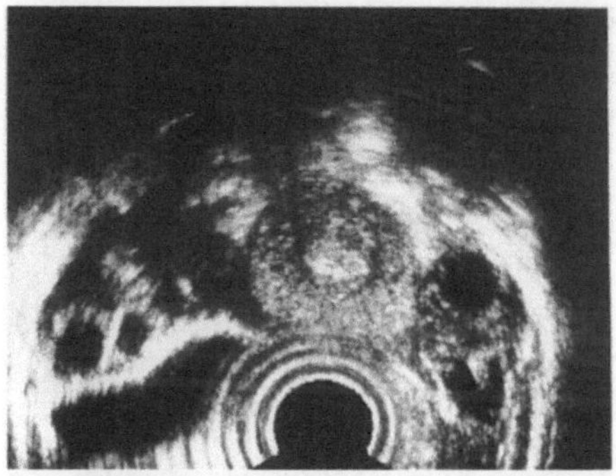

6.95
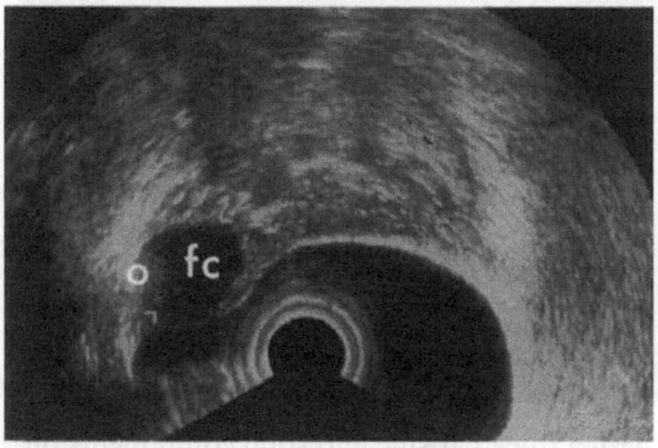

6.96
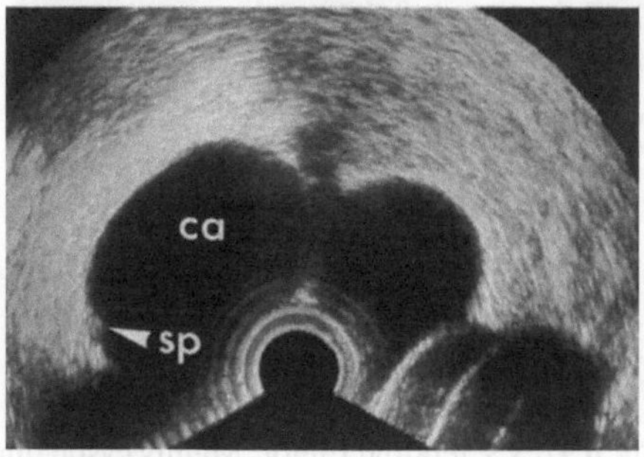

Fig. 6.93. VS: normal ovaries. Follicle (*f*) in the right ovary (*o*)

Fig. 6.94. VS: multiple follicular cysts. Both ovaries are enlarged; the cysts are smooth with no solid components

Fig. 6.95. VS: follicular cyst. The residual ovary (*o*) is seen on the lateral border of the cyst (*fc*)

Fig. 6.96. VS: serous cystadenoma. Multilocular cyst with smooth borders. Only on the right side is there a tiny solid part (*sp*). *ca*, cystadenoma

detect. Malignancy is suspected, if VS shows irregular enlargement of the ovaries with cystic and solid components. The more irregular the appearance of the solid elements, the higher is the probability of malignant degeneration. Secondary signs of malignancy are ascites and peritoneal carcinosis. No specific histologic diagnosis may be achieved with VS (Figs. 6.93–6.99).

Ovarian Abscesses. Ovarian abscesses are relatively rare. Vaginosonographically they are characterized by irregular enlargement of the ovary with secondary necrotic areas. The appearance may be identical to that of carcinomas but the clinical situation is quite different (Fig. 6.100).

6.5.6.9 Salpingitis

Inflammation of the fallopian tubes may be acute or chronic, unilateral or bilateral. Vaginosonographic criteria for salpingitis are thickening of the tubes and, in case of hydrosalpinx or pyosalpinx, fluid retention. The diagnosis of sal-

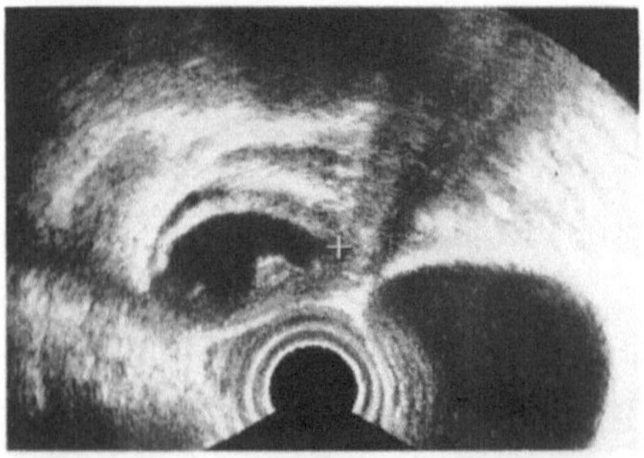

6.97

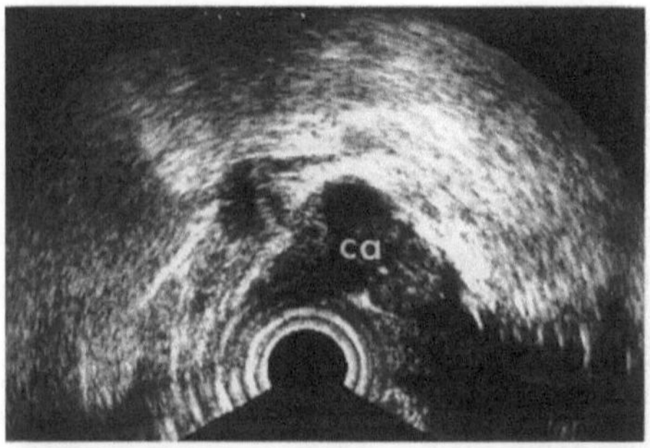

6.98

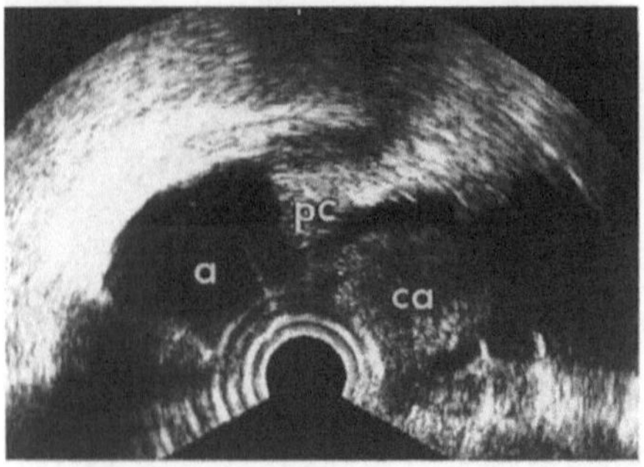

6.99

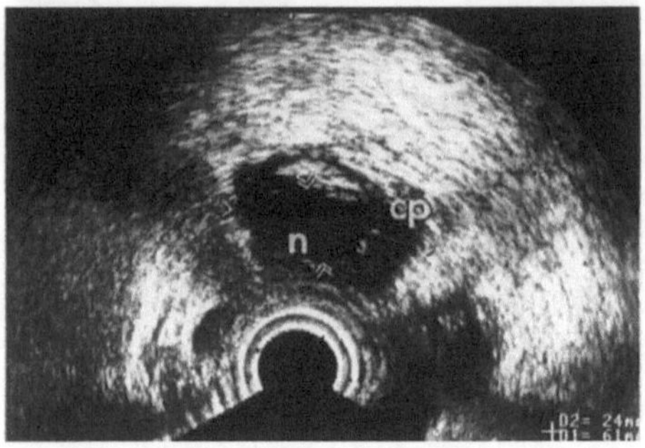

6.100

Fig. 6.97. VS: teratoid tumor. Mainly cystic tumor with a thick capsule and solid components on the anterior wall. Solid tumor masses like these suggest malignancy

Fig. 6.98. VS: adenocarcinoma of ovary. Typical irregular structure with solid and cystic elements suggesting malignancy. *ca*, carcinoma

Fig. 6.99. VS: ovarian carcinoma (*ca*) with ascites (*a*) and peritoneal carcinosis (*pc*)

Fig. 6.100. VS: ovarian abscess. Centrally anechoic necrotic tissue (*n*) with an irregular capsule (*cp*)

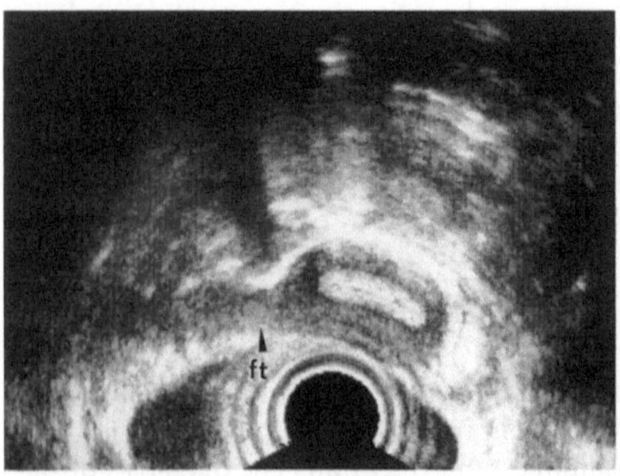

Fig. 6.101. VS: right salpingitis. Massive thickening of the fallopian tube (*ft*) but no fluid retention

pingitis can only be established in conjunction with clinical examination (Fig. 6.101).

6.5.6.10 Status After Hysterectomy

After hysterectomy the rectum or small bowel comes into direct contact with the cranial portion of the vagina (Fig. 6.102). This is the reason why every space-occupying lesion at this location after hysterectomy is suspicious. Hematomas are not infrequent in the postoperative period, but later the most common lesions at this site are local recurrences. Whatever their histologic type, these local recurrences normally do not differ greatly in their appearance on VS, showing varying degrees of hypoechoicity. Therefore histologic verification is necessary (Figs. 6.103, 6.104).

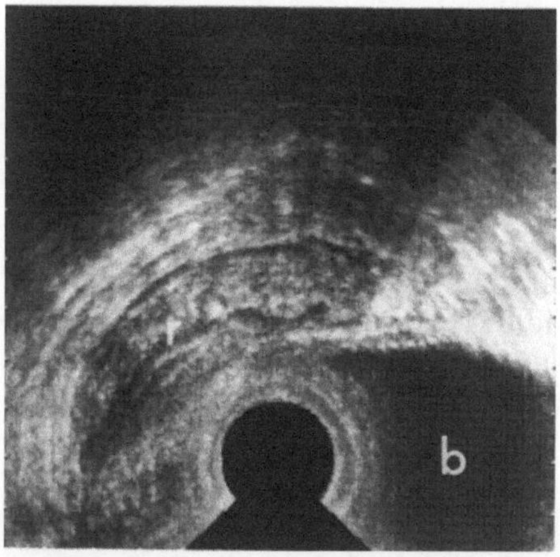

Fig. 6.102. VS: status after hysterectomy with no evidence of local recurrence. *b*, bladder; *r*, rectum

6.103
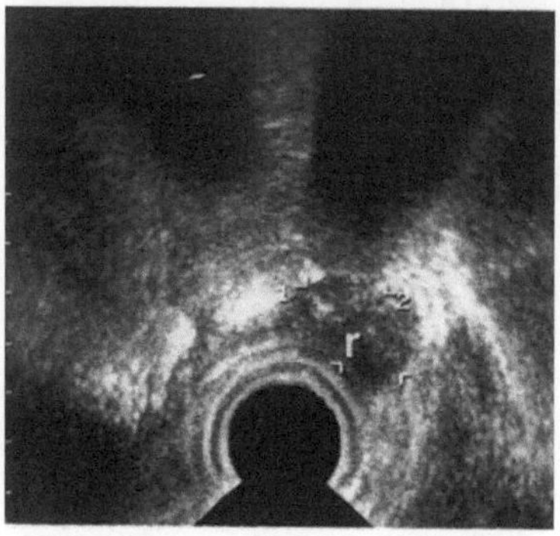

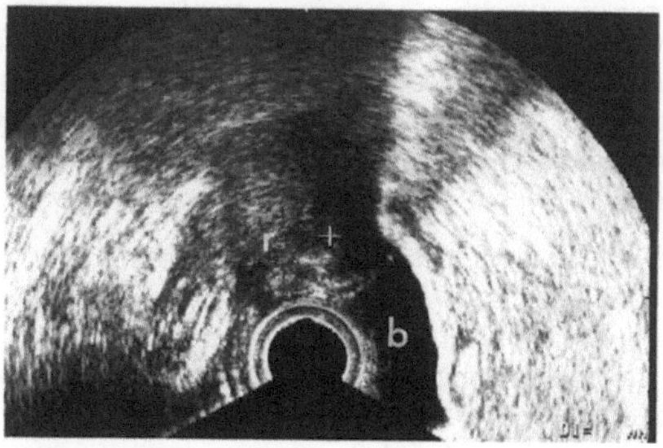

6.104

Fig. 6.103. VS: small local recurrence (*r*) 5 years after extended hysterectomy for carcinoma of cervix stage Ib

Fig. 6.104. VS: large local recurrence (*r*) of adenocarcinoma with infiltration of dorsal wall of bladder (*b*)

6.105
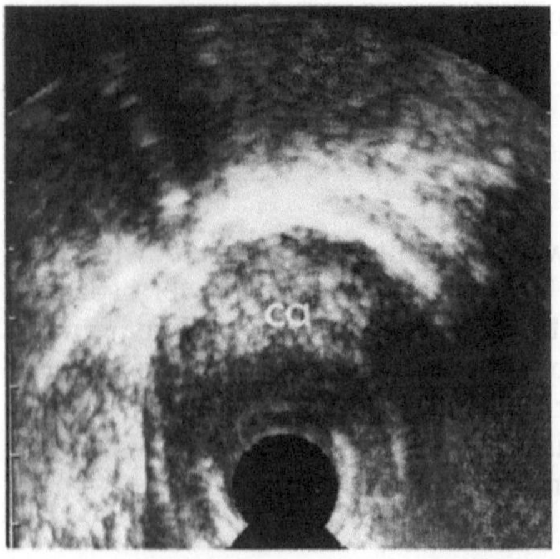

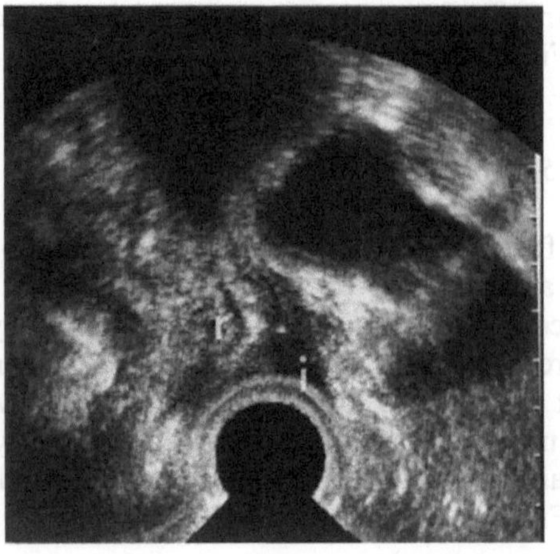

6.106

Fig. 6.105. VS: large solid carcinoma (*ca*) of urethra

Fig. 6.106. VS: carcinoma of rectum (*r*) with infiltration (*i*) of vagina

6.5.6.11 Further Applications

Vaginosonography is able to deliver much additional information on space-occupying lesions within the lesser pelvis that do not originate from the internal female genitalia. The indication for VS should be determined individually in light of the clinical problem. As an example, Fig. 6.105 shows a case of a large carcinoma of the urethra (Fig. 6.105) and the rectum (Fig. 6.106).

6.5.7 Vaginosonography in Obstetrics

6.5.7.1 Fetal Biometry

Although the physiologic variability of the size of the fetus makes it difficult to calculate the date of birth by means of ultrasound in the second or third trimester, ultrasonic biometry of the embryo/fetus is possible in the first trimester. The high resolution of VS allows particularly accurate measurement [32]:

Early 5th week after menstruation (p.m.):
- chorionic sac 0.2–0.5 cm
- yolk sac 0.2 cm
- deciduotrophoblastic complex ringlike

Late 5th week p.m.:
- chorionic sac 0.5–1.0 cm
- yolk sac 0.3 cm (Fig. 6.107)

Early 6th week p.m.:
- yolk sac 0.4 cm (remains constant in size and serves as "biological indicator")
- embryo 0.2 cm with detectable cardiac activity

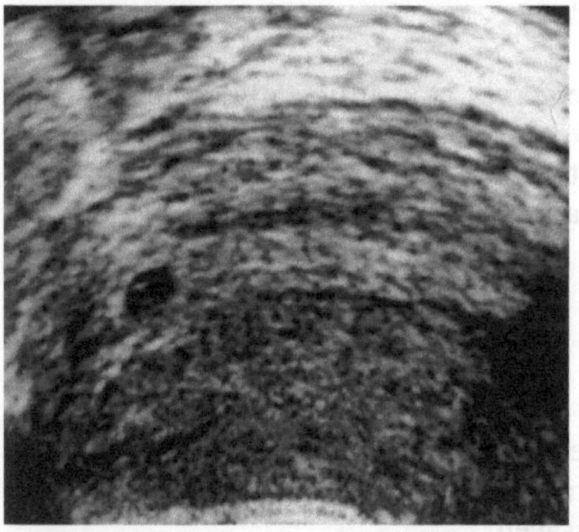
6.107

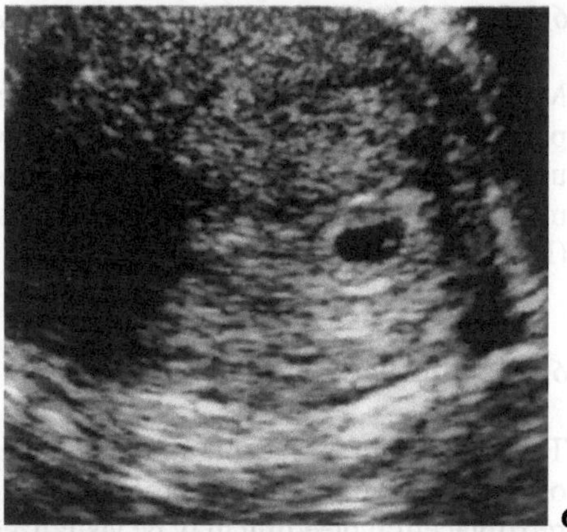
6.108

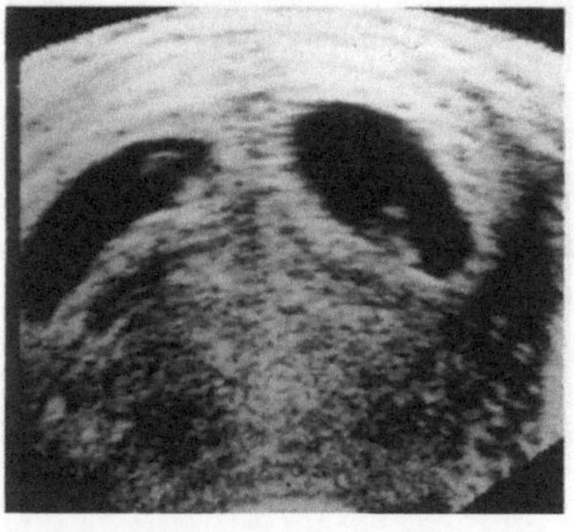
6.109

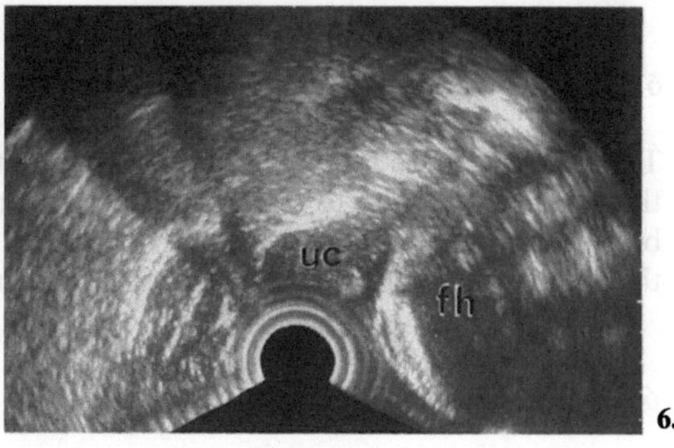

6.110

Fig. 6.107. VS: pregnancy, 5th week p.m.

Fig. 6.108. VS: pregnancy, 6th week p.m.

Fig. 6.109. VS: twin pregnancy, 8th week p.m.

Fig. 6.110. VS: cervix in third trimester of pregnancy. The internal os uteri is closed. *uc*, uterine cervix; *fh*, fetal head

Late 6th week p.m.:
- chorionic sac 1.5 cm
- embryo 0.4 cm (Fig. 6.108)

Early 7th week p.m.:
- amniotic cavity same size as yolk sac

Late 7th week p.m.:
- amniotic cavity twice as big as yolk sac

Early 8th week p.m.:
- amniotic cavity half as big as chorionic sac

Late 8th week p.m.:
- head of fetus as big as yolk sac (Fig. 6.109)

6.5.7.2 Measurement of the Length of the Cervix

Measurement of the length of the uterine cervix is insufficiently accurate with percutaneous ultrasound. With VS, however, not only the length of the pregnant uterine cervix but also the width of the internal os can be measured. At the moment the therapeutic relevance of these additional data is not clearly defined (Fig. 6.110) [32].

6.5.7.3 Diagnosis of Placenta Previa

The location of a placenta previa can be determined simply and exactly by means of VS at any time during pregnancy. Premature separation of the placenta and retroplacental bleeding may be visualized as well.

6.5.7.4 Evaluation of the Fetal Membranes

The relation of the fetal membranes to the internal os is of great importance in the period leading up to birth. The detection of a separation of both fetal membranes seems possible with VS. In such cases the whole hydrostatic pressure of the pregnancy is on the chorion laeve and the thin capsular decidua.

6.5.7.5 Pelvimetry

The true conjugate, the obstetric conjugate, the diagonal conjugate, the greatest anteroposterior diameter of the pelvis, the diameter of the midpelvis and the transverse diameter can all be measured with VS (Figs. 6.111, 6.112) [32].

6.5.7.6 VS During Delivery

Little experience of VS during delivery has yet been reported. Some additional information concerning the relation of the fetal head to the maternal pelvis seems to be gained.

6.5.7.7 Ectopic Pregnancy and Abortion

Differentiation between ectopic and intrauterine pregnancy may be difficult with percutaneous ultrasound. This distinction is made much more readily with VS, as the biometric parameters of normal early pregnancy are clearly defined (see Sect. 6.5.7.1). A reliable sign of ectopic pregnancy is the absence of myometrium around the embryo/fetus together with the presence of specific endometrial changes (Fig. 6.113). In the case of an incomplete abortus, ill-defined remnants of the chorionic sac are seen (Fig. 6.114).

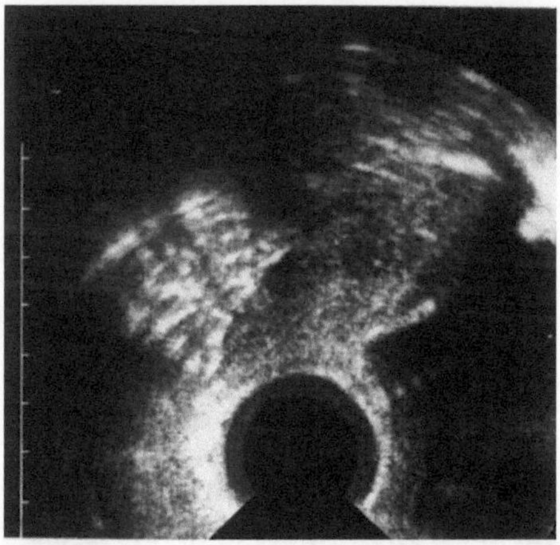

6.111

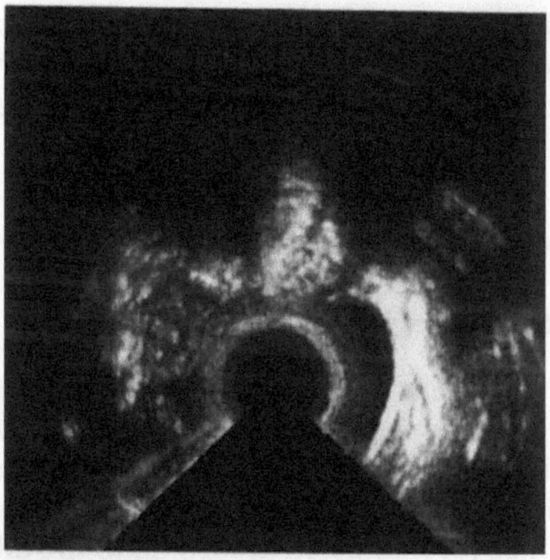

6.112

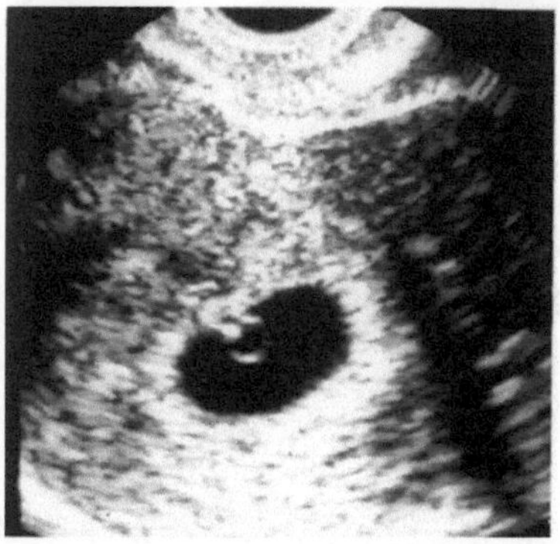

6.113

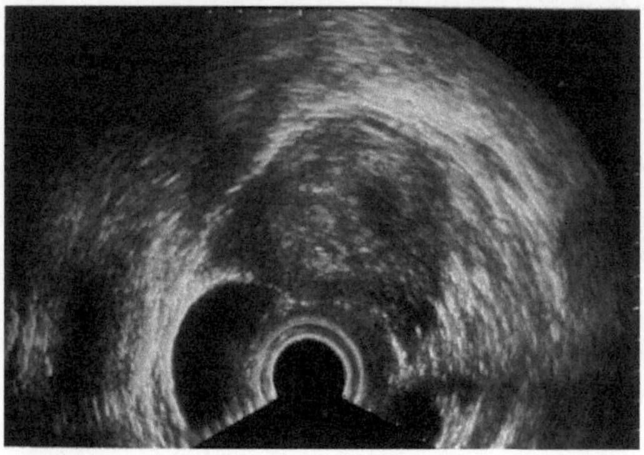

6.114

Fig. 6.111. VS: greatest anteroposterior diameter of pelvis

Fig. 6.112. VS: transverse diameter of bony pelvis

Fig. 6.113. VS: ectopic pregnancy. Typical nonvisualization of the myometrium around the chorionic sac

Fig. 6.114. VS: incomplete abortus with ill-defined remnants of chorionic sac

6.5.7.8 Specific Gynecological Indications

Measurements of Follicles. VS is able to follow the growth of normal follicles and of follicles stimulated for in-vitro fertilization [29].

Transvaginal Puncture of Follicles. Transvaginal follicular puncture for IVF seems to be superior to percutaneous puncture [9, 10]. Various techniques have been suggested [32].

Biopsy of the Trophoblast. Trophoblast sampling is an established procedure which seems to be safer and more accurate if performed under vaginosonographic guidance [12].

Evaluation of the Circulation of the Trophoblast. VS, especially if combined with the Doppler technique, seems to deliver some additional information about the circulation between uterus and trophoblast [39].

6.6 Computed Tomography

6.6.1 Principle

A thin sclice of tissue perpendicular to the body axis is imaged according to the principle expounded by Hounsfield [21]. The X-ray attenuation of a definite number of projections lying in a plane is measured, and these single attenuation coefficients are correlated using a mathematical algorithm [38]. Thus an image can be reconstructed according to the different absorption values of tissues in the slice.

6.6.2 Method

CT scanning may be done without or with contrast medium. Contrast medium may be administered orally or intravenously – both are routine. Sometimes it seems useful to introduce a tampon into the vagina in order to improve the visualization of the vaginal wall.

6.6.3 Radiation Exposure

In a CT examination involving about 20 slices of the lesser pelvis the radiation dose to the ovaries is about 7.5 mGy, to the whole body, 5 mGy [44].

6.6.4 Indications and Limitations

CT has a great advantage over ultrasonographic procedures in that it yields transverse sectional images which are easily reproducible. Moreover, not only the lesser pelvis may be visualized, but also the whole abdomen and the thorax.

CT diagnosis of a pathologic process is based on alterations in size, contours and X-ray attenuation in comparison with normal tissue. Thus CT may give a false-negative result if these criteria cannot be evaluated. In addition, irradiation of the patient, though slight, is unavoidable.

6.6.5 Findings

6.6.5.1 Carcinoma of the Cervix

Superficial carcinomas of the cervix are missed with CT. The CT diagnosis of cervical cancer rests on alterations in the size appearance and X-ray attenuation of the cervix. The primary CT criteria for cervical carcinoma are a necrotic cervical

a

b

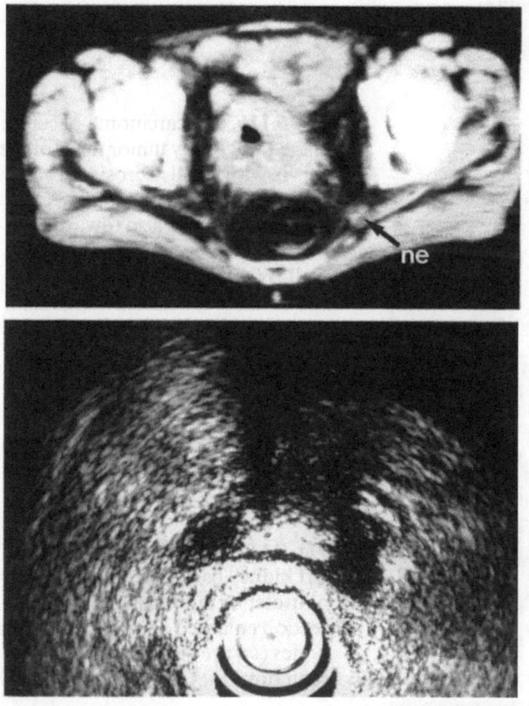

Fig. 6.115 a, b. CT and RS: carcinoma of cervix stage IIIb. **a** CT shows a bulky tumor mass with central necrosis and irregular contrast enhancement with nodular tumor extension (*ne*) to the left pelvic wall. **b** RS demonstrates the central portion of the tumor with a necrotic area, but the nodular spread to the left pelvic wall is missed

canal, irregular contrast enhancement and a bulky tumor of the cervical region [43]. A secondary sign is fluid retention within the uterine cavity.

Infiltration into the vagina causes irregular thickening of the vaginal wall.

Early *infiltration into the parametrium* is missed with CT in most cases. In later stages either bulky or nodular infiltration is visualized. In stage IIIb extension to the pelvic wall can be ascertained on bimanual gynecologic examination, but CT is needed to find out whether the internal obturator muscle is involved. This is usually not the case, as infiltration of this muscle is uncommon (Fig. 6.115) [50].

Tumor extension to the urinary bladder and the rectum is diagnosed easily, in some cases, but in others it may be impossible to differentiate, with CT, between mere edematous swelling of the bladder or rectal wall and early infiltration. Endoscopy and biopsy are necessary in these cases. The CT appearance of massive infiltration with bulky tumor masses within the bladder or the rectum is conclusive, however (Fig. 6.116).

Signs of *secondary urinary obstruction* caused by tumor growth are easily detectable with CT. Even in the case of a nonfunctioning kidney, a dilated renal pelvis or a dilated ureter can be identified. Endosonographic procedures usually miss such lesions because of their limited field of view (Fig. 6.117).

Metastatic lymph nodes may be diagnosed with CT if they are enlarged. The minimum detectable size varies with location, but the node must be at least 0.5 cm in diameter. In most cases no differentiation between metastatic and hyperplastic enlargement is possible. It is difficult to visualize lymph nodes along

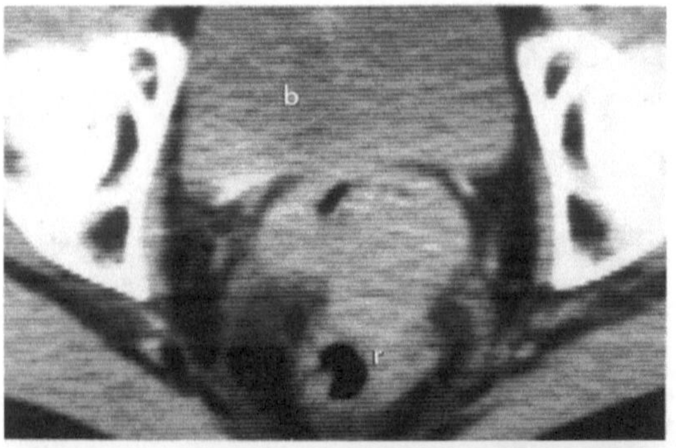

Fig. 6.116. CT: carcinoma of cervix stage IVb. Bulky tumor mass of the cervix with small necrosis. Broad infiltration of the rectum (*r*). Tumor extension also towards the bladder (*b*), reaching its dorsal wall. Whether there is already infiltration or not must be clarified with cystoscopy and biopsy

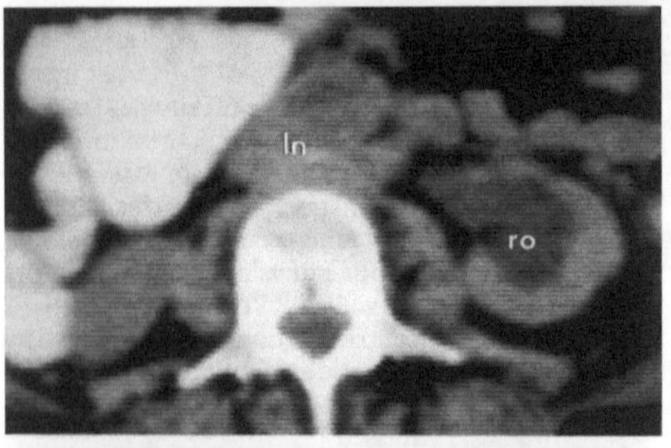

Fig. 6.117. CT: dilation of pelvis of left kidney because of obstruction of ureter by lymph nodes. In this section enlarged para-aortic lymph nodes (*ln*) are visible. *ro*, renal obstruction

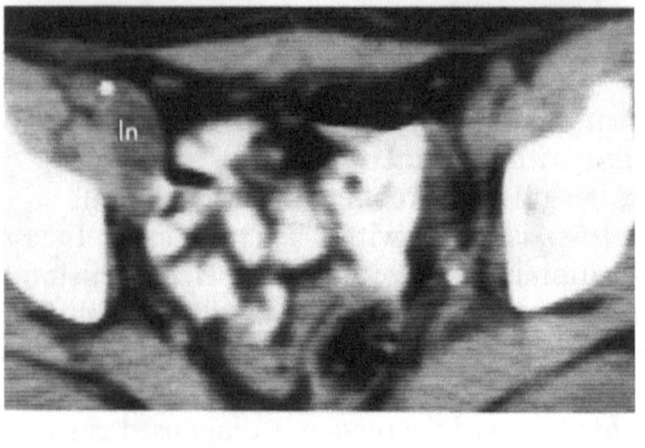

Fig. 6.118. CT: cystic lymph node metastasis along external iliac vessels on right side. *ln*, lymph nodes

the internal iliac vessels, whereas those along the external iliac vessels, on the pelvic wall and in the para-aortal region may be well visualized (Fig. 6.118) [49].

CT seems to be useful for the determination of tumor extension in late stages, where far advanced local penetration and high lymph node metastases can be visualized more reliably than with endosonography.

6.6.5.2 Myomas

CT is not used for routine diagnosis of myomas. These lesions cause enlargement (sometimes eccentric) of the uterus. Myomas may be isodense to myometrium, but may also appear hypodense or hyperdense, depending upon their consistency.

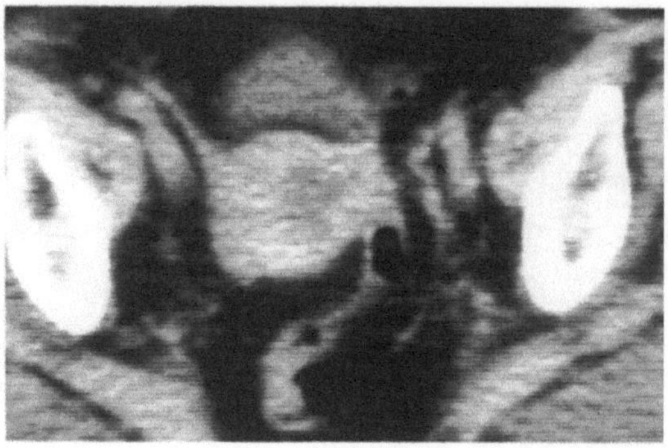

Fig. 6.119. CT: carcinoma of endometrium. Slightly enlarged uterine corpus with central irregular hypodense area

6.6.5.3 Carcinoma of the Endometrium

The CT criterion for carcinoma of the endometrium is thickening of the uterine wall, which sometimes appears irregular. In the case of extensive growth the tumor penetrates the uterine wall. An indirect sign of tumor is hypodense tissue (retention of fluid) within the uterine cavity. It is difficult with CT to identify the exact location, extension and depth of infiltration into the myometrium. Tumor growth is sometimes better delineated with the aid of intravenously administered contrast medium (Fig. 6.119) [17]. In contrast, tumor extension beyond the natural organ borders is easily accessible to CT diagnosis. The CT appearance of invasion of the urinary bladder, bowel or lymph nodes does not differ from that described for carcinomas of the cervix in Sect. 6.6.5.

6.6.5.4 Ovarian Tumors

The ovary is an ovoid, flattened, solid organ that varies in size but generally measures around 1.5 × 3.5 × 3.5 cm. It is located in the ovarian fossa between the external and the internal iliac artery. Ovarian tumors are divided according to the WHO classification [41].

CT permits differentiation by consistency into cystic, solid and mixed ovarian tumors. Criteria for malignancy are a thickened, irregular wall, nodular components, irregular enhancement of contrast medium, signs of tumor growth beyond the organ borders and metastatic disease. Calcifications are suspect for malignancy if they have an irregular appearance (Fig. 6.120).

The sensitivity of CT for ovarian tumors is high, exceeding 90% [3]. Predictions concerning malignancy were correct in 81% of the cases in the study reported by Steinbrich and Rhode [36]. Staging of carcinomas was correct in 62% of cases, with overstaging in 11% and understaging in 27%.

In contrast to endosonography, CT provides information not only about local tumor extension, but also about any existing metastatic disease. Several pos-

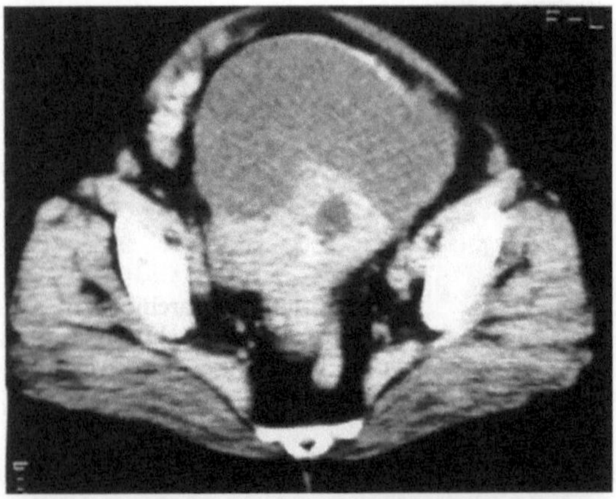

6.120

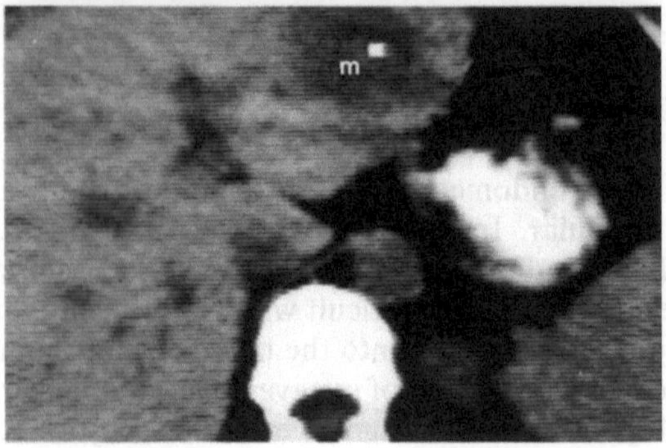

6.121

Fig. 6.120. CT: ovarian carcinoma. Extensive tumor growth within the small pelvis with cystic and irregular solid elements suggesting malignancy

Fig. 6.121. CT: liver metastasis (*m*) from ovarian carcinoma

sibilities must be considered: invasion through the capsule, infiltration of the small or large bowel, ascites, peritoneal carcinosis, involvement of the greater omentum, metastasis to lymph nodes and to the liver (Fig. 6.121).

6.6.5.5 Recurrences of Gynecologic Carcinomas

Recurrences of gynecologic carcinomas after operation or radiotherapy may develop locally, at other sites within the lesser pelvis or as distant metastasis. CT diagnosis is based on recognition of newly developing tissue formations, in most cases with the aid of contrast enhancement (Figs. 6.122, 6.123). To be detected with CT a recurrence must have a minimum diameter of 2 cm. Sensitivity for recurrences of carcinomas of the cervix has been reported as 89%, specificity 91% [3].

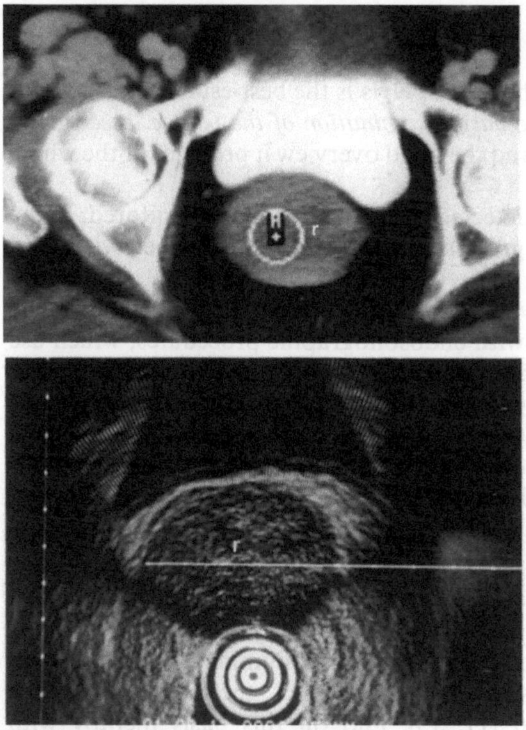

a

b

Fig. 6.122 a, b. CT and RS: local recurrence (*r*) after hysterectomy for carcinoma of endometrium

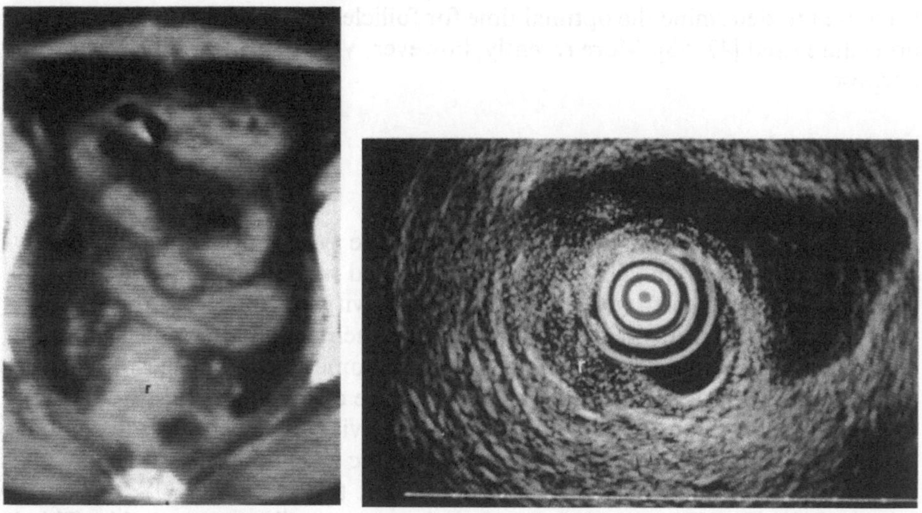

a b

Fig. 6.123 a, b. CT and RS: local recurrence (*r*) after hysterectomy and ovariectomy for carcinoma of ovaries with extension into rectum

6.7 Percutaneous Ultrasound

Percutaneous ultrasound (US) of the lesser pelvis is the best-established application of this modality. *US is still the basic examination of the female lesser pelvis* because of its lack of intrusiveness and the good overview it provides of the whole pelvis.

In *obstetrics*, pregnancy can be detected early and its course monitored. In the second and third trimesters fetal growth is depicted well, together with fetal anatomy and pathology.

In *gynecology*, US allows the evaluation of the internal female genitalia. The spatial resolution is not as high as with endosonographic procedures, which use higher frequencies, but on the other hand the depth of penetration is higher, permitting a good overview of the whole area of the lesser pelvis. One has to consider, however, that US is more sensitive to artifacts produced by overlying loops of bowel, a poorly filled bladder or obesity. This fundamental *disadvantage* of US cannot be avoided even by an experienced examiner.

6.7.1 Normal Anatomy

US is able to visualize the uterus, the ovaries and the abdominal great vessels but only seldom the fallopian tubes. Cyclic changes of the ovaries and the endometrium have been described [11, 15], and on this basis therapy with gonadotropin or Clomifen can be monitored. For in-vitro fertilization, US has been used to determine the optimal time for follicle puncture and in the puncture procedure itself [47, 53]. More recently, however, VS has proved superior for this purpose.

6.7.2 Pathology

Abnormalities of the uterus are diagnosed by the typical appearance of the hyperechoic endometrium. They are often combined with other abnormalities [52]. Myomas are diagnosed with US with a sensitivity of about 60% [14]. Single myomas are often difficult to visualize because their echo pattern does not differ significantly from that of normal myometrium. Sometimes a nonspecific enlargement of the uterus is the only sign of the presence of myomas (Fig. 6.124). Large myomas causing mass effects within the lesser pelvis can be demonstrated in their entirety better with US than with endosonographic techniques (Fig. 6.125).

Although normal *fallopian tubes* are difficult to detect with US, thickening because of salpingitis or a tubo-ovarian abscess is easily demonstrable. This is important for the differential diagnosis of ovarian enlargement [46].

US is useful in the diagnosis of *ovarian tumors*. The size of the tumor can be accurately monitored, as can its structure, which may be cystic, solid or mixed. A lot of studies have attempted to establish reliable sonographic criteria for malignancy, but all have failed. Findings highly suggestive of malignancy include ir-

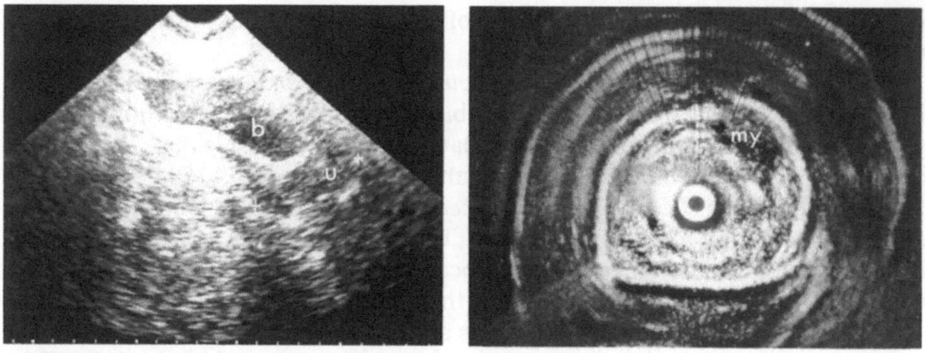

Fig. 6.124 a, b. US and HS: small subserous myoma. **a** The myoma (*my*) is not visualized on US because of inadequate filling of the bladder (*b*). **b** With HS the myoma is clearly defined as a hypoechoic area of the anterior wall. *u*, uterus

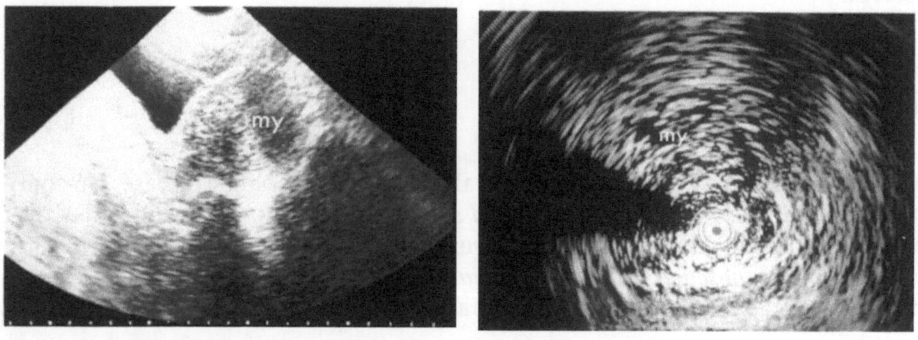

Fig. 6.125 a, b. US and HS: large myoma. **a** US gives a good overview of the whole organ. **b** With HS only the inner portions of the myoma (*my*) are visualized

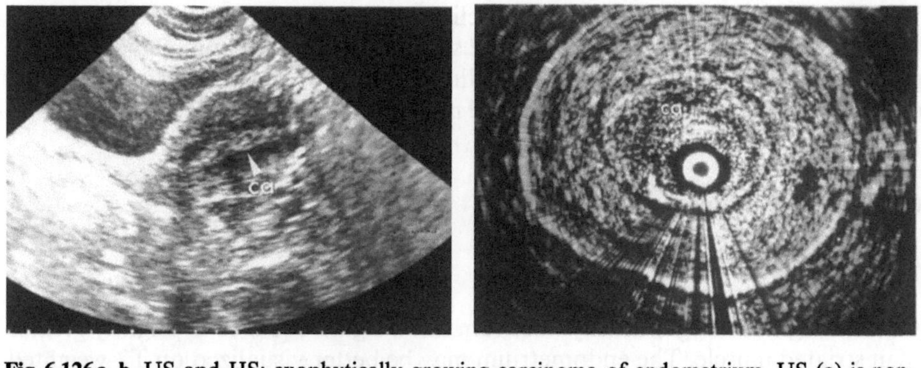

Fig. 6.126 a, b. US and HS: exophytically growing carcinoma of endometrium. US (**a**) is non-specific, while HS (**b**) clearly shows the exophytic tumor (*ca*) which fills the whole uterine cavity. No signs of invasion into the myometrium

regular solid parts or secondary signs of metastasis such as ascites or pelvic peritoneal carcinosis [27].

There is little literature on US of *carcinomas of the endometrium*. The fact is that no reliable primary diagnosis is possible with US, with one exception: a highly built-up endometrium in a postmenopausal woman is suspicious. The tumor extension within the myometrium is difficult to evaluate (Fig. 6.126).

The early stages of *carcinoma of the cervix* are missed with US. Later stages are characterized by huge tumor masses. The exact extension of the tumor into the parametrium cannot be evaluated. Local recurrences, especially on the pelvic wall, can be diagnosed by US, confirming the findings on bimanual examination.

Secondary signs of malignancy such as ascites, pleural effusion, metastases in the liver or metastatic enlargement of lymph nodes are detectable with US. With the exception of ascites these secondary tumor signs are missed on endosonography.

As US is nonintrusive it may be applied even in patients who do not tolerate endosonographic procedures because of posttherapeutic changes of the vagina or rectum.

6.8 Magnetic Resonance Imaging

MRI is increasingly being used in the evaluation of gynecologic diseases. In comparison with CT, MRI shows *improved soft tissue contrast*, allowing better discrimination among tissues. Another advantage of MRI over CT is its *multiplanar capability*. The *absence of ionizing radiation* and the lack of any other known hazards makes MRI attractive to physicians and patients alike.

6.8.1 Technical Considerations

Patients should fast for about 4 h before the study. The vagina is usually marked with a tampon. Normally *T1- and T2-weighted spin-echo images* are obtained. The choice of section depends upon the clinical findings: the axial plane forms the basis of every examination, but a second section in an orthogonal plane is always performed. Sometimes the contrast medium *Gd-DTPA* is given intravenously or orally. *Fast field sequences* are being used more frequently.

6.8.2 Normal Anatomy

6.8.2.1 Uterus

On T1-weighted images the myometrium has a signal equal to or slightly greater than striated muscle. The endometrium may be better visualized on T2-weighted images, where *three zones* are identified within the uterus. The outermost area of intermediate signal represents the *myometrium*. The middle zone, showing up as a dark ring, is known as the *junction zone*. The innermost zone has a high signal and represents the *endometrium* (both stratum basale and stratum functionale). The thickness of the endometrium depends upon the hormonal stimulation: it varies from between 1 and 3 mm during the proliferative stage to between 5 and 8 mm during the midsecretory phase [5]. The cervix shows up as an area of decreased signal intensity on all pulse sequences, because of the presence of more fibrous tissue than in the myometrium.

6.8.2.2 Ovaries

On T1-weighted images the ovaries have a signal approximately equal to muscle, sometimes with areas of lower signal. On T2-weighted images they may show focal areas of higher signal, representing follicular or functional cysts. The ovaries are detected easily on coronal planes by following the course of the broad ligament and the fallopian tubes. They are situated on the posterior surface of the broad ligament with the fallopian tubes lying superior and medial [7].

6.8.2.3 Vagina

The vagina is best visualized in the axial or the sagittal plane. The thickness of the vaginal wall may be better appreciated if a tampon has been inserted.

6.8.2.4 Vessels, Ureter, Bladder, Bowel

The uterine vessels arise from the internal iliac vessels and approach the uterus via the base of the broad ligament. The ureter lies medial to the iliac vessels and passes the cardinal ligament caudal to the uterine arteries. The ureter may be differentiated from the blood vessels due to flow artifacts. The urinary bladder and the rectum are well delineated anterior and posterior to the uterus.

6.8.3 Pathology

6.8.3.1 Leiomyoma of the Uterus

Uncomplicated myomas have a lower signal intensity than myometrium on all sequences. Their signal intensity may increase or decrease depending on secondary changes [28].

6.8.3.2 Carcinoma of the Endometrium

Carcinomas of the endometrium have a signal intensity higher than myometrium and lower than endometrium in most cases. Endometrial carcinomas appear as irregular areas within the uterine cavity. In early stages the outer contour of the

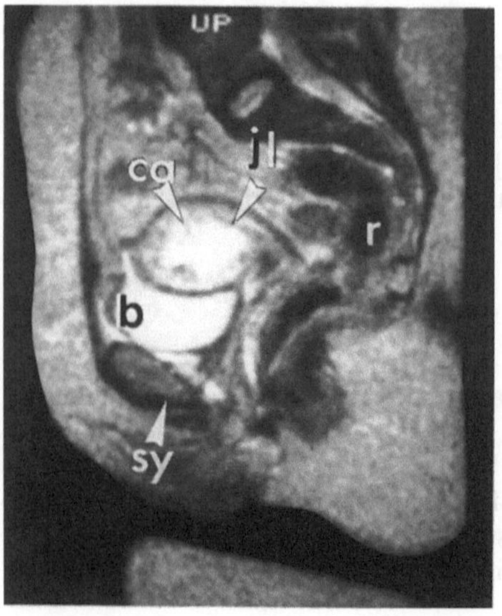

Fig. 6.127. MRI: infiltrating carcinoma of endometrium. Typical irregular appearance of the carcinoma (*ca*). Destruction of the junction line (*jl*) in the fundus. *b*, bladder; , rectum; *sy*, symphysis

uterus remains intact. A sign of myometrial invasion may be an alteration of the junction zone, which disappears in cases of myometrial invasion. Early infiltration may be missed with MRI, however (Fig. 6.127) [22, 54].

6.8.3.3 Carcinoma of the Cervix

In most cases cervical cancer is characterized by increased signal intensity of the carcinoma in comparison with normal cervical tissue. The tumor may have an irregular appearance depending on the extent of necrotic areas within it. Tumors within the natural cervical borders are better delineated than with CT. Early parametrial infiltration is diagnosed with accuracy equal to that of CT, as are further tumor stages with deep involvement of the parametrium.

Multiplanar projections, especially those including the sagittal plane, are superior for visualization of involvement of the urinary bladder or the rectum (Fig. 6.128) [37].

6.8.3.4 Ovaries

Simple ovarian cysts appear on MRI as well-circumscribed, homogeneous masses with smooth walls. On T1-weighted images their intensity is similar to or slightly higher than that of urine, while on T2-weighted images they show high signal intensity (Fig. 6.129). Hemorrhagic cysts have an increased signal intensity in all pulse sequences. MRI is able to delineate normal ovaries as well as ovarian enlargement. The criterion of malignancy is the presence of irregular solid tumor masses with a varying cystic component. Both the detection rate and the specificity concerning malignancy are better than with CT [31].

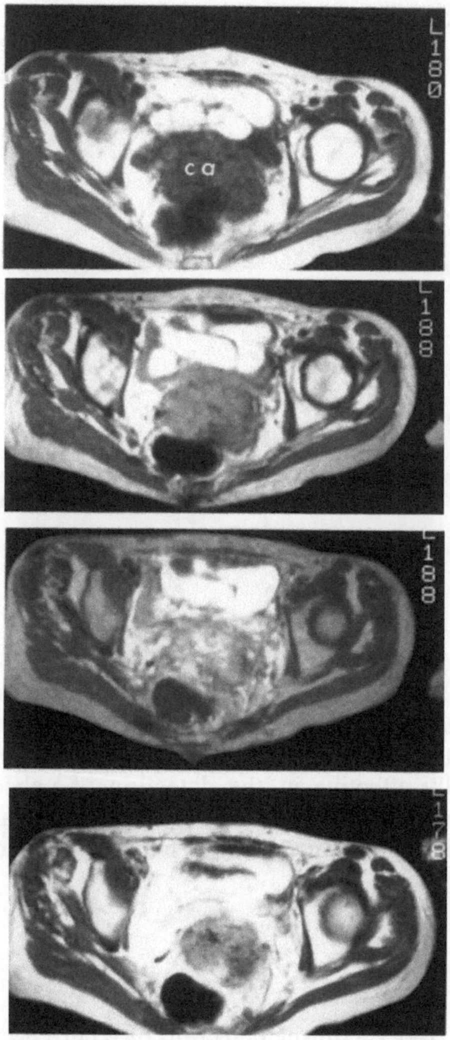

a b c d

Fig. 6.128 a–d. MRI: carcinoma of cervix stage IIb. **a** SE 500/20, **b** SE 2000/20, **c** SE 2000/80, **d** SE 500/20 after Gd-DTPA i.v. (0.1 mmol/kg/body weight). Note the irregular appearance of the carcinoma (*ca*), which is best visualized with T2 weighting and after administration of contrast medium

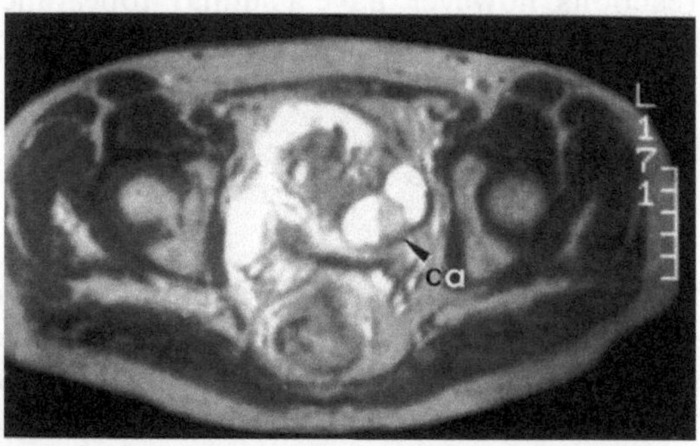

Fig. 6.129. MRI: cystadenoma of left ovary. The T2-weighted image clearly shows a central solid part of the tumor, whereas the liquid parts have a high signal intensity. *ca*, cystadenoma

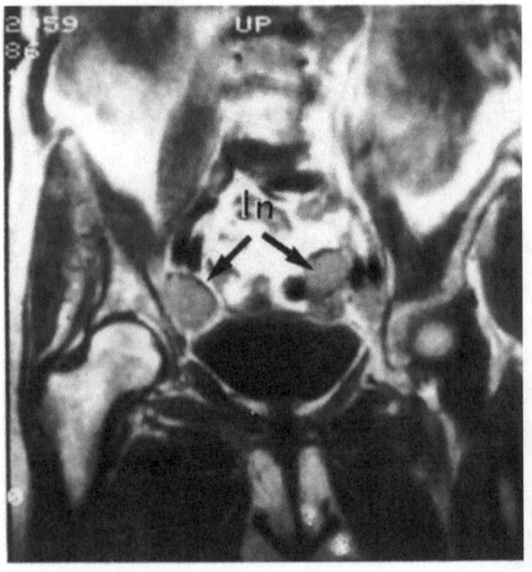

Fig. 6.130. MRI: enlarged iliac lymph nodes (*ln*) after Wertheim's operation

6.8.3.5 Lymph Nodes

Lymph nodes may be identified with MRI from a diameter of 5 mm. On T1-weighted images they appear as round or oval, low-signal areas in the iliac or para-aortic region. On T2-weighted images the signal intensity of the lymph nodes increases relative to fat, making their identification difficult (Fig. 6.130). Thus MRI and CT seem to be equally effective in the detection of pelvic lymphadenopathy. One major disadvantage of MRI should be kept in mind: at present there is no means of differentiating between benign hyperplasia and metastatic disease [6].

6.8.3.6 Recurrences

It seems that MRI has some advantage over CT in the detection of recurrences within the lesser pelvis. With MRI the separation of fibrosis from recurrence is possible in those cases where fibrosis has a decreased signal on T2-weighted images (Fig. 6.131). Acute radiation reactions, however, have a similar appearance to neoplasms. At the moment it is not clear how long following radiation therapy such changes persist [13].

6.8.4 Obstetrics

MRI is being increasingly utilized to examine fetal and maternal anatomy and pathology, especially in the USA. The reasons are its lack of adverse effects and its potential for better tissue characterization. The fetal head, lungs, liver and heart are routinely visualized on MRI in the third trimester, and congenital ab-

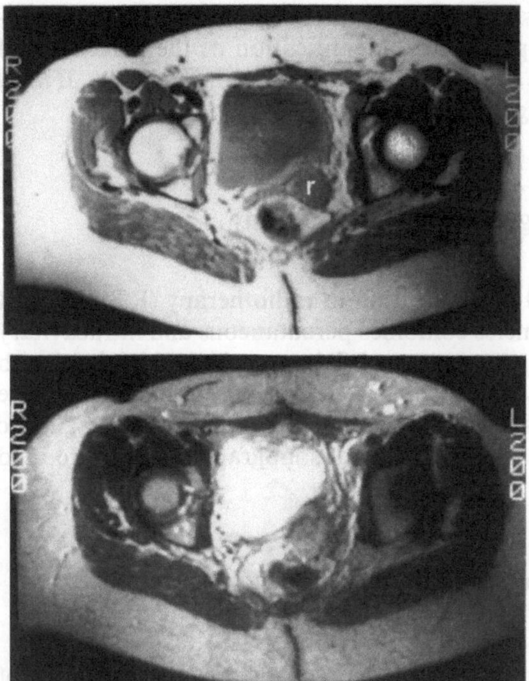

a

b

Fig. 6.131 a, b. MRI: local recurrence after Wertheim's operation. **a** SE 2000/20, **b** SE 2000/80. Left-sided recurrence (*r*) with reactive swelling of the adjacent wall of the bladder

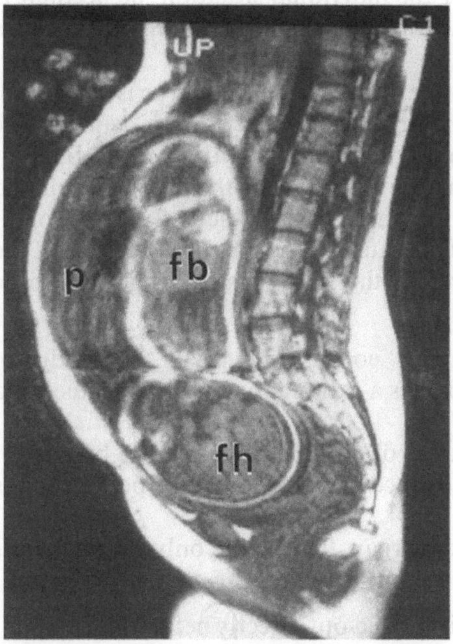

Fig. 6.132. MRI: late pregnancy with fetal head and body well delineated. Placenta (*P*) located at the anterior wall of the uterus. *fh*, fetal head; *fb*, fetal body

normalities such as hydrocephalus have been identified (Fig. 6.132). Potential applications of MRI are maternal pelvimetry, identification of the placenta and measurement of the length of the cervix [51]. At the moment, however, *MRI in obstetrics seems to have no advantage over ultrasound.*

6.9 Applications of Endosonography in Radiotherapy

Endosonography has a wide field of application in radiotherapy (RT). In most cases, RT of gynecologic malignancies combines percutaneous and intracavitary irradiation. Whereas planning of percutaneous RT has reached a high level with CT [16], planning of intracavitary and interstitial RT has been difficult because of the lack of adequate imaging systems. With endosonography this diagnostic gap has been closed successfully. The specific endosonographic procedure used depends on the clinical situation.

6.9.1 Hysterosonography in the Planning of Intracavitary RT of Endometrial Cancer

Intracavitary RT forms a substantial part of the radiotherapeutic treatment of endometrial carcinomas. It is accomplished either by conventional application of radium or, increasingly, by means of the afterloading technique [4]. The dose distribution is calculated in relation to the point A [45] 2 cm laterally and cranially to the external os uteri. This method has the advantage of good reproducibility and comparability, but does not consider the individual situation: no account is taken of the location and the extent of the tumor or the depth to which it invades the myometrium.

With HS, however, the macroscopic fine structure of the uterus is visualized, i.e., the macroscopic extent of an endometrial carcinoma can be defined. The depth of tumor infiltration into the myometrium can be clearly shown. In addition, with HS the size of the whole organ, the thickness of the myometrium and the diameter of the uterine cavity can be measured under exactly the same conditions that obtain during intracavitary RT, because of the identical position of the uterus during the two procedures. Therefore the following information can be gained from HS:

1) The diameter of the uterus at the fundus, corpus and cervix. Knowledge of the diameter of the uterine cavity provides a rational basis for the choice of a single or a double applicator.
2) The thickness of the myometrium. Areas of diminished resistance because of thinness of the wall are detected in advance and the danger of perforation is minimized.
3) The extent of the carcinoma within the organ. This is the only rational basis for the definition of the target volume for intracavitary RT.

The HS procedure lasts about 3 min and is carried out directly before RT.

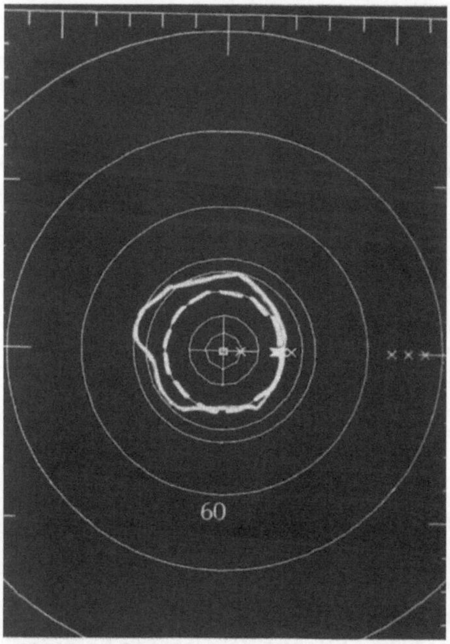

6.133

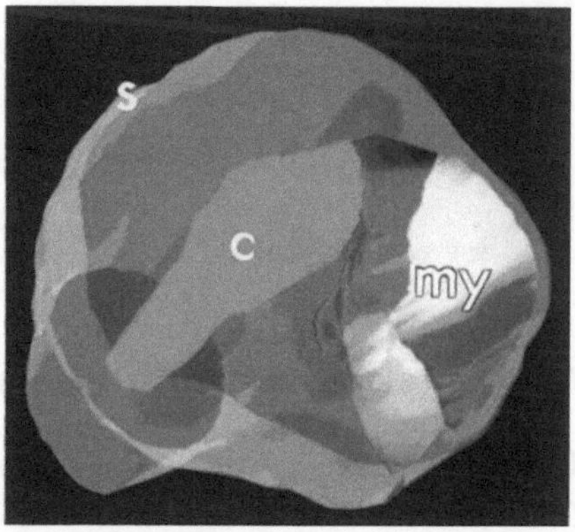

6.134

Fig. 6.133. Direct overlay of hysterosonogram and isodose distribution at 60 mm cranial from external os uteri. (—), outer contour of the uterus; (--), intended isodose curve

Fig. 6.134. Pseudo-three-dimensional presentation of hysterosonograms. Centrally the uterine cavity (*c*), on the left an intramural myoma (*my*); the outer contour is the serosa (*s*)

Hysterosonographic data may be used for RT without any digital postprocessing, by direct overlay of the hysterosonogram over the intended isodose distribution. Thus a direct correlation of the outer organ contours, the macroscopic extent of the carcinoma and the intended isodose curve can be established. Of utmost importance is the fact that there is an instant decision as to whether or not the whole carcinoma is covered by the intended isodose curve (Fig. 6.133) [18].

A mathematical computer program has been developed which allows digital postprocessing of hysterosonographic pictures [8]. This program permits the automatic detection of the outer organ contour, the uterine cavity and pathologically altered areas of the myometrium. The results may be demonstrated pseudo-three-dimensionally (Fig. 6.134).

The pseudo-three-dimensional presentation may be extended to cover not only the presentation of the hysterosonographic information but also the visualization of the overlying isodose curves together with the isodose curves from the external irradiation.

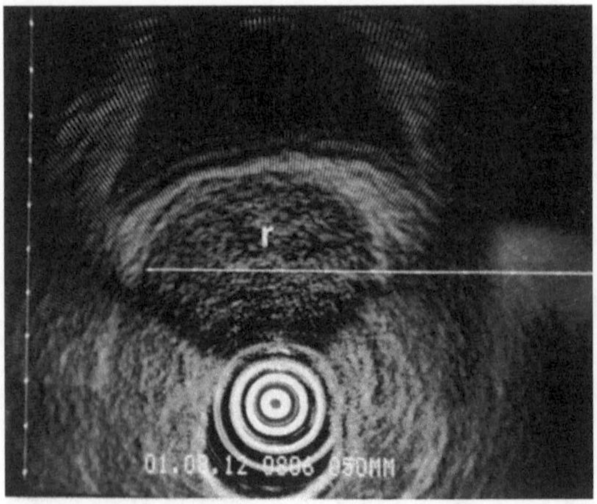

Fig. 6.135. RS: local recurrence (*r*) after hysterectomy at cranial end of vagina

6.9.2 Rectosonography in the Diagnosis and RT of Local Recurrences

Local recurrences of gynecologic tumors after operative or radiologic treatment present major problems of early diagnosis and effective treatment.

CT criteria for recurrences have been described [3], but RS seems to be superior for the early diagnosis of local recurrences [19]. The rectosonographic criteria for a local recurrence are a mass effect at the cranial portion of the vagina, low echogenicity, sometimes irregular borders and the observation of a growth tendency on control examinations (Fig. 6.135).

The most important differential diagnosis is scarring, which most often is noticed after irradiation. Scars have a typical rectosonographic appearance: in contrast to recurrences, which are hypoechoic, they have the same echogenicity as normal tissue.

6.9.3 Interstitial RT of Gynecologic Recurrences

Local recurrences of gynecologic tumors are difficult to manage. In most cases operative treatment is impossible and percutaneous RT is only palliative. Interstitial RT, however, seems promising. Either of two methods is used: ^{125}I can be implanted and left in place continuously [30], or ^{192}Ir can be employed in the afterloading technique [40]. We prefer the afterloading technique because it involves no exposure of medical and paramedical personnel to radiation.

6.9.3.1 Needle Placement

For interstitial RT of gynecologic recurrences we use needles with an outer diameter of 2.2 mm and a length of 20 cm. These needles are placed into the recurrence via the transvaginal route during brief general anesthesia. Optimal positioning of the needles is critical: without it, homogeneous isodose distribu-

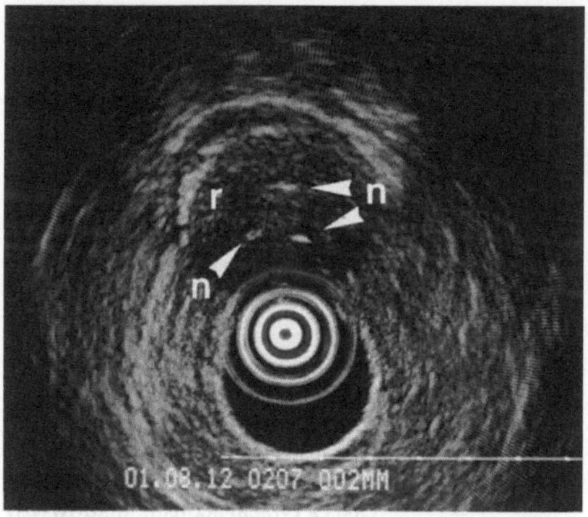

Fig. 6.136. RS: local recurrence (*r*) with three afterloading needles (*n*) placed centrally

tion within the tumor mass cannot be achieved. For this reason blind puncture cannot be advocated. Conventional imaging techniques like US or CT do not allow continuous monitoring of the puncture procedure; only with RS is this uninterrupted monitoring possible.

The puncture procedure with RS has been standardized. First, the rectal probe is introduced. RS follows the insertion of the afterloading needle into the recurrence, thus enabling the radiotherapist to alter the position of the needle at once if it is placed incorrectly. The number of needles used depends upon the size of the recurrence, but the placement of each needle is monitored in the same manner (Fig. 6.136).

6.9.3.2 *Irradiation*

After the correct placement of the afterloading needles the interstitial RT may be carried out. We use ^{192}Ir in a high-dose-rate remote afterloading technique, with single doses of 10–15 Gy. The individual isodose distribution may be laid directly over the rectosonogram as described for HS and intracavitary RT of endometrial carcinoma in Sect. 6.9.1, the needles seen in their actual location. In most cases we administer three or four doses.

6.9.3.3 *Follow-up*

Acute reactions to interstitial irradiation are relatively severe. Inflammation of the vaginal mucosa is the most common complication seen. However, with conservative treatment these reactions last only a short time.

Late reactions occur in about 10% of cases. The most severe side effect is the formation of a fistula, which we saw in 3% of our patients. The danger of fistula formation is greater with higher single fractions.

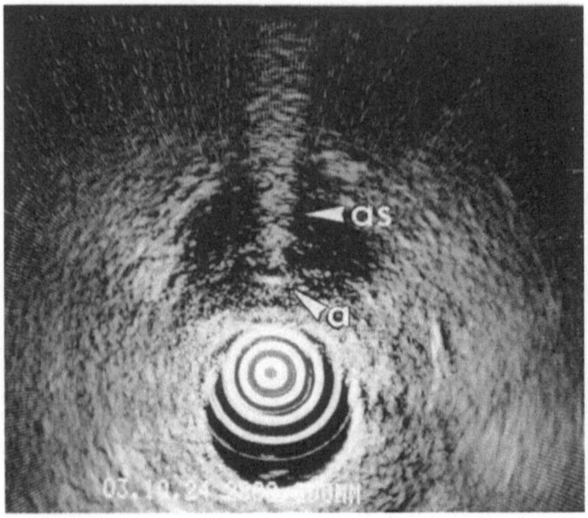

Fig. 6.137. RS cervical carcinoma stage IIb with applicator tube within cervical canal. Central positioning of the tube (*a*), which casts a typical acoustic shadow (*as*)

Results are promising. Of our 32 patients with a minimal follow-up of 2 years, 16% are free of disease and 54% exhibited a partial response. Only 30% did not show tumor regression.

6.9.4 Rectosonography to Check the Placement of Afterloading Applicators

Checking the placement of an afterloading applicator for intracavitary RT with X-ray simulators delivers information on its position in relation to the bony pelvis, but not to the uterine structures. This gap is filled with RS. After positioning of the applicator, RS shows its location within the uterine cavity (Fig. 6.137). The aim is central placement of the applicator in order to ensure homogeneous, symmetrical isodose distribution. If this cannot be achieved the degree of asymmetry must be evaluated and modification of the percutaneous irradiation considered.

References

1. Bernaschek G, Janisch H (1983) Eine Methode zur Objektivierung des Parametrienbefundes beim Zervixcarcinom. Geburtshilfe Frauenheilkd 43:498–503
2. Bernaschek G, Bartl W, Janisch H (1984) Erste Ergebnisse eines echographischen Staging beim Zervixkarzinom. Wien Klin Wochenschr 96:286–291
3. Breit A, Rohde U (1983) Computertomographie gynäkologischer Tumoren. Thieme, Stuttgart
4. Busch M, Makoski B, Schulz U, Sauerwein K (1977) Das Essener Nachlade-Verfahren für die intracavitäre Strahlentherapie. Strahlentherapie 153:581–588
5. Demas BE, Hricak H, Jaffer RB (1986) Uterine MR imaging: effects of hormonal stimulation. Radiology 159:123–126
6. Dooms GC, Hricak H, Crooks LE, Higgins CB (1984) Magnetic resonance imaging of the lymph nodes: comparison with CT. Radiology 153:719–728

7. Dooms GE, Hricak H, Tscholakoff D (1986) Adnexal structures: MR imaging. Radiology 158:639–646
8. Englmeier K-H, Hecker R, Hötzinger H, Pöppl S, Thiel H (1985) Reconstruction and pseudo-3-dimensional presentation of the uterus from automatic segmented transversal ultrasound slices – a fundamental precondition for optimizing the individually adjusted therapy planning in case of a carcinoma of the body of the uterus. In: Lemke HU, Rhodes ML, Jaffee CC, Felix R (eds) Computer assisted radiology. Springer, Berlin Heidelberg New York
9. Feichtinger W, Kemeter P (1984) Laparoscopic or ultrasonically guided follicle aspiration for in vitro fertilization? J In Vitro Fert Embryo Transfer 1:244–248
10. Feichtinger W, Kemeter P (1986) Erste Ergebnisse der transvaginalen Follikelpunktion mit Hilfe eines vaginalen Ultraschallsectorscanners mit Punktionsnadelführung. In: Popp LW (ed) Gynaekologische Endosonographie. Klemke, Quickborn, pp 147–151
11. Fleischer AC, Pittaway DE, Beard L (1983) Sonographic depiction of endometrial changes in spontaneous and stimulated cycles. 28th annual meeting, American Institute for Ultrasound in Medicine, New York
12. Ghirardini G, Poll LW, Gualerzi C, Spreafico L, Fochi F, Agnelli P (1986) Chorionskopische and vaginosonographisch gezielte Trophoblastbiopsie. In: Popp LW (ed) Gynaekologische Endosonographie. Klemke, Quickborn, pp 133–142
13. Glazer HS, Lee IKT, Levitt RG et al. (1985) Radiation fibrosis: differentiation from recurrent tumor by MR imaging. Radiology 156:721–726
14. Gross BH, Silver TM, Jaffe MH (1983) Sonographic features of uterine leiomyomas. Ultrasound Med 2:401–406
15. Hackelöer BI, Fleming R, Robinson HP et al. (1979) Correlation of ultrasonic and endocrinologic assessment of human follicular development. Am J Obstet Gynecol 135:122–128
16. Hackl A, Krispel F (1980) Neue Wege der Dosisplanung bei primärer Strahlentherapie von Uterusmalignomen. Strahlentherapie 156:519–523
17. Hamlin DJ, Burgener FA, Beecham JB (1981) CT of intramural endometrial carcinoma: contrast enhancement is essential. AJR 137:551–554
18. Hötzinger H (1984) Durch Intrauterinsonographie optimierte intracavitäre Strahlentherapie bei Korpuskarzinomen. Strahlentherapie 160:600–604
19. Hötzinger H, Atzinger A, Ries G (1983) Transrektale Ultraschalltomographie des weiblichen Genitales: erste Ergebnisse. Röntgenpraxis 36:387–391
20. Hötzinger H, Becker H, Becker V (1984) Intrauterine Ultraschalltomographie (IUT): Vergleich mit makroskopischen Präparatschnitten. Geburtshilfe Frauenheilkd 44:219–224
21. Hounsfield GN (1973) Computed transverse axial scanning (tomography). Part 1. Description of system. Br J Radiol 46:1016–1022
22. Hricak H, Stern JL, Fisher MR, Shapeero LG, Winkler ML, Lacey CG (1987) Endometrial carcinoma staging by MR imaging. Radiology 162:297–305
23. Kratochwil A (1969) Ein neues vaginales Schnittbildverfahren. Geburtshilfe Frauenheilkd 28:379–385
24. Kratochwil A (1986) Ultraschalldiagnostik in Geburtshilfe und Gynäkologie. Thieme, Stuttgart
25. Kratochwil A, Grasser G, Mar HG (1970) Die Ultraschalldiagnostik in der Urologie. Wien Klin Wochenschr 82:795–800
26. Kratochwil A, Störger H, Zaibekis N (1971) Die Darstellung von Beckenwandrezidiven im Ultraschalltomogramm. Geburtshilfe Frauenheilkd 34:742–747
27. Lawson T, Albarelli J (1977) Diagnosis of gynecologic pelvic masses by gray scale ultrasonography: analysis of specificity and accuracy. Am J Roentgenol 128:1003–1006
28. Lee JKT, Gessell DJ, Balfe DM, Worthington JL, Picus D, Gapp G (1985) The uterus: in vitro MR-anatomic correlation of normal and abnormal specimens. Radiology 157:175–179
29. Martin J (1986) Follikulometrie mit Hilfe der Vaginosonographie. In: Popp LW (ed) Gynaekologische Endosonographie. Klemke, Quickborn, pp 143–146
30. Martinez A, Herstein P, Portnuff J (1983) Interstitial therapy of perineal and gynecological malignancies. Int J Radiat Oncol Biol Phys 9:409–416
31. Mitchell DG, Minta MC, Spritzer CE et al. (1987) Adnexal masses: MR imaging observations at 1.5 T with US and CT correlation. Radiology 162:319–324

32. Popp LW (1986) Vaginosonographie mit dem Panoramasektor- und dem Fingertipscanner. In: Popp LW (ed) Gynaekologische Endosonographie. Klemke, Quickborn, pp 91–98
33. Popp LW (1986) Möglichkeiten der vaginosonographisch gezielten Punktion in einem in-vitro-Fertilisationsprogramm. In: Popp LW (ed) Gynaekologische Endosonographie. Klemke, Quickborn, pp 153–162
34. Popp LW, Lemster S (1986) Vaginosonographische Detailbefunde der Frühschwangerschaft: erlebte Embryologie. Klinische Anwendung. In: Popp LW (ed) Gynaekologische Endosonographie. Klemke, Quickborn, pp 107–126
35. Popp LW, Mueller-Holve W (1983) Die Indikationsstellung zur Vaginosonographie. In: Lutz H, Reichel L (eds) Ultraschalldiagnostik 83. Thieme, Stuttgart, pp 74–76
36. Popp LW, Lueken RP, Lindemann H-J (1982) Hysterosonographie. Diagn Intensivther 15:69–73
37. Powell MC, Worthington BS, Sokal M, Wastie M, Buckley J, Symonds EM (1986) Magnetic resonance imaging: its application to cervical carcinoma. Br J Obstet Gynecol 93:1276–1285
38. Radon J (1917) Über die Bestimmung von Funktionen durch ihre Integralwerte längst gewisser Mannigfaltigkeiten. Ber Math Phys Kais Saechs Ges Wiss 59:262–277
39. Schaaps J-P, Mustin J, Lambotte R (1986) Vaginosonographie Aspekte der Uterus – Trophoblastzirkulation. In: Popp LW (ed) Gynaekologische Endosonographie. Klemke, Quickborn, pp 127–132
40. Schulz M, Busch M, Bamberg M, Schmitt G (1984) Die interstitielle Afterloading-Therapie: Prinzip, Praxis und erste klinische Erfahrungen. Strahlentherapie 160:85–89
41. Serov SF, Scully RE, Sobin LH (1973) Histologic typing of ovarian tumours. International typing of ovarian tumours. International histologic classification of tumours, no 9. World Health Organization, Geneva
42. Steinbrich W, Rohde U (1982) Präoperative Klassifikation von Ovarialtumoren mit der Computertomographie. Strahlentherapie 158:722–725
43. Steinbrich W, Rohde U, Friedmann G (1982) Wert der Computertomographie für die Diagnostik von Uterustumoren und ihrer Rezidive. Radiologe 22:154–161
44. Thomasz E, Alott VD, Nollmann CE, Kunst JJ (1980) Determination of absorbed doses in a computerized tomography scanner. Nucl Instrum Methods 175:196–197
45. Tod MC, Meredith WJ (1953) Treatment of cancer of the cervix uteri – a revised Manchester method. Br J Radiol 26:252–257
46. Ulrich PC, Sanders RC (1976) Ultrasonic characteristics of pelvic inflammatory masses. J Clin Ultrasound 4:199–204
47. Vargyas J, Marrs R, Kletzky O, Mishell DR (1982) Correlation of ultrasonic measurements of ovarian follicle size and serum estradiol levels in ovulatory patients following clomiphene citrate for in-vitro fertilization. Am J Obstet Gynecol 144:569–573
48. von Micsky LI (1966) Transvesical pelveosonography – a new theoretical and experimental approach to the investigation of gynecological cancer. Obstet Gynecol 27:597–598
49. Walsh JW, Amendola MA, Konerding KF, Tisuado J, Hazra TA (1980) Computed tomographic detection of pelvic and inguinal lymph-node metastases from primary and recurrent pelvic malignant disease. Radiology 137:157–166
50. Walther HE (1948) Krebsmetastasen. Schwabe, Basel
51. Weinreb JC, Lowe TW, Santos-Ramos R, Cunningham FG, Parkey R (1985) Magnetic resonance imaging in obstetric diagnosis. Radiology 154:157–161
52. White JL, Lawson TL (1978) Congenital uterine anomaly with renal agenesis. J Clin Ultrasound 6:117–121
53. Wood C, Trounson A, Leeton J et al. (1981) A clinical assessment of nine pregnancies obtained by in vitro fertilization and embryo transfer. Fertil Steril 35:502–508
54. Worthington JL, Balfe DM, Lee JKT et al. (1986) Uterine neoplasms: MR imaging. Radiology 159:725–730

Subject Index

MIX
Papier aus verantwortungsvollen Quellen
Paper from responsible sources
FSC® C105338

If you have any concerns about our products,
you can contact us on
ProductSafety@springernature.com

In case Publisher is established outside the EU,
the EU authorized representative is:
Springer Nature Customer Service Center GmbH
Europaplatz 3, 69115 Heidelberg, Germany

Printed by Libri Plureos GmbH
in Hamburg, Germany